Restrictive Cardiomyopathy and Arrhythmias

Cardiomyopathy Update

Cardiomyopathy Update 3

Restrictive Cardiomyopathy and Arrhythmias

Editors
Eckhardt G. J. Olsen and Morie Sekiguchi

UNIVERSITY OF TOKYO PRESS

Published in association with the Japan Research Promotion
Society for Cardiovascular Diseases

In cooperation with International Society and Federation of Cardiology

© Japan Research Promotion Society for Cardiovascular Diseases, 1990
Published by University of Tokyo Press

ISBN 0-86008-458-2
ISBN 4-13-068154-0

Printed in Japan

Production of this book was supported by the promotion fund of the Japan Keirin Association.

Contents

Foreword

Cardiomyopathies are defined as heart muscle diseases of unknown cause. Clinically they may become manifest as congestive heart failure, arrhythmias, conduction disturbances, embolic phenomena or sudden death. It is often difficult to determine the exact nature or mechanism of the disease process. In another group of diseases, referred to as specific heart muscle diseases, interaction between a general disease process and concomitant cardiac involvement is well recognized although the actual mechanisms are still ill understood.

An immense amount of scientific and clinical activity is being undertaken throughout the world, and contributory factors to pathogenetic mechanisms are slowly emerging, among which viruses, immunological idiosyncrasy and electrolytic imbalance may be cited. The role that alcohol may play is also being defined.

This annual monograph series, *Cardiomyopathy Update*, will cover all aspects of heart muscle diseases. Special care will be taken to include both clinical and basic research as well as day-to-day clinical cardiology. Topics, volume editors and authors will be selected by the series editors in close collaboration with the scientific committee and editorial board.

Publication of this series was proposed by Dr. Hiroto Yoshioka, Chairman of the Board of Trustees of the Japan Research Promotion Society for Cardiovascular Diseases, during the first International Symposium on Cardiomyopathy (ISCM), which was held in Tokyo in December 1984. We are greatly indebted to the society for its support, and to the International Society and Federation of Cardiology (ISFC) for its cooperation in effective scientific communication.

The series editors hope that these publications will provide a wealth of information not only from research but also from clinical work.

Morie Sekiguchi
Eckhardt G. J. Olsen

Preface

Hypertrophic or dilated cardiomyopathies have been studied by many investigators. This does not apply to the restrictive form of cardiomyopathy which is not well defined or understood.

Hypereosinophilia, ventricular thickening with or without the deposition of an abnormal substance, and myocardial disarray or fibrosis may play an important role in the loss of compliance of the myocardium, although no consistent clinico-pathologic correlation has been identified.

Another important problem is to confirm the causal relationship between arrhythmias or conduction disturbances and heart muscle diseases. Viral myocarditis and sarcoidosis, for example, have been proven to be important agents in the development of intraventricular conduction disturbances or ventricular arrythmias.

In view of these two important topics, the Second International Symposium on Cardiomyopathy and Myocarditis took place in Tokyo in September 1988 under the sponsorship of the Japan Research Promotion Society for Cardiovascular Diseases in cooperation with International Society and Federation of Cardiology (ISFC). About 100 distinguished investigators from all parts of the world participated at this meeting, and important findings were reported and discussed.

This monograph is the compilation of the papers presented at that meeting; it contains comprehensive reviews by experts in their fields and new insights into restrictive cardiomyopathy and certain heart muscle diseases. Wherever possible our aim has been to leave the style of the individual contribution as closely as feasible to the original text without distorting the scientific content.

The editors hope that this volume will be helpful to both clinical cardiologists and those engaged in basic research in cardiology. It is further hoped that postgraduate students may find useful information in these papers.

At the time of this symposium, various subjects related to this volume were presented by posters, and these are included in *Heart and Vessels* Supplement 3.

E. G. J. Olsen and M. Sekiguchi

Definitions of Cardiomyopathies and Specific Heart Muscle Diseases

Olsen, E. G. J.

Department of Histopathology, Royal Brompton and National Heart Hospital, London, U.K.

The definition and classification of cardiomyopathies and heart muscle diseases has resulted in much confusion, which has led in the past to misunderstanding, misinterpretation, and misconception.

In order to overcome these misunderstandings, the World Health Organization and the Scientific Council of Cardiomyopathies of the International Society and Federation of Cardiology set up a Task Force which made the following recommendations[1] based on Goodwin's and Oakley's original concepts.

DEFINITION

Cardiomyopathies are defined as "heart muscle diseases of unknown cause" and classified into three major groups: dilated cardiomyopathy, hypertrophic cardiomyopathy, and restrictive cardiomyopathy.

DILATED CARDIOMYOPATHY

Dilatation of the left, of the right, and of both ventricles is recognized. The term "dilated" is preferred to "congestive" as congestion may or may not supervene, despite severe dilatation. Dilatation may be severe with impairment of systolic ventricular function. Disturbances of ventricular or atrial arrhythmias are frequent. Death may occur at any stage.

Morphologically, severe dilatation of all cardiac chambers is striking in longstanding cases, with evidence of a hypertrophied, dilated myocardium on microscopic examination. The changes are non-specific. By means of the bioptome, myocarditis has also been found in up to 63 % of patients with dilated cardiomyopathy, resulting in immunological consequences.

HYPERTROPHIC CARDIOMYOPATHY

Disproportionate hypertrophy of the left ventricle, and occasionally of the right ventricle, is typical with asymmetric hypertrophy of the interventricular septum. Concentric hypertrophy is now well recognized. Left ventricular volume is normal or reduced. Systolic gradients are frequent, but whether true obstruction is present is debatable. The underlying mechanism is believed to be failure of diastolic compliance.

Characteristic morphologic changes are well recognized, but whether disarray alone makes diagnosis possible is problematic. Familial incidence is well recognized, and an autosomal dominant gene with incomplete penetrance has been established.

RESTRICTIVE CARDIOMYOPATHY

Under this title endomyocardial fibrosis and Loffler's endocarditis parietialis fibro-plastica (associated with eosinophilia) are included. Obliteration of the affected ventricular cavities (right, left, or both) may be found. Persuasive evidence has been accumulating that the underlying disease process is attributable to eosinophilia with at least 15% of eosinophils degranulated, irrespective of the geographic origin. It is usual to refer to these conditions, which at one time were thought to be separate, collectively as eosinophilic endomyocardial disease.

Necrotic, thrombotic or fibrotic stages are recognized depending on the average length of the patient's history (5 weeks, 10 months, and 2.5 years, respectively). The first stage is characterized by eosinophilic myocarditis, the last by immense endocardial thickening, typically arranged in layers. Filling is restricted. The atrioventricular valves and papillary muscles are frequently involved, but the outflow tract is usually not affected. The atria may not be spared.

In view of the established association of eosinophilia, it has been proposed that this form of cardiomyopathy be reclassified under specific heart muscle diseases.

There is, however, an increasingly recognized group of patients showing signs and symptoms of restriction without consistent morphologic changes, to which the clinical manifestations can be attributed.

SPECIFIC HEART MUSCLE DISEASES

Definition

Specific heart muscle diseases are defined as "heart muscle diseases of known cause or association of other systems." It should be noted that disorders caused by systemic or pulmonary hypertension, coronary artery disease, valvular heart disease, or congenital heart disease are excluded; inclusion of these entities would render such a classification meaningless.

Classification

1. Infective Diseases

Infective myocarditis including viral myocarditis. This condition is now recognized as a pathogenetic pathway of dilated cardiomyopathy.

2. Metabolic Diseases

(a) Metabolic diseases, including those with endocrine causes

(b) Familial storage disease and infiltrations

(c) Deficiency conditions e.g., disturbances of potassium metabolism

(d) Kwashiorkor, anemia, and beri-beri

(e) Amyloidosis: "primary," "secondary," "familial," and senile forms

3. General System Diseases

(a) Connective tissue disorders: systemic lupus erythematosus, polyarteritis nodosa, rheumatoid arthritis, scleroderma dermatomyositis

(b) Infiltrations and granulomas: sarcoidosis and leukemia

4. Heredofamilial Disorders

(a) Muscular dystrophies: Duchenne, dystrophia myotonica

(b) Neuromuscular disorders: Friedreich's ataxia

5. Sensitivity and Toxic Reactions
Toxic reactions including alcohol abuse.

MISCELLANEOUS COMMENTS

Most of the specific heart muscle diseases are associated with non-specific hypertrophy and dilatation of the ventricles; but in conditions such as Pompe's disease, hemochromatosis, Fabry Anderson's disease, amyloidosis, and sarcoidosis, diagnostic features are discernible. Exceptions to the non-specific changes also include localized infiltrations leading to rhythm disturbances or conduction defects without generalized myocardial dysfunction. Amyloidosis is associated with a unique hemodynamic fault, and this, like glycogen storage disease, may be associated with clinical manifestations of hypertrophic cardiomyopathy.

Heart failure due to alcohol abuse or peripartal heart disease is similar to dilated cardiomyopathy.

Toxins in carcinoid heart disease affect the endomyocardium.

Heredofamilial disorders, such as Noonan's syndrome, lentiginosis, and Friedreich's ataxia, may mimic or be associated with hypertrophic cardiomyopathy.

Unclassified conditions include endocardial fibroelastosis, an infantile form of cardiomyopathy (histiocytoid) and right ventricular arrhythmogenic dysplasia, characterized by fatty infiltration predominantly of the right ventricle.

No definitions or classifications are perfect, but the nomenclature presented here is well proven. Adherence to these guidelines will minimize misinterpretations and will lead to better understanding and a uniform approach to research.

REFERENCES

1. WHO/ISFC Task Force Report on the Definition and Classification of Cardiomyopathies. *Br. Heart J.* **44**: 672–673, 1980.

Morphological Overview and Pathogenetic Mechanism in Endomyocardial Fibrosis Associated with Eosinophilia

E.G.J. Olsen

National Heart Hospital, London, U.K.

ABSTRACT

The controversy as to whether or not endomyocardial fibrosis and Loffler's endomyocarditis parietalis fibroplastica are separate disease entities or the same disease process is analyzed. In a large retrospective study of cases associated with eosinophilia from patients in the temperate zones, progressive changes from necrotic to thrombotic to fibrotic phase were found. The fibrotic phase from this retrospective study was compared with endomyocardial fibrosis from the tropics, and no differences were found. These observations formed the basis of the unitarian theory.

The conclusion that degranulated eosinophils are closely linked to the pathogenesis of this disease has been substantiated through monoclonal studies.

According to the WHO/ISFC Task Force recommendations on the nomenclature of cardiomyopathies and specific heart muscle diseases, endomyocardial fibrosis (EMF) is classified as restrictive cardiomyopathy.[1] This entity must be differentiated from specific heart muscle diseases that may present with restrictive signs and symptoms, such as amyloid heart disease.

EMF was first described clinically in 1946[2] and the first detailed account of the pathology by Davies in 1948.[3] For several years, it was believed that EMF was confined to Uganda and the African continent. Subsequently, it was considered to be essentially a tropical disease in distribution, corresponding to a belt extending 5° north and south of the equator. It soon became evident that this was by no means the case following reports from West Africa, India, Brazil, Sri Lanka, and other countries.[4]

A similar disease, for several years considered to be a separate entity, was described by Loffler in 1936[5] and referred to as Loffler's endocarditis parietalis fibroplastica associated with eosinophilia. This condition has been renamed Loffler's endomyocardial disease, following the suggested nomenclature of the WHO/ISFC Consultative Committee (London, December 1978). The likelihood that EMF and Loffler's endomyocardial disease represent in fact one disease entity, was predicted in 2 patients[6] and also simultaneously from workers in West Africa.[7]

A comprehensive, retrospective study was undertaken of 30 cases with Loffler's endomyocardial disease, drawn from the literature of well-documented cases in which full post mortem examination has been carried out and comparison made with 6 nontropical cases without eosinophilia and 26 patients with EMF from Nigeria, Uganda, Brazil, and Europe (the total number with tropical EMF was subsequently increased to 75 patients).[8] The initial predictions by other workers were confirmed and the conclusion

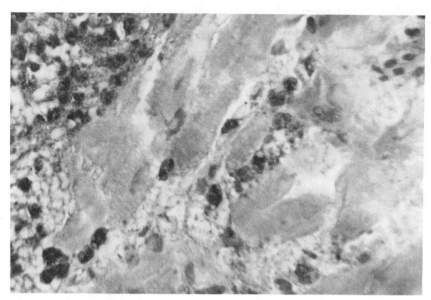

Fig. 1. Necrotic phase of endomyocardial disease associated with eosinophilia. Active myocarditis is clearly seen along with abnormal eosinophil morphology. Chromotrope 2R; × 1000.

reached that both entities belonged to the same disease process, the origin of which
could be traced to the presence of eosinophils in the myocardium.[8] This conclusion
was based on the following findings:

Active myocarditis, often with severe inflammatory cell infiltrates consisting mostly
or entirely of eosinophils, was found after the disease history had lasted for 5 weeks on
average. The interstitial cellular infiltrate was often limited to the inner third of the
myocardium and was frequently confluent in distribution; not infrequently, necrosis of
adjacent myocardial fibers was noted, indicating that an active process was present.
For that reason, this phase of the disease process was referred to as the necrotic phase
(Fig. 1). In addition, intramyocardial vessels showed fibrinoid necrosis of the wall with
interruption of the internal elastic lamina, and were surrounded by an inflammatory
cell infiltrate. This vasculitis was not confined to the arteries and arterioles in the heart
alone, but also affected small vessels of other organs examined.

When EMF had continued for an average of 10 months, the thrombotic phase was
noted, characterized by thrombus superimposition on the already thickened endocardium (Fig. 2), occasionally so severe as to completely obliterate the entire affected ventricular cavities. Nonspecific endocardial thickening was also identified at this stage.
In the myocardium itself, the inflammatory cell infiltrate had largely abated, but a
widened vascular interstitium with varying degrees of eosinophilic infiltrates was always
identified. The small intracardiac vessels showed fragmentation of the elastic lamina,
fibrosis of the previously damaged media, and intravascular thrombi.

The third and final major phase, designated the fibrotic phase, was reached after an
average history of 2.5 years. At this stage, the lesions appeared to be mainly confined to
the endocardium, which was immensely thickened. Measurements exceeding 5,000 μ m
were not unusual (the normal thickness of the left ventricular endocardium is 20 μm).
In agreement with the original description,[3] the sites most frequently involved were the

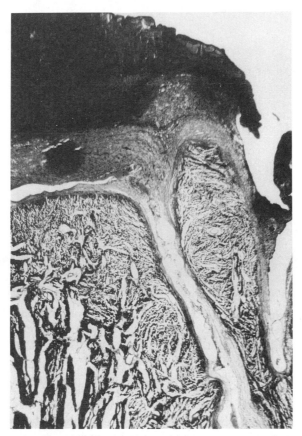

Fig. 2. Thrombotic phase of endomyocardial disease. The endocardium is already thickened; dark area at the top of the photomicrograph is superimposed thrombus. Note the septum extending into the underlying myocardium. Haematoxylin and eosin staining; × 25.

left ventricular inflow tract, the apex, and part of the left ventricular outflow tract. The thick endocardium ended abruptly in a thick rolled edge[9] in the region of the anterior mitral valve leaflet. In addition, the posterior mitral valve leaflet and the papillary muscles were also involved. Septa extending from the thickened endocardium could clearly be seen extending sometimes through the entire ventricular wall. Fibrin or thrombus frequently lined the ventricular cavity.

In cases of right ventricular involvement, the apex and an area beneath the posterior valve leaflet of the tricuspid valve were affected, frequently drawing the apex progressively toward the atrioventricular valve ring, resulting in a W-shaped contour of the ventricle. Commonly, massive lesions developed involving the outflow tract, ending just below the pulmonary valve cusps. This resulted in a shallow, saucer-shaped right ventricular cavity with involvement of the tricuspid valve, as well as the posterior papillary muscle. Rarely did the process start in the vicinity of the apex alone, which became separated as the disease progressed, resulting in a small pouch-like apical sack lined by the characteristic thickened endocardium.[10]

Irrespective of the ventricle involved, histological changes were identical. Beneath the superficial layer of fibrin or thrombus, a band of dense collagen tissue was present

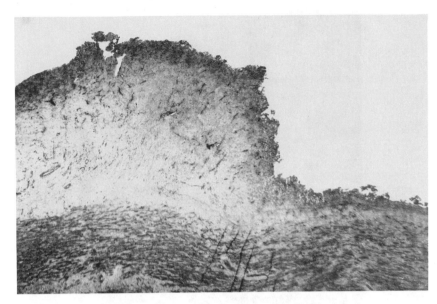

Fig. 3.   Photomicrograph of the fibrotic phase showing a typical arrangement
of thick endocardium in layers. Superficially, fibrin is superimposed and in the
deepest layer vascular channels can be seen. Note the abrupt start of the thickening. Elastic van Gieson staining; × 25.

with varying degrees of elastic tissue. Occasionally, some inflammatory cells in a
band-like distribution could be identified beneath the fibrin and thrombus layer. The
deepest layer, referred to as "the granulation tissue layer," was composed of loose connective tissue in which numerous vascular channels were prominent (Fig. 3). Even at
the late stage in the natural history of the disease process, inflammatory cells could be
identified, occasionally including eosinophils. The granulation tissue layer extended to
varying degrees into the underlying myocardium and formed the septa noted on naked-
eye inspections of slides or when the whole heart was available for examination. These
septa also consisted of loose vascular connective tissue and inflammatory cells. They
are believed to be the sites of previous damage resulting from myocarditis (the necrotic
phase). At this stage, the intramyocardial vessels showed nonspecific changes consisting
only of intimal fibroelastic thickening of varying severity.

In the study mentioned above, 16 cases were from the fibrotic phase[8] where evidence
of associated eosinophilia was clearly established. These 16 cases were initially compared
with 6 cases of nontropical EMF without eosinophilia and 26 cases (subsequently increased to 75 cases) of EMF from hearts received from Uganda, Brazil, and Nigeria.
Many measurements and all possible counts were taken, and no differences could be
established. This was why Brockington and Olsen[8] concluded that EMF and Loffler's
endocarditis belonged to the same disease spectrum, the origin of which could be traced
to the presence of eosinophils in the myocardium.

This work formed the basis of the previously suggested but refuted,[10] unitarian
concept of this disease, irrespective of the geographical origin of the patients. Controversy concerning this unitarian concept has been largely based on two factors. First,
Loffler's endomyocardial disease involves many organs and is not confined to the
heart; second, there is a causal relationship with eosinophilia.[11] In Loffler's en-

domyocardial disease arteritis is widespread, involving many organs of the body other than the heart. It would seem reasonable to suggest that when patients have reached the end-stage of the disease, vascular changes are nonspecific. This stage is usually reached when death occurs in tropical regions. As described above, when the necrotic phase is diagnosed in the heart, arteritis is found in other organs.

The association of eosinophilia with EMF in the tropics had long been noted, but possible causal links had not. In Daviess' original description, 12 of 24 cases had eosinophilia.[12] Subsequently, cases of eosinophilia and endomyocardial fibrosis were reported from Nigeria[13] with filariasis, but the resulting eosinophilia was not linked with the disease process. Eosinophilia has also been reported from Zaire, Uganda, and Venezuela, as well as Britain, Denmark, Switzerland, Japan, and other countries.[4] It must be remembered that in Loffler's original report of 2 patients, high eosinophilic counts diminished significantly as the disease progressed, and it is therefore not surprising that at the fibrotic stage eosinophils are scarce. The transitory nature of eosinophilia was also commented upon subsequently.[14] Eosinophils have also been found more recently in African cases and in EMF on endomyocardial biopsy examination of cases in southern India (Olsen, personal observation).

Clinically, numerous similarities between Loffler's endomyocardial disease and EMF exist and have been emphasized.[15] Some differences do, however, exist. In the tropics, right ventricular involvement (11%), pure left ventricular involvement (38%), and involvement of both ventricles (51%) have been noted,[16] whereas in the temperate zone biventricular involvement is typical.[17] The mean age of patients is also higher in the temperate zone compared to that in the tropics. Thrombotic and embolic complications are common in the temperate zones.[18] Common in all regions in the world, cardiac involvement is heralded by a constitutional illness. The differences observed in embolic complications (especially in the temperate zone) could be that EMF represents a milder form of the disease process and greater chronicity. Alternatively, it may be that the earlier phases goes undetected.[19] There is therefore ample evidence that the unitarian concept is correct.

Returning to the eosinophilia, closer studies of the morphology of these cells have shown significant abnormalities in the form of vacuolation and degranulation. Further studies have shown that if over 20% of eosinophils contained vacuoles ($>1.5 \times 10^9$/l) and over 15% showed degranulation ($>1 \times 10^9$/l), endomyocardial disease was confirmed at endomyocardial biopsy, even if cardiac disease had at this early stage not been manifest.[4] The severity of the eosinophilia was not important. Even with normal eosinophil counts, if a significant percentage of degranulated cells was exceeded, endomyocardial disease was present, explaining endomyocardial fibrosis in patients with normal eosinophil counts.

The causes of eosinophilia were in the majority of patients idiopathic,[8] but causal relationships with polyarteritis nodosa, status asthmaticus, sensitivity to antitubercular drugs and parasites,[8,11] myeloproliferative diseases, acute eosinophilic leukemia, hypereosinophilia and granulomatous angiitis, acute T lymphocyte leukaemia, Hodgkin's disease, melanoma, and carcinoma have also been found in association with endomyocardial disease and eosinophilia.[4]

The likely principal mechanism involved and the sequence of events have been suggested to take place as follows: Consequent upon stimulation, either due to idiopathic causes or as a result of the associated conditions mentioned above, the eosinophil is stimulated, resulting in an unmasking of the Fc receptors, and exocytosis of the granular content occurs after they have bound to IgG or C3B-coated particles or parasites.[4]

This results in the morphological changes of vacuolation and degranulation. The activated cells reach the inner layers of the myocardium through the microcirculation and with additional toxic substances, such as hydrogen peroxide, form an intense inflammatory cell infiltrate, *i.e.*, myocarditis rich in eosinophils (the necrotic phase). It has been shown that cationic proteins are thrombogenic.[4] Exposure of these proteins results in thrombus superimposition (the thrombotic phase). Finally, the fibrotic phase is the healed phase of the previous two phases. Studies with purified eosinophil granule basic proteins have shown that the damage in cardiac cells is the result of a specific toxic effect of eosinophil cationic proteins on the plasma membrane and two enzyme complexes, pyruvate dehyrogenase and oxoglutarate dehyrogenase, important systems involved in mitochondrial respiration.[20]

Deposition of eosinophilic granule protein in cardiac tissue obtained by endomyocardial biopsy or post mortem examination in acute and chronic lesions has been demonstrated by preparing sections for eosinophil major proteins for indirect immunofluorescence and for eosinophil cationic protein, eosinophil protein X, and activated eosinophils by means of alkaline phosphatase-linked monoclonal antibodies. Results showed that activated proteins were particularly evident in the earlier phases (necrotic and thrombotic phases) and in areas of tissue necrosis in the endocardium and in the wall of small blood vessels. These findings therefore confirmed that eosinophilic granule proteins are involved in cardiac injury leading to the development of EMF.[21]

How do these findings fit in with the general concept of hypereosinophilic syndromes? Chusid[22] found that at least 95% of patients with hypereosinophilic syndrome suffered from some form of myocardial disease. The endomyocardial disease (Loffler's endomyocardial disease or endomyocardial fibrosis) can therefore be looked upon as a complication of the hypereosinophilic syndrome. Several different types have been recognized. Myocarditis in conjunction with eosinophilia can occur in several disease entities, such as eosinophilic endomyocardial disease, tropical endomyocardial disease, parasitic infection, vasculitis and granulomatous disease (Churg-Strauss syndrome), eosinophilic necrotizing myocarditis, drug-induced reactions, and transplantation rejection.[23] Whether or not endomyocardial disease develops appears to be due to the discharge of cationic proteins, *i.e.*, degranulation. Many patients with hypereosinophilia do not develop endomyocardial disease. The possible explanation for this may lie in the intrinsic mechanisms inhibiting the release of a granule protein or neutralizing the effects of release by substances such as heparin,[24] which along with other strongly charged molecules can bind to cationic proteins. Work is in progress to study the events that occur at the level of the cell membrane which induce discharge of granule protein.[25-27]

Concerning the disease classification, with the association of eosinophils, by definition restrictive cardiomyopathy can be considered to be a specific heart muscle disease, and should therefore be reclassified under this heading. It will, however, be realized from the descriptions above that much work remains to be done to explain regional differences in incidence and seasonal variations. Genetic factors, individual predisposition, and immunological factors may also play important roles. As there are so many unanswered questions, it is at present inappropriate to regroup this disease entity.

It can be concluded that Loffler's endomyocardial disease and EMF belong to the same disease spectrum, the cornerstone of which is the abnormal eosinophil. The therapeutic agents that have been shown to inhibit eosinophilic granule protein release are corticosteroids,[28] explaining the rationale for medical treatment. Encouraging results from surgical intervention in the late phases of the disease process have been reported.[29]

REFERENCES

1. WHO/ISFC. Report of the task force on the definition and classification of cardiomyopathies. *Br. Heart J.* **44**: 672–673, 1980.
2. Bedford, D.E. and Konstam, G.L.S. Heart failure of unknown aetiology in Africans. *Br. Heart J.* **8**: 236–237, 1946.
3. Davies, J.N.P. Endocardial fibrosis in Africans. *East Afr. Med. J.* **25**: 10–14, 1948.
4. Olsen, E.G.J. and Spry, C.J.F. The pathogenesis of Loffler's endomyocardial disease, and its relationship to endomyocardial fibrosis. In: Progress in Cardiology, Yu, P.N. and Goodwin, J.F. (eds.), Lea & Febiger, Philadelphia, 1979, vol. 8, pp. 281–303.
5. Loffler, W. Endocarditis parietalis fibroplastica mit Bluteosinophilie, ein eigenartiges Krankheitsbild. *Schweiz. Med. Wochenschr.* **66**: 817–820, 1936.
6. Roberts, W.C., Liegler, D.G., and Carbone, P.P. Endomyocardial disease and eosinophilia. A clinical and pathologic spectrum. *Am. J. Med.* **46**: 28–42, 1969.
7. Brockington, I.F., Luzzaro, L., and Osunkoya, B.O. The heart in eosinophilic leukaemia. *Afr. J. Med. Sci.* **1**: 343–352, 1970.
8. Brockington, I.F. and Olsen, E.G.J. Loffler's endocarditis and Davies' endomyocardial fibrosis. *Am. Heart J.* **85**: 308–322, 1973.
9. Davies, J.N.P. The ridge in endomyocardial fibrosis.*Lancet* **1**: 631–632, 1968.
10. Davies, J.N.P. African endomyocardial fibrosis. In: Cardiomyopathy, Brest, A.N. (ed.), F.A. Davis Company, Philadelphia, 1972, vol. 4.1, pp. 349–359.
11. Oakley, C.M. and Olsen, E.G.J. Eosinophilia and heart disease. *Br. Heart J.* **39**: 233–237, 1977.
12. Davies, J.N.P. Endomyocardial necrosis. A heart disease of obscure aetiology in Africans. *Bristol University, M.D. Thesis*, 1948.
13. Ive, F.A., Willis, A.J.P., Ikeme, A.C., and Brockington, I.F. Endomyocardial fibrosis and filariasis. *Quart. J. Med.* **36**: 495–516, 1967.
14. Weiss-Carmine, S. Endocarditis parietalis fibroplastica mit Bluteosinophilic (Loffler) und ihre Stellung im Rahmen der Parietalendokardifibrosen. *Schweiz. Med. Wochenschr.* **87**: 890–898, 1957.
15. Bell, J.A., Jenkins, B.S., and Webb-Peploe, M.M. Clinical haemodynamic, and angiography findings in Loeffler's eosinophilic leukaemia. *Am. J. Med.* **30**: 310–322, 1969.
16. Shaper, A.G., Hutt, M.S.R., and Coles, R.M. Necropsy studies of endomyocardial fibrosis and rheumatic heart disease in Uganda 1950 to 1965. *Br. Heart J.* **30**: 391–401, 1968.
17. Davies, J., Spry, C.J.F., Sapsford, R., Olsen, E.G.J., De Perez, G., Oakley, C.M., and Goodwin, J.F. Cardiovascular features of 11 patients with eosinophilic endomyocardial disease. *Quart. J. Med. New series LII*, **205**: 23–39, 1983.
18. Spry, C.J.F., Davies, J., Tai, P.C., Olsen, E.G.J., Oakley, C.M., and Goodwin, J.F. Clinical features of fifteen patients with the hypereosinophilic syndrome. *Quart. J. Med. New series LII*, **205**: 1–22, 1983.
19. Patel, A.K., D'Arbela, P.G., and Somers, K. Endomyocardial fibrosis and eosinophilia. *Br. Heart J.* **39**: 238–241, 1977.
20. Spry, C.J.F., Tai, P.C., and Davies, J. The cardiotoxicity of eosinophils. *Postgrad. Med. J.* **59**: 147–151, 1983.
21. Tai, P.C., Spry, C.J.F., Olsen, E.G.J., Ackerman, S.J., Dunnette, S., and Gleich, G.J. Deposits of eosinophils granule proteins in cardiac tissues of patients with eosinophilic endomyocardial disease. *Lancet* 643–648, 1987.
22. Chusid, M.J., Dale, D.C., West, B.C., and Wolff, S.M. The hypereosinophilic syndrome: analysis of fourteen cases with review of the literature. *Medicine* **54**: 1–27, 1975.
23. Spry, C.J.F., Take, M., and Tai, P.C. Eosinophilic disorders affecting the myocardium and endocardium: A review. In: Myocarditis and Related Disorders, Sekiguchi, M., Olsen, E.G.J., and Goodwin, J.F. (eds.) Springer-Verlag, Tokyo, 1985, pp. 240–242.
24. Davies, J., Spry, C.J.F., Vijayaraghavan, G., and de-Souza, J.A. A comparison of the clini-

cal and cardiological features of endomyocardial disease in temperate and tropical regions. *Postgrad. Med. J.* **59**: 179–183, 1983.

25. Tai, P.C., Spry, C.J.F., Bakes, D.M., and Barkans, J.R. Eosinophil membrane antigens: Phenotypic frequencies in normal individuals and in patients with the hypereosinophilic syndrome. *Int. Arch. Allerg. Appl. Immunol.* 249–251, 1985.

26. Tai, P.C., Bakes, D.M., Barkans, J.R., and Spry, C.J.F. Plasma membrane antigens on light density and activated human blood eosinophils. *Clin. Exp. Immunol.* 427–436, 1985.

27. Lopez, A.F. and Vadas, M.A. Stimulation of human granulocyte function by monoclonal antibody WEM-G1. *Proc. Natl. Acad. Sci. USA* **81**: 1818–1822, 1984.

28. Winqvist, I., Olofsson, T., and Olsson, I. Mechanisms for eosinophil degranulation; release of the eosinophil cationic protein. *Immunology* **51**: 1–8, 1984.

29. Moraes, C.R. Surgical intervention in patients with EMF. (in press)

Endomyocardial Fibrosis in India: An Overview

G. Vijayaraghavan,* S. Sadanandan,** and George Cherian***

* Department of Cardiology, Medical College and Hospital, Kerala, India, and Consultant in Cardiology, Faculty of Medicine, Kuwait University, Kuwait
** Lecturer in Cardiology, Medical College and Hospital, Trivandrun, India
*** Department of Cardiology, Faculty of Medicine, Kuwait University, Kuwait

ABSTRACT

Endomyocardial fibrosis (EMF) is the most common (58%) form of cardiomyopathy at our center in South India. Over a 10-year period from 1975 we investigated 142 patients with EMF. The clinical, radiologic, hemodynamic, and angiographic features were similar to those reported from Africa. Echocardiographic studies using conventional and color-coded images revealed the pathologic anatomy of the disease, which enabled us to confirm the diagnosis of EMF noninvasively. Patchy endocardial thickening was observed in 22 siblings (29%) of EMF patients. The role of medical and surgical management is discussed.

INTRODUCTION

The state of Kerala on the the southwestern coast of peninsular India is well known to demographers for its very high population density (650 to 1,000 per sq km). The coastal districts of this state are hyperendemic for filariasis. High incidences of certain rare diseases like endomyocardial fibrosis (EMF), chronic relapsing pancreatitis, and oral submucous fibrosis have been reported from this state. Kerala State, like Uganda, Nigeria, the Ivory Coast, and Brazil where a high incidence of EMF have been reported, is located 120° in latitude from the equator. During the 1950s and early 1960s autopsy reports of EMF were reported from various parts of India.[1-5] Gopi,[6] while working at the Medical College Hospital at Trivandrum, Kerala, reported a very high incidence of EMF in this part of the country. He found that 8% of all cardiac admissions to that hospital, had cardiomyopathies, of whom 85% had EMF. Later, reports on clinical, hemodynamic, angiographic, and echocardiographic studies[7-10] as well as a comparative study of endomyocardial disease found in Kerala, Brazil, and the U.K.[11] were published. The present authors investigated 142 patients with EMF over a 10-year period, and the results form the basis of this paper.

PATIENTS AND METHODS

During the 10-year period from 1975 to 1985 at the Christian Medical College Hospital, Vellore (Tamil Nadu, South India) and at the Trivandrum Medical College Hospital (Kerala), 266 patients were referred with a clinical diagnosis of restrictive cardiomyopathy, of whom 142 were found to have EMF. There were 101 male and 41 female patients. Their ages varied from 4 to 43 years (mean $\pm$ SD 24$\pm$13 years). Seventyfour patients (52%) were from 10 to 20 years age group. During the earlier part of the study

9

diagnosis was confirmed by cardiac catheterization and angiography (29 patients). With the availability of two-dimensional echocardiography (2-DE) we found that the pathologic anatomy of EMF could be clearly delineated by this technique.[12] In 113 patients the diagnosis was mainly based on 2-DE studies, among whom 24 underwent cardiac catheterization and angiography. Twelve patients underwent transvenous cardiac biopsy. Autopsy material from 18 patients was available for study. The 2-DE studies were complemented by regional echo intensity studies[12] using a Brompton Colour Encoder.[13] Sera from 28 patients and 26 controls were analyzed in the immunology laboratory of the Royal Postgraduate Medical School, London. Immunoglobulin levels, eosinophilic immunologic studies, filarial antibody titers, and antibodies against the heart and other organs were determined. Like other workers in this field, we found a familial incidence of EMF[14] in some patients. Hence we surveyed 75 siblings of EMF patients. In addition to a detailed clinical evaluation they underwent conventional and color-coded echocardiography to detect areas of high echo intensity indicating intracardiac fibrosis.

OBSERVATIONS

The hospital incidence of EMF remained high in the late 1970s and early 1980s, corroborating the earlier observation of Gopi.[6] It was the most common form of cardiomyopathy (6% of all cardiac admissions) found in our wards. This apparently very high incidence is partly due to a policy of admitting all patients with EMF for evaluation and aggressive medical management. Toward the end of our study period we could identify 3 different forms of clinical presentations of EMF. Fifty-three patients (37.3%) presented with features of dominant right ventricular disease, while in 43 patients (30.3%), features of left ventricular disease were predominant. On detailed investigation many of these patients were found to have some evidence of involvement of the other ventricle. Forty-six patients (32.4%) presented with features of involvement of both ventricles. Thus we classified our patients into dominant right ventricular, dominant left ventricular, and biventricular EMF groups. During our study period 3 patients with dominant right ventricular disease and 6 patients with dominant left ventricular disease developed significant disease of the other ventricle and moved to the biventricular group.

The onset of disease was very slow in all our patients. The "initial illness" described by Parry and Abrahams[15] was not present in any of our patients. Except for 2, all our patients came from the poor socioeconomic strata. Sixty-six percent of them were from the coastal districts. None came from the hilly terrain which occupies one third of the state of Kerala.

RIGHT VENTRICULAR ENDOMYOCARDIAL FIBROSIS

There were 53 patients with dominant right ventricular disease and 46 patients in whom the right ventricle was involved as part of biventricular disease. Symptoms were often mild, in spite of advanced heart disease. In 14 patients EMF was suspected by physicians when the patients attended hospital for noncardiac problems. Four patients were referred to the gastroenterology department for treatment of ascites.

Presenting Symptoms

Table 1 lists the presenting symptoms of our patients, which were similar to those reported by other workers.[16] Dyspnea when present was related to the severity of ab-

TABLE 1. Presenting Symptoms and Physical Signs of Patients with Right Ventricular EMF ($N=99$)

Symptom	No. of patients	%
Puffiness of face	99	100
Ascites	99	100
Dyspnea	79	80
Palpitation	82	83
Ankle edema	48	48
Oliguria	14	14
Joint pain	14	14
Primary amenorrhea	8	8
Growth retardation	67	68
Proptosis	40	40
Parotid enlargement	51	52
Hepatomegaly	87	88
Splenomegaly	51	52
Central cyanosis	10	10
Atrial fibrillation	44	44
Elevated JVP	99	100
Cardiomegaly	99	100
Pericardial effusion	10	10
RV 3rd heart sound	91	92
Tricuspid regurgitation	75	76
Tricuspid diast. murmur	32	32

dominal distension. A striking feature is a protuberant abdomen with minimal or no ankle edema.

Physical Signs (Table 1)

The triad of engorged jugular veins, ascites, and hepatomegaly were observed in all patients. Dependent edema was observed only in patients with a long history of illness and irregular treatment. Hepatomegaly was firm, smooth, and often nonpulsatile. Proptosis and parotid enlargement were common in malnourished children with hepatic or pancreatic disorders. Central cyanosis when present was very mild except in one patient who was later found to have an associated secundum atrial septal defect.

Forty-five patients were in sinus rhythm and 44 had atrial fibrillation. Jugular venous pressure showed very prominent "a" waves in 24 patients. Massive cardiomegaly with heart borders extending from the right midclavicular to the left posterior axillary line was quite common. Tricuspid regurgitation murmur when present was of low grade and high pitched. Patients below 20 years showed growth retardation, and in those in whom the disease had an early onset secondary sexual characteristics did not develop. Late-onset patients complained of the loss of axillary and pubic hair. Forty-six patients had anemia with hemoglobin less than 12.5 Gms%. Erythrocyte sedimentation rate was more than 30 mm in 42 patients. Peripheral blood eosinophilia of $>1,500$ cells/mm³ was observed in 23% of patients, but abnormal eosinophils were not found.

Electrocardiographic Signs (Table 2)

A characteristic qR pattern in lead V_1 was observed in 79 patients (80%), and this sign helped to differentiate EMF from pericardial diseases. Simultaneous recordings of

TABLE 2. Electrocardiographic Features in Patients with Right Ventricular EMF ($N = 99$)

Feature	No. of patients	%
Sinus rhythm	53	54
Atrial fibrillation	44	44
Right atrial "P" waves	44	44
Low-voltage QRS	95	96
qR pattern in lead V_1	79	80

V_1 and V_6 showed that the q waves in V_1 occurred later than in V_6, indicating this to be right atrial cavity potential appearing in the surface electrocardiogram due to right atrial dilatation.

Radiological Signs

Massive cardiomegaly with a cardiothoracic ratio of more than 75% was seen in 34 patients. Fluoroscopy revealed dilated hyperdynamic outflow tract of the right ventricle in 38 patients (72%). Myocardial calcification was evident in 9 (18%) and pericardial effusion in 8 (15%).

Hemodynamic Findings

Right atrial mean pressure was always elevated and was higher in patients with atrial fibrillation (average 16.6 mmHg), compared to those in sinus rhythm (average 12.3 mmHg). Moderate elevations of right atrial pressure were associated with prominent "a" waves. With increasing severity of the disease "v" waves appeared to dominate. The right ventricular pressure pattern was characterized by an elevated earlydip diastolic with prominent end diastolic "a" wave impression (Fig. 1). Only in patients with

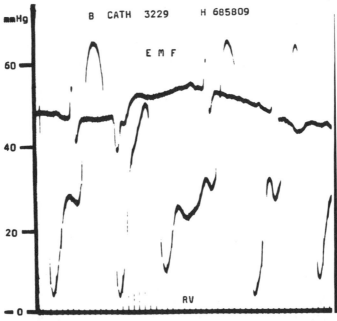

Fig. 1. Right ventricular pressure tracing from a patient with right ventricular EMF. Note the prominent "a" waves and high end diastolic pressure.

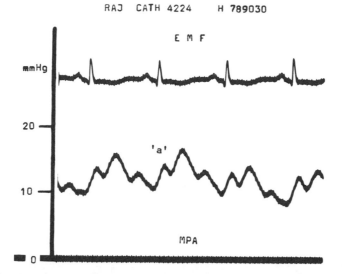

Fig. 2. Pulmonary artery pressure tracing recorded using catheter tip transducer, from a patient with right ventricular EMF. Note the rise of pressure at
end diastole. This "a" wave follows the "P" wave of the electrocardiogram (see
text).

atrial fibrillation was a "dip and plateau" pattern observed. In all patients with dominant
right ventricular disease the right ventricular end diastolic pressure was more than 50%
of the peak systolic pressure. Mean right ventricular end diastolic pressure was 14.2
(SD±4.1) mmHg. Mean pulmonary artery pressure was normal in all cases. The most
striking feature of the pulmonary artery pressure curve was a distinct positive pressure
wave in late diastole (Fig. 2). This coincided with the "a" wave of the right atrial pressure tracings. It was obvious that the strong right atrial contractions were forcing the
pulmonary valve to open in diastole. The right atrium and right ventricular outflow
tract formed the main pumping chambers, while the fibrosed inflow tract could contribute little towards right ventricular ejection. The cardiac index was normal (mean±
SD = 2.56+0.45 l/mt/M2).

Angiographic Features

Angiography demonstrated a dilated right atrium, a normal tricuspid anulus, a
diminutive right ventricular inflow region, and a dilated, hyperdynamic outflow tract.
Tricuspid regurgitation was present in all patients but difficult to assess in 14 patients
as the right atrium and ventricle formed a common chamber.

Echocardiographic Features (Table 3)

The large right heart displaced the left ventricle posteriorly, making imaging difficult.
The most striking features were ankylosed tricuspid valves and echo-dense, thinned-out
noncontractile right ventricular free walls. In 15 patients the apex appeared thickened
due to dense fibrosis. In 20 patients the tricuspid leaflets were completely fibrosed and
the right atrium and ventricle formed a common chamber. A dimple could clearly be
seen in 70 of our patients (89%) over the right ventricular apex (Fig. 3). The presence
of pericardial effusion in these patients made the detection of the dimple easy. This 2-D

TABLE 3.   Echocardiographic Features of Right Ventricular EMF ($N = 79$)

Feature	No. of patients	%
Small left venticle	64	81
Paradoxical IVS movement	70	89
Dimunitive RV inflow	72	91
Thin RV free wall	56	71
Dimple over RV apex	70	89
Tricuspid ankylosis	77	98
Dilated RV outflow	79	100
RV calcification	32	41
RA/RV thrombus	21	27
Aneurysmal RA	65	82
Pericardial effusion	79	100
Dilated inferior vena cava	63	80

IVS: interventricular septum, RV: right ventricle, RA: right atrium.

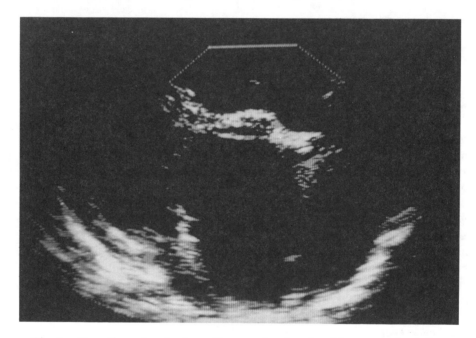

Fig. 3.   Two-dimensional echocardiogram showing the right ventricular inflow view from a patient with right ventricular EMF. The right atrium and ventricle have become a common chamber. Top center shows interventricular groove with echo-dense fibrosis. To the right of it there is another epicardial depression over the right ventricular apex. This is the "right ventricular apical dimple."

echo sign corresponds to the pathologic description of an apical dimple, pathognomonic of EMF. Crescentic calcification of the free wall was observed in 18 patients. Slowing of the bloodstream in the right cardiac chambers could be demonstrated by the slow passage of injected contrast medium as well as by the presence of dynamic intracavitary echoes. Large thrombi were seen occupying the common right atrial and ventricular chambers in 16 patients, and smaller ones in 5 other patients. Thrombus formation and calcification were seen only in patients with a history of symptoms for more than 5 years. Contrast echocardiography demonstrated right-to-left shunt across the patent foramen ovale in 13 patients with central cyanosis.

LEFT VENTRICULAR ENDOMYOCARDIAL FIBROSIS

There were 43 patients with dominant involvement of the left ventricle. In 46 patients left ventricular disease was part of biventricular EMF. These patients presented with symptoms of left heart failure (Table 4). Twenty-four patients had congestive heart failure. Peripheral pulses were normal. Cardiomegaly, when present (56%), was only of mild to moderate degree. Left parasternal heave and palpable shock of the second sound were present in 36 patients (88%). A loud 3rd heart sound over the apex was a constant finding. Mitral regurgitation murmurs were heard in 34 patients; these were only of grade 2 or 3 and tapered off toward the end of systole. We consider the possibility of EMF in all patients who present with severe symptoms of left heart failure, but show mild cardiomegaly, mild to moderate mitral regurgitation, and pulmonary hypertension.

Electrocardiograms showed sinus rhythm with left atrial enlargement in all, left ventricular hypertrophy in 6, and left axis deviation in 8. Four patients developed atrial fibrillation while under observation, with marked deterioration of their clinical status. Skiagram of the chest showed myocardial calcification in 12 patients. In 18 patients calcification could be demonstrated by fluoroscopy. Lung fields showed evidence of pulmonary venous congestion in every case. Classic features of pulmonary arterial hypertension were not seen.

Hemodynamic Features (Table 5)

Severity of involvement of the left ventricle was reflected in marked elevation of the left-ventricular-end-diastolic pressure. From the early diastolic dip the pressure continued to rise until end diastole without forming a plateau. It was not uncommon to find the left ventricular end diastolic pressure as high as one-quarter to one-third of peak systolic pressure. In 3 patients it remained above 30 mmHg. Mean right atrial pressure was normal in patients with isolated left ventricular disease. With the exception

TABLE 4. Presenting Symptoms of Patients with Left Ventricular EMF ($N = 89$)

Symptom	No. of patients	%
Effort dyspnea	88	99
Paroxysmal nocturnal dyspnea	10	11
Dependent edema	24	27
Systemic embolism	4	4
Asymptomatic	1	1

TABLE 5. Hemodynamic Features of Left Ventricular EMF ($N = 11$)

Feature	Mean	±SD
Left ventricular end diastolic pressure	24	9.6 mmHg
Pulmonary artery pressure	48	15.7 mmHg
Pulmonary vascular resistance index	8	6.3 units/M²
Cardiac index	2.4	0.8 l/min/M²

TABLE 6.   Echocardiographic Features of Left Ventricular EMF ($N = 69$)

Feature	No. of patients	%
Left ventricle: Small	36	52
Normal	19	28
Dilated	24	35
LV ejection fraction: Low	21	30
Normal	48	70
Posterior leaflet adherent to posterior wall of LV	60	87
LV aneurysm	24	35
LV thrombus	12	17
LV calcification	30	43
Left atrial enlargement	69	100

LV: left ventricle.

of one patient, all had pulmonary hypertension with elevation of pulmonary vascular resistance. The cardiac index was low in 6 patients.

Angiographic Features

The left ventricular cavity was enlarged in one and small in 2 patients. End systolic volume was large in all. The ventricular configuration was altered by obliteration of the apex in all, and formation of aneurysmal areas had occurred in 4 patients. Apical and inferior wall dyskinesia was seen in 8. Mitral regurgitation of trivial degree was observed in 2, mild degree in 4, and moderate degree in 2 patients. One patient had a large apical thrombus.

Echocardiographic Features (Table 6)

Normal or small left ventricle with left atrial enlargement was characteristic of left ventricular EMF (Fig. 4). The posterior mitral leaflet was thickened, echo-dense, and adherent to the posterior left ventricular wall in 60 patients (87%). Calcification extending from the base of the posterior leaflet to the base of the posterior papillary muscle was seen in 18 patients. In 6, calcific nodules over the base of the posterior papillary muscle could be identified. Areas of high echo density with dyskinesia were commonly observed over the inferior wall and apex. Thrombus occupying the apex of the left ventricle was seen in 8, and over the apex and inferior wall in 4 patients. Thrombi were seen only in patients with severe disease, who were in the low-output stage. Systemic heparinization did not decrease the size of the thrombi.

Color-coded echocardiography   Amplitude-processed, color-coded, 2-dimensional echocardiograms were used for the study of areas of abnormal echo intensity.[9,13] The distribution of areas with high echo intensity is shown in Table 7. The values corresponded with those observations obtained using conventional 2-D echocardio graphy.

Immunological studies   Both patients and control subjects had elevated immunoglobulin levels, although a higher proportion of patients had markedly raised serum IgG, IgA, IgM, and IgE levels. A large number of patients (60%) also had elevated filarial antibody titers. A combination of markedly elevated IgE and high titers of filarial antibodies appeared characteristic of this disease. Our patients did not show anti-heart

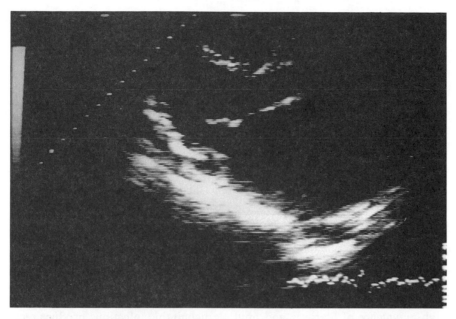

Fig. 4. Two-dimensional echocardiogram from a patient with left ventricular EMF showing the parasternal long-axis view. Note the thickened posterior mitral leaflet adherent to the posterior left ventricular wall. A long shelf of myocardial calcification can be seen extending from the base of the posterior cusp to the base of the papillary muscle.

TABLE 7.   Distribution of Abnormal Echo-Dense Areas in the Heart ($N=86$)

Heart area	No. of patients	%
Interventricular septum,		
Basal	19	22
Apical	26	30
Posterior LV wall	62	72
Posterior papillary muscle	33	38
Mitral anterior leaflet	9	10
Mitral posterior leaflet	83	97
Left ventricular apex	36	42
Base of anterior tricuspid		
leaflet	53	62
Right ventricular apex	69	80
Right ventricular anterior		
wall	69	80

LV: left ventricle.

antibodies or antibodies to gastric parietal cells or thyroid as was observed in Uganda.[17] Eosinophilic immunologic studies were inconclusive.

Echocardiographic study of siblings (Table 8)   None of the siblings showed clinical signs of EMF nor had any disability. Skiagrams of the chest and electrocardiograms were within normal limits. Endocardial thickening was highly echodense and dis-

TABLE 8.   Echocardiographic Abnormalities Seen in Siblings of Patients with EMF ($N=75$)

Abnormality	No. of subjects	%
Left ventricular posterior wall endocardial thickening	21	28
Left ventricular apical endocardial thickening	6	8
Thickening of base of posterior mitral leaflet	7	9
Right ventricular apical endocardial thickening	7	9

crete. However, there were no dyskinetic myocardial segments or mitral regurgitation. We are following up those patients to determine whether they are in the early or burnt-out phase of disease. None has shown any progression of lesions so far.

ETIOLOGICAL FACTORS

A high prevalence of filariasis and multiple helminthic infections produce recurrent peripheral blood eosinophilia in 16% of the general Kerala population. However, efforts to demonstrate eosinophilic toxic damage to the myocardium of our patients have not been fruitful. The hypothesis that thorium excess in tropical regions in conjunction with magnesium deficiency may damage the endocardium lacks proof.[18]

PROGNOSIS UNDER MEDICAL MANAGEMENT

Since 1979, we have followed the natural history of EMF in 98 patients. Sixty-eight of them remained asymptomatic until 1985. Six patients were operated on after failure of medical management. Twenty-four patients (24%) died during the study period; they progressively failed to respond to medical treatment, developed large intracardiac thrombi with occasional systemic and/or pulmonary emboli, and died in the low-output stage. With the availability of powerful diuretics and better techniques of control of cardiac failure, the prognosis of these patients under medical management is different from the often-quoted 44% mortality within one year of onset of disease.[19]

SURGERY FOR ENDOMYOCARDIAL FIBROSIS

Three centers in India are actively involved in surgery for EMF patients who are symptomatic and experience significant valval regurgitation. John *et al.*[20] and Cherian *et al.*[8] in Vellore have found that endocardiectomy with valve replacement considerably ameliorates symptoms in such patients. Valiathan and colleagues[21] in Kerala, after operating on 62 patients, have reported that surgery is associated with a 29.5% operative mortality, mainly due to low-output state or a failure to come off bypass. In addition, there were 6 late deaths due to prosthetic valve problems or postoperative complete heart block. Even though surviving patients showed considerable symptomatic improvement, postoperative hemodynamic studies in 17 patients showed only limited benefit.[22] Mean right ventricular end diastolic pressure decreased from 16.71 ± 6.56 to 10.82 ± 5.31 ($P < 0.05$), and the left ventricular end diastolic pressure changed from

19.22 ± 6.04 to 12.17 ± 3.08 ($P < 0.025$). Angiographic studies showed an increase in both right and left ventricular dimensions. Cherian et al.[23,24] in Madras, India, operated on 8 patients without any operative mortality, by careful patient selection and conservative endocardiectomy over the interventricular septum.

CONCLUSIONS

EMF is a severely disabling cardiovascular disease commonly affecting young individuals in the southern districts of Kerala State in South India. We could not identify any etiologic factors that would suggest preventive measures. Early diagnosis and aggressive medical management gives patients long periods of symptomatic relief. However, those who fail to respond to medical treatment, especially those patients with significant atrioventricular valve regurgitation, benefit from surgical treatment.

REFERENCES

1. Samuel, I. and Anklesaria, X.J. Endomyocardial fibrosis in South India. *Indian J. Pathol. Bacteriol.* **3**: 157, 1960.
2. Shah, V.V., Goodluck, P.L., and Mehtha, A.C. Cardiomyopathy. *Indian Heart J.* **14**: 70, 1962.
3. Mehrothra, A.N., Maheswari, H.B., Khosla, S.N., and Kumar, S. Endomyocardial fibrosis. *J. Assoc. Phys. India* **12**: 845, 1964.
4. Kinare, S.G., and Deshpande, D.H. Endomyocardial fibrosis. *Indian J. Med. Sci.* **19**: 63, 1965.
5. Reddy, D.J., Omer, S., Prabhaker, V., Rao, P.S.S., and Rao, K.S. Endomyocardial fibrosis. *J. Indian Med. Assoc.* **45**: 440, 1965.
6. Gopi, C.K. Endomyocardial fibrosis. *Bull. WHO*, **38**: 939, 1968.
7. Vijayaraghavan, G., Cherian, G., Krishnaswami, S., and Sukumar, I.P. Left ventricular endomyocardial fibrosis in India. *Br. Heart J.* **39**: 563, 1977.
8. Cherian, G., Vijayaraghavan, G., Krishnaswami, S., Sukumar, I.P., John, S., Jairaj, P.S., and Bhaktaviziam, A. Endomyocardial fibrosis: Report on the haemodynamic data in 29 patients and review of the results of surgery. *Am. Heart J.* **105**: 659, 1983.
9. Vijayaraghavan, G., Davies, J., Sadanandan, S., Spry, C.J.F., Gibson, D.G., and Goodwin, J.F. Echocardiographic features of tropical endomyocardial fibrosis. *Br. Heart J.* **50**: 450, 1983.
10. Vijayaraghavan, G. Endomyocardial fibrosis: Clinical, electrocardiographic and radiological features. In: Endomyocardial Fibrosis in India, Sapru, R.P. (ed.), Indian Council of Medical Research, New Delhi, India, 1983, pp. 22.
11. Davies, J., Spry, C.G.F., Vijayaraghavan, G., and De Souza, T.A. A comparison of the clinical and cardiological features of endomyocardial disease seen in temperate and tropical regions. *Postgrad. Med. J.* **59**: 179, 1983.
12. Vijayaraghavan, G., Davies, J., Sadanandan, S., Spry, C.J.F., Gibson, D.G., and Goodwin, J.F. 2-D echocardiographic diagnosis of endomyocardial fibrosis. Abnormalities of regional echo intensity. *Circulation* 66, Suppl. **11**: 122, 1982.
13. Logan-Sinclair, R., Wong, C.M., and Gibson, D.G. Clinical application of amplitude processing of echocardiographic images. *Br. Heart J.* **45**: 621, 1981.
14. Patel, A.K., Ziegler, J.L., D'Arbela, P.G., and Somers, K. Familial cases of endomyocardial fibrosis in Uganda. *Br. Med. J.* **4**: 331, 1971.
15. Parry, E.H.O. and Abrahams, D.G. The natural history of endomyocardial fibrosis. *Quart. J. Med.* **44**: 383, 1965.
16. Somers, K., Brenton, D.P., and Sood, N.K. Clinical features of endomyocardial fibrosis of the right ventricle. *Br. Heart J.* **30**: 309, 1968.

17. Shaper, A.G. Cardiovascular disease in the tropics—endomyocardial fibrosis. *Br. Med. J.* **3**: 743, 1972.
18. Valiathan, M.S., Kartha, C.C., Pandey, V.K., Dang, H., and Sunta, C.M.A. Geochemical basis for endomyocardial fibrosis. *Cardiovasc. Res.* **20**: 679, 1986.
19. D'Arbela, P.G., Mutazindwa, T., Patel, A.K., *et al.* Survival after first presentation with endomyocardial fibrosis. *Br. Heart J.* **34**: 403, 1972.
20. John, S., Mani, G.K., Muralidharan, S., Krishnaswami, S., and Cherian, G. Endomyocardial fibrosis from a surgical standpoint. *J. Thorac. Cardiovasc. Surg.* **80**: 437, 1980.
21. Valiathan, M.S., Balakrishnan, K.G., Sankarkumar, R., and Kartha, C.C. Surgical treatment of endomyocardial fibrosis. *Ann. Thorac. Surg.* **43**: 68, 1987.
22. Balakrishnan, K.G., Venkatachalam, C.G., Pillai, V.R.K., Subrahmonyam, R., and Valiathan, M.S. Postoperative evaluation of endomyocardial fibrosis. *Cardiology* **73**: 73, 1986.
23. Cherian, K.M., John, T.A., and Abraham, K.A. Endomyocardial fibrosis: Clinical profile and role of surgery in management. *Am. Heart J.* **105**: 706, 1983.
24. Cherian, K.M. Personal communication, 1988.

The Relationship of Microfilaria and Other Helminthic Worms to Tropical Endomyocardial Fibrosis (EMF): A Review

Joseph J. Andy

Department of Medicine, College of Medical Sciences, University of Calabar, Calabar, Nigeria

ABSTRACT

Observations of migrants and prospective observations of indigenous patients in EMF-endemic areas have associated helminthic parasitic infections (particularly filariasis) and eosinophilia with causation of tropical EMF. Pathologic, histochemical, and immunologic studies have indicated that: 1) EMF is a pancarditis with severe damage to epi- and endomyocardium; and 2) the mechanism of cardiac damage may involve allergy and "activated" eosinophils.

A review of organ damage reported during larval migration of some helminthic worms associated with induction of endomyocardial necrosis or EMF is presented and evidence is advanced that endomyocardial necrosis/fibrosis is caused by such larval migration. The mechanism of endomyocardial damage is probably basically allergic with added eosinophilic cytotoxicity.

INTRODUCTION

Extensive endomyocardial fibrosis (EMF) in Africans, affecting one or both ventricles and occurring usually without, but sometimes with, blood eosinophilia was first mentioned in 1946 among idiopathic cardiomyopathies seen in West African soldiers serving in the Middle East.[1] Davies,[2] working in Uganda, clearly defined its unique clinical and cardiac morphologic features in 1948, and his work was to stimulate much research into the clinical features, pathology, epidemiology, and etiology of this disease entity. EMF, initially thought to be unique to Africa, has now been shown to be frequent in South India,[3-6] Thailand,[7] Colombia,[8] Venezuela,[9] Brazil,[10] and the Middle East.[11] Occasional cases have been reported in Europe and North America.[13-16] The cardiac morphologic features of EMF, which consist of extensive fibrosis affecting the inflow tract, the apex, and the papillary muscles of one or both ventricles, are easily recognized when well developed. However, less severe and less extensive cardiac morphologic expression of the disease cannot easily be identified.[17] The typical clinical features of EMF, which generally consist of clinical and hemodynamic features of restrictive heart disease in association with features of atrioventricular valvular regurgitation, render the disease relatively easy to diagnose.[18] However, the typical clinical features of EMF are present only when the cardiac pathologic features are extensive and chronic.

Although the clinical and hemodynamic features of established EMF are well described and the diagnosis of the late stage of disease is relatively easy, the clinical and hemodynamic features of early EMF have received very limited attention,[5,19] and remain difficult to recognize. The failure to diagnose EMF at its inception has greatly hindered investigations into its etiology and pathogenesis. The difficulty in identifying early EMF results partly from a lack of a clinical or laboratory marker capable of separating early EMF from other causes of acute heart failure.

Although EMF has occasionally been induced by drugs and anticancer agents,[20-22] the geographic distribution of endemic tropical EMF in humans, which is limited mainly to the rain forest belt of Africa, South India, Brazil, Venezuela, and Thailand and which is very different from the distribution of dilated cardiomyopathies, suggests on epidemiologic grounds that multifactorial causation is unlikely unless the causes operate through a common pathway.

The purpose of this paper is to summarize the considerable amount of evidence now available associating EMF with infective agents, particularly helminthic worms and filariasis, with or without eosinophilia. A second objective is to examine possible mechanisms by which these parasites are associated with endomyocardial damage.

Significant Clinical and Pathologic Leads to Etiology and Pathogenesis of Tropical EMF

One indication that EMF is caused by an infective agent is the fact that most patients of European ancestry[23] and some African patients[18,19,23] have febrile illness and malaise at the onset. Also, IgM levels are generally raised in Nigerian[24] and Ugandan[25,26] EMF patients. Osunkoya and colleagues in 1972[27] reported a much higher frequency of granulomatous lesions in the liver, lungs, and spleens of Nigerian EMF patients compared with matched controls with rheumatic heart disease.

The cardiac morphology of EMF has now been shown to be indistinguishable from the cardiac morphology of the eosinophilic endomyocardial diseases.[28,29] In addition, hypereosinophilia has been present in the early stages of EMF of nearly all European residents in Africa[24,30,31] and hypereosinophilia in some,[18,19] although absent[32] in most African EMF patients. Moreover, in some cases with eosinophilic endomyocardial damage, the eosinophilia may return to normal in the later stages of the disease.[12,33] These observations led to the suggestion that tropical EMF is most likely the burnt-out phase of eosinophilic heart disease.[29]

In studies of the vascular pattern in normal and abnormal hearts from Uganda, using dye injection, microradiograph, and histologic techniques, Farrer-Brown and colleagues commented on myocardial scarring in EMF hearts.[17,34] Myocardial scarring was found throughout the width of the myocardium in all parts of the heart, and the distribution resembled that seen in healed cases of myocarditis, rather than the pattern associated with myocardial ischemia. The same authors described one case of EMF from Uganda with typical endomyocardial fibrosis and mural thrombus, but with a more extensively affected entire myocardium by myocarditis than is usually reported in EMF.[17] They suggested the concept of EMF as a pancarditis in the majority of hearts, but with more severe changes in the endomyocardium and pericardium. In EMF, pericarditis occurs in about 70% of cases and mural thrombi in up to 45%.[35]

Farrer-Brown and colleagues[17,34] also pointed out that when endocardial scarring or massive thrombosis associated with fibrosis occupies the inflow tract or apex in a patient with idiopathic cardiomegaly, neither the histopathology nor the vascular pattern was useful for differentiating the case from EMF.

Using a wide variety of histologic staining methods, Connor and his colleagues[36] found that in early EMF cardiac connective tissue, especially that of the endocardium, is swollen with acid mucopolysaccharide (AMP) and the endocardium is covered by a layer of fibrin. In later lesions, the involved areas had resolved as hard white scars composed of collagen and elastic fibers. They also reported peculiar and characteristic foci of collagen necrosis in the scar tissue at the endomyocardial junction. The consistent mucinous swellings of the cardiac "ground substance" and vessels as well as the focal nonsuppurative disintegration of collagen suggested to the authors that hypersensitivity is the underlying mechanism in EMF.[36]

Becker's heart disease reported from South Africa is characterized by focal subendocardial necrosis or fibrosis and mural thrombi.[37,38] A thin rippled layer of fibrinous coagulum may cover the entire endocardial surface of the ventricles, but always occurs in relation to areas of mucinous exudate.[37,38]

The earliest lesion was characterized by focal swelling of the mural endocardium due to acid mucopolysaccharide deposition with rare and scanty infiltration of subendocardial tissues with mononuclear cells. The lesion in Becker's heart disease was also thought to be induced by hypersensitivity based on histochemical staining techniques. Becker's heart disease confirms the existence of an allergic mural heart disease. It is probable that this disease represents a morphologically milder expression of the same process as tropical EMF.

The recent report of glomerular lesions including capillary wall thickening, basement membrane duplication, mesangial expansion and interposition, intraluminal fibrin, and dense, subendothelial deposits in EMF patients from India suggests that in tropical EMF a more diffuse organ involvement than previously recognized does occur.[39] This glomerular involvement was attributed to deposition and organization of immune complexes. The occurrence of diffuse neurologic manifestations including headache, meningoencephalitis, delirium, drowsiness, hemiplegia, and coma in some Nigerian patients[18,40] as well as some European patients with EMF[23] also indicates diffuse organ involvement in EMF. In most of the European patients and our Nigerian patients, diffuse neurologic features either predated clinical heart disease by some days, months, or years or it occurred during the early stages of the heart disease.[18,40]

Thus clinical and pathologic evidence indicates: i) that EMF is induced by an infective agent; ii) that the cardiac damage is usually part of a diffuse organ system damage; iii) that EMF is usually a pancarditis with more severe damage to epi- and endomyocardium; and iv) that the mechanism of cardiac damage is most likely allergic.

EPIDEMIOLOGIC OBSERVATIONS

European Workers in EMF-endemic Areas Who Developed EMF

The first report incriminating *Acanthocheilonema perstans* and eosinophilia in causation of EMF was of a French colonial officer resident in West Africa, by Morenas in 1929, i.e., 7 years before Loffler identified the characteristics of eosinophilic heart disease and 19 years prior to the description by Davies of tropical EMF.[41] Other isolated reports of European migrant workers in Africa who developed EMF were summarized by Gerbaux and colleagues in 1957,[42] and by Brockington and colleagues in 1967.[23] To our knowledge 26 European residents in Africa have been reported with EMF,[23,30,31] including the recent report (1986) of EMF associated with *Loa loa*-induced hypereosinophilia in an American Peace Corps worker in West Africa.[31] White cell counts and differentials were available in 23, and eosinophilia was severe in 20 of them; microfilaria was diagnosed in 16 of 26 patients.[23,30,31] Those European residents in Africa who were reported to have EMF lived in Gabon (5 cases), Nigeria (3 cases), Zaire (8 cases), Cameroon (6 cases), the Central African Republic (2 cases), and "West Africa" (2 cases).

Experience from these European patients suggested that once severe heart disease had occurred, reversal of eosinophilia to normal[23,43] with cortisone[42,44] or with antiparasitic agents[31,44] did not appear to affect significantly the course of the heart disease.

The other helminthic worms that have been associated with eosinophilia and EMF in an emigrant to an endemic area are *Ascaris lumbricoides* and hookworm.[45]

Epidemiologic Evidence from EMF-endemic Areas

The first attempt to study seriously the association of microfilaria, eosinophilia, and EMF in an endemic area was reported by Ive and colleagues from Nigeria in 1967.[46] Their study reported that: i) many Nigerian EMF patients had elevated eosinophil counts; ii) the area of endemicity of EMF in Nigeria was similar to the area of endemicity of *Loa loa*; and iii) most EMF patients were rural dwellers in the tropical rain forest belt of Nigeria. Their study did not define the normal limits and distribution of eosinophilia, which is very common in Nigeria. Also, they studied only established cases of EMF, some of whom had had the disease for many years. But since it is well known that helminth-induced eosinophilia usually runs a self-limiting course, it was not surprising that their association of EMF with eosinophilia was not sustained when their initial observations were extended.[47] In another effort to test the association of EMF with eosinophilia in Nigeria, we assumed that such an association would best be evaluated early in the course of heart disease, and that it could best be assessed in cases with very high eosinophil counts.[18] The distribution of eosinophilia in the locality was determined on 1956 patients with or without helminthic infestations. We used 4 hospitals, 2 each in 2 towns 20 miles apart, and studied eosinophil counts in all patients below 20 years of age who had presented with acute idiopathic heart failure with symptoms of less than 6 months' duration. We identified 13 such patients who had eosinophil counts greater than the 97 percentile value for our locality during a 2-year period. *Loa loa* was identified in 5 of them; 2 others had noticed a worm crossing their eyes, but diethylcarbamazine had returned eosinophil counts to normal in all cases. During a mean follow-up period of 2 years, 8 of 11 patients (73%) had developed clinical and some hemodynamic features of endocardial restrictive disease. EMF was confirmed at necropsy in one of them. This particular patient, who had previously been in good health, was seen on the 10th day of an illness characterized by fever, chills, periorbital swelling, urticarial rash, dyspnea on exertion, abdominal swelling, and eosinophilia caused by *Loa loa*. He died 25 1/2 months later[48] and EMF was confirmed at necropsy.

We later extended these observations to include other organ damage associated with helminthiasis and eosinophilia.[40] We observed that neurologic features including drowsiness, headache, acute confusional state with vomiting, hemiplegia with cranial nerve palsy, and meningoencephalitis with or without coma were frequent,[40] and usually occurred abruptly. Other associated conditions were skin urticaria, lymphadenopathy, and one case with pulmonary infiltration. Five patients had CNS features associated with cardiac enlargement, and 3 of these developed features of restrictive heart disease long after the neurologic features had subsided.

One 18-year-old patient[18,40] was admitted on the 7th day of an illness characterized by fever, severe headache, pleuritic type chest pain, signs of meningitis, and generalized itching and urticarial rash. Cerebrospinal fluid was normal except for slight elevation of protein. There was clinical and radiologic evidence of cardiomegaly and a tricuspid regurgitation murmur, and the ECG showed atrial tachycardia with 2:1 A-V block as well as symmetrical T inversion. Hemoglobin was normal, and white count was 9,900/ml with eosinophil count of 3,120/ml. No microfilaria were identified by thick film only, but Banocide returned the eosinophil counts to normal. Thirteen months later, he had developed typical clinical features of endocardial restrictive disease confirmed by cardiac catheterization.

Zilberg and colleagues[49,50] in Zimbabwe reported some patients with Katayama fever caused by schistosomiasis, who had diffuse encephalitis and myocarditis. One of the cases, a 9-year-old girl, had fever, eosinophilia (30% of 9,700/ml WBC), and clinical as well as ECG and EEG evidence of myocarditis and encephalitis.[50] The eosinophilia was controlled by a 6-week course of ambilhar. But 4 months after the onset of illness, she developed dyspnea and predominant features of restrictive heart failure with gross edema and a low-voltage ECG. Right heart catheterization revealed a restrictive pattern with normal pulmonary artery pressures (RV 32/17; PA 30/21). Thoracotomy for pericardectomy, carried out 9 months after first symptoms, excluded constrictive pericarditis and revealed a dilated right atrium and ventricle. Right atrial biopsy revealed chronic myocarditis, and lung biopsy showed extensive bilharzial tubercles and chronic bronchopneumonia. The patient appeared to have developed endocardial restrictive disease from schistosomiasis. Schistosomiasis with skin rash, eosinophilia, and hepatic granulomata in association with EMF have been recorded in Nigeria[51] and Brazil.[52]

In Uganda, EMF has an unusually high incidence in poor migrant laborers from Rwanda and Burundi compared with the Ganda people indigenous to the Kampala region.[35] Rheumatic fever, on the other hand, affects the Ganda group more than expected and the Rwanda people less than expected.[35] The Ganda people of Uganda live in an area holoendemic for malaria, whereas the Rwandans migrated from a mountainous area where malaria transmission is absent or seasonal. When in Uganda, the Rwandans had much heavier spleens than the Gandans from the age of 15 years and also had higher IgM and higher titers of malarial antibody.[35] Many of the Rwandans were born in Uganda of immigrant parents. There are a number of interpretations to which these very useful data have been subjected, but there is a possibility that a vector that transmits an agent capable of inducing EMF may share a similar habitat with the mosquito transmitting malaria. The interpretation of the present author is that emigrants from Rwanda to Uganda are mainly engaged as farmhands where they may be more exposed to such vectors, as well as to mosquitos bearing malaria. The experience in Nigeria is that EMF is more common in lower socioeconomic groups and in particular among peasant farmers and their children.[19]

Endomyocardial Damage in Trichinella Spiralis *and Other Helminthic Worms*

Among helminthic worms, cardiac pathology has been best studied in trichinosis, where 42 fatalities with 35 cardiac pathologic reports had been made by 1977.[53] Of those 35 cases, 4 showed evidence of endomyocardial necrosis, which was extensive in 3 who also had mural thrombi (Table 1).[53-56]

One patient died suddenly on the 13th day of an illness marked by fever, headache, neck stiffness, myalgias, pleuritic chest pain, and periorbital swelling. There was extensive necrosis of the endomyocardium of left and right ventricles with a fibrin thrombi overlay, as well as pericarditis. The endomyocardial necrotic lesion and fibrin thrombi were infiltrated by eosinophils and round cells. The patient had eosinophilia, and *Trichinella spiralis* was found at necropsy in the tongue and diaphragmatic muscle.[53] Trichinosis is a known cause of endomyocardial thrombosis in experimental animals,[57] of thrombosis in small vessels,[58] and sometimes of thromboembolism of large arteries.[59,60] Other helminthic worms associated with eosinophilia and EMF include *Giardia lamblia*[61] and fasciolae.[62]

TABLE 1.   Mural Endocarditis and Mural Thrombosis Induced by Trichinosis

Authors	Year	Age	Sex	Peak eosinophilia	Parasite	Total duration of illness	Cardiac pathology
Gruber and Gamper	1927	38	F	Eosinophilia	*Trichinella spiralis* in brain and skeletal muscle	5 weeks	Heart not enlarged. Endocardium of LV destroyed. A large adherent mural thrombus in LV, smaller thrombus in RV. Ventricular endothelium thickened with increased connective tissue in the subendocardium. Pericardial effusion.
McCabe and Zatuchni	1951	19	F	600/mm³	*Trichinella spiralis* in muscle	20 days	Clinical pericardial rub. Heart 180 g. Numerous petechial hemorrhages into pericardium and myocardium. Ventricles moderately dilated. Myocardial degeneration and diffuse polymorphic infiltration of myocardium. Endocardial surface swollen and coagulation of this layer of the ventricle.
Terplan, Kraus, and Barnes	1957	6	M	0% eosinophils	*Trichinella spiralis* in brain	8 days	Edema of LV endocardium with rare infiltrates of histocytes. Clusters of recent, adherent thrombi in RV consisting largely of fibrin and leukocytes adherent to the endocardium and completely blending with the heart wall as if forming a part of it, though apparently free of organizing cells and capillaries. No eosinophils seen in this thrombi.
Andy, O'Connell, Daddario, and Roberts	1977	46	F	9890/mm³	*Trichinella spiralis*	13 days	Heart weighed 260 g. Endocardium of both ventricles extensively destroyed and covered by fibrin deposits. The fibrin thrombi and endomyocardium infiltrat-

ed by eosinophils and round cells. Inflammatory changes particularly severe in the endomyocardium.

LV: left ventricle, RV: right ventricle, RA: right atrium.

MECHANISM OF CARDIOVASCULAR AND OTHER ORGAN SYSTEM DAMAGE IN HELMINTHIC DISEASES

The helminthic worms associated with EMF, including filariae, schistosomes, ascarides, hookworm, and *Trichinella spiralis*, usually induce organ damage distant from the site of localization of their adult forms during their phases of larval migration. Eosinophilia usually appears for the first time and often reaches its peak value during this phase of larval migration.[40,63] The current problem appears to be to determine whether eosinophil cytotoxicity alone,[64] allergic damage alone,[36,40] or a combination of both processes is important in cardiac damage in EMF induced by helminthic worms.

Evidence for Eosinophilic Cytotoxicity

The striking association of severely elevated eosinophilia with endomyocardial disease in the hypereosinophilic syndrome has led most investigators to the view that eosinophils themselves are intimately involved in the pathogenesis of this form of the disease.[64,65] In the hypereosinophilic conditions with organ damage, the eosinophils have been reported to lose some or all of their granules.[66] Also antibody-dependent killing of Chang and Girardi heart cells, and antibody-dependent lyses of human and chicken red blood cells by eosinophils from patients with hypereosinophilic syndrome have been reported.[67] Such studies demonstrated that eosinophils had cytotoxic properties that were less striking than for other phagocytic cells. But when eosinophil granule basic proteins were isolated and incubated with rat heart cells they were found to be highly toxic to these cells *in vitro*.[68] In addition, serial sections of tissues taken at necropsy or at cardiac biopsy from eosinophilic endomyocarditis showed that "activated" eosinophils and secreted eosinophil granule proteins were most evident within the necrotic and later-stage thrombotic lesions and were found mainly within the areas of acute tissue damage in the endocardium and in the walls of small blood vessels.[69]

Many patients with elevated blood eosinophil counts do not develop endomyocardial disease, but those with more than $1 \times 10^9/l$ degranulated eosinophils have been observed upon endocardial biopsy to have heart disease.[64] Also 2 patients with tropical EMF from Venezuela were found to have degranulated blood eosinophils,[70] and degranulated eosinophils have been observed in cardiac biopsies from patients with tropical EMF in India.[64] A prospective study of 14 patients with helminthic-related eosinophilia who were followed up clinically and by echocardiography for a mean of 14.5 months failed to show the presence of heart disease in those patients.[70] The highest level of eosinophilia (84% of 38,000/ml, WBC) that we have observed in loiasis occurred in a patient who died in progressive renal failure, severe hypertension, and hypertensive heart failure. At autopsy he had granular contracted kidneys, hypertensive heart disease, and uremic pericarditis. There was no evidence of acute tissue damage by eosinophilia and loiasis. It is therefore probable that when eosinophilia causes tissue damage, the eosinophils must first be "activated" to discharge their granules at the location of damage.[64]

Evidence for Allergic Tissue Damage Caused by Helminthic Larvae

During larval migration of the helminthic worms associated with EMF, organ damage, including to the skin, kidneys, lungs, central and peripheral nervous systems, liver, heart, and lymph nodes has been reported.[40] Diffuse central nervous system dysfunction including coma, delusion, confusion, psychosis, diffuse EEG changes, cerebellar dysfunction, cranial nerve palsy, and peripheral neuropathy have been described in tropical EMF,[23,40] filariasis,[71-73] trichinosis,[74] ascariasis,[75,76] and schistosomiasis.[49,50] The encephalopathy seen in tropical EMF,[23,40] loiasis,[40,71-73] and trichinosis[74] appears to develop in bursts. In acute fatal filariasis, detailed histopathologic changes occurring in the central nervous system have been reported by Van Bogaert and colleagues,[76] by Toussaint and Dannis,[72] and by Kivits,[77] The changes consist of granulomatous reactions with a variable necrotic component and lesions indicative of acute, diffuse edema with lymphocytic sheathing of some of the main vessels. The initial cellular infiltrates in the brain in trichinosis consist mainly of lymphocytes, glial cells, and a variable amount of eosinophils.[74]

An asthma-like syndrome with or without pneumonic infiltrates may occur during larval migration in ascariasis,[78] trichinosis,[40] and schistosomiasis.[79] Tropical pulmonary eosinophilia is now thought to be induced by an immediate type hypersensitivity response to microfilarial antigen.[80] Acute diffuse neurologic complications[81] and acute cardiac failure[82] may sometimes complicate cases of tropical eosinophilia.

Cardiac dysfunction and myocarditis, with or without pneumonia and/or encephalitis, is the leading cause of death in trichinosis[53] and in acute fatal filariasis.[71,72] Myocarditis has also been reported in human and experimental infection with ascariasis,[83] and in human infection with schistosomiasis.[49,50] The initial damage to the heart in trichinosis,[84] ascariasis,[83] and filariasis[40,71,77] appears to consist of focal cellular necrosis with dominant infiltration by round cells and by a variable amount of eosinophils. Fediyanina reported focal myocardial necrosis as well as infiltration with lymphocytes and rare eosinophils with a first-dose infection with 600 *Ascaris suum* eggs.[83] Superinfection with a second and third dose of 600 *A. suum* eggs worsened the cardiac injury, and the infiltrates became more marked, particularly in the endomyocardium and epimyocardium. Vasculitis with collagen swelling then developed and eosinophilic infiltrates increased. She concluded that ascariasis myocarditis is allergic.[83] Thus during larval migration, myocardial damage that is not mediated by eosinophilis occurs early but eosinophil-mediated damage may follow later. In filariasis an acute pericardial effusion teaming with microfilaria was described by Foster in 1959.[85] That patient had dyspnea and a systolic murmur at onset of symptoms, probably suggesting more extensive cardiac damage than pericarditis alone. In fulminant trichinosis the myocardial damage may be more severe in the endomyocardium and epimyocardium.[53,55,56,86]

The experience with European residents in Africa who developed EMF[23] and our experience with African patients with early tropical EMF[19,48] indicate that once the heart has been severely damaged, reversal of eosinophilia to normal or eradication of the infective agents does not appear to alter the course of the disease. In operated cases with eosinophilic heart disease, the general experience seems to be that there is no evidence of recurrence of endomyocardial lesions or of progression of heart damage,[64] although in a few cases surgical treatment in the thrombotic stage may be complicated by recurrent thrombi.[87] The cardiac damage in tropical EMF may also be phasic. In the few patients observed as early as 7 days, 10 days, and 3 weeks, cardiac damage had occurred abruptly.[19]

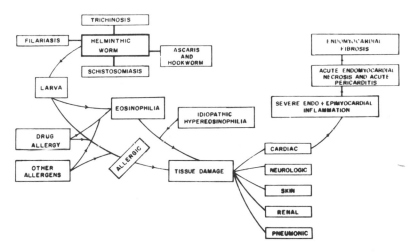

Fig. 1.   Proposed pathogenesis of EMF

Proliferative glomerulonephritis has been described in tropical EMF,[39] trichinosis,[88] schistosomiasis,[89,90] and filariasis.[91-94] In clinical,[93] and experimental,[94] filarial infection as well as clinical[90] and experimental[89] schistosomiasis infection, the glomerulonephritis was found to be due to immune complex deposition. Hepatic enlargement, lymphadenopathy, skin urticaria, and itching are described in filariasis,[40] ascariasis,[78] trichinosis,[53] and Katayama fever.[79]

Organ Damage Reported in Drug Allergy

Organ damage induced by severe allergic reaction to various drugs includes skin urticaria, itching, periarteritis nodosa with glomerulonephritis, pulmonary infiltrations with eosinophilia, peripheral neuritis, hemorrhagic encephalitis, and liver damage.[95] Cardiovascular damage induced by allergic reaction to various drugs includes vasculitis, focal myocarditis with eosinophilic and lymphocytic infiltrations, fibrinoid degeneration, pericarditis, and pericardial effusion.[96] Extensive endomyocardial necrosis/fibrosis has been described in severe allergic reaction to arsenicals,[97] to bismuth and penicillin,[98] and to antituberculous medications.[99] Endomyocardial necrosis was associated with diffuse encephalitis in the reaction to arsenic and antituberculosis therapy.

Mechanism of Cardiac Damage in Tropical EMF Associated with Worms

A proposed mechanism of cardiac damage in filariasis, other helminthic worms, and other allergens is presented in Fig. 1. These worms appear to induce allergic myocarditis, which in fulminant cases may be more severe in the epi- and endomyocardium, during their phase of larval migration. Lymphocytes, the initial cellular response, infiltrate the heart early. Eosinophilia appears a little later, and eosinophils are attracted to the myocardium where they become activated and lose their granules, thus extending the initial damage. In fulminant cases endomyocardial necrosis with fibrin thrombi overlay may result. Healing of the endomyocardial necrosis and organization of the endomyocardial fibrin thrombi probably result in EMF. Most of these stages appear to have been documented in *Trichinella spiralis*[53] and in severe allergic reaction to various drugs.[95-99]

CONCLUSIONS

Helminthic worms (especially filariae) have been most frequently associated with tropical EMF both in European and non-European emigrants to EMF-endemic areas of West Africa, as well as in indigenous patients in such areas.

Loa loa, the filarial worm associated with perhaps the most intense allergic response, is also the most frequently associated with EMF in European emigrants, as well as in African patients from West Africa. Other helminthic worms are capable of causing identical damage. But the same helminth need not be responsible for causing EMF in the different regions where this disease exists. Clinically, the abrupt onset of neurologic and cardiac damage, the association with skin urticaria, as well as the recent association with immune deposit glomerulonephritis, suggest an allergic type of cardiac damage. Histopathologic reports of initial cellular damage during helminthic larval migration appear to indicate that eosinophil infiltration and eosinophil-related cardiac damage occur later. There is, however, good evidence now for eosinophil cytotoxicity to cardiac cells. There is also good histochemical evidence that tropical EMF is an allergic myocarditis. It now appears that the cardiac damage in tropical EMF is initiated by severe allergic reaction and is made worse by the cytotoxic effects of "activated" eosinophils. While eosinophil-mediated cardiac damage may be dominant in eosinophilic cardiomyopathy, the evidence currently available on tropical EMF appears to favor a dominant role for allergy.

REFERENCES

1. Bedford, D.E. and Konstam, G.L.S. Heart failure of unknown aetiology in Africans. *Br. Heart J.* **8**: 236–237, 1946.
2. Davies, J.N.P. Endocardial fibrosis in Africans. *East Afr. Med. J.* **25**: 10–14, 1948.
3. Davies, J., Spry, C.J., Vijayaraghavan, G., and De Souza, J.A. A comparison of the clinical and cardiological features of endomyocardial disease in temperate and tropical regions. *Postgrad. Med. J.* **59**: 179–185, 1983.
4. Cherion, G., Vijayaraghavan, G., Krishnaswami, S., Sukumar, I.P., John, S., Jairaj, P.S., and Bhaktaviziam, A. Endomyocardial fibrosis: Report on the haemodynamic data in 29 patients and review of the results of surgery. *Am. Heart J.* **105**: 659–666, 1983.
5. Sasidharan, K., Kartha, C.C., Balakrishnan, K.G., and Valiathan, M.S. Early angiographic featues of right ventricular endomyocardial fibrosis. *Cardiology* **70**: 127–131, 1983.
6. Balakrishnan, K.G., Venkitachalam, C.G., Pillai, V.R., Subramanian, R., and Valiathan, M.S. Postoperative evaluation of endomyocardial fibrosis. *Cardiology* **73**: 73–84, 1986.
7. Sueblinvong, V. and Sandpradit, M. Endomyocardial fibrosis in Thai children. *J. Med. Assoc. Thailand* **67**: 334–340, 1984.
8. Correa, P., Restrepo, C., Garcia, C., and Quiroz, A.C. Pathology of heart diseases of undetermined aetiology which occur in Cali, Colombia. *Am. Heart J.* **66**: 584–596, 1963.
9. Puigho, J.J., Combellas, I., Acquatella, H., Marsigha, I., Tortolede, F., Casal, H., and Suarez, J.A. Endomyocardial disease in South America—report on 23 cases in Venezuela. *Postgrad. Med. J.* **59**: 162–169, 1983.
10. Carvalho, F.R., Matos, S., Victor, E.G., Saraiva, L., Brindeiro, F.D., Maranhao, E., and Moraes, C.R. Phonomechanocardiographic findings in endomyocardial fibrosis. *Angiology* **35**: 63–70, 1984.
11. Fawzy, M.E., Ziady, G., Halim, M., Guindy, R., Mercer, E.N., and Feteih, N. Endomyocardial fibrosis: Report of eight cases. *J. Am. Coll. Cardiol.* **5**: 983–988, 1985.
12. Loffler, W. Endocarditis parietalis fibroplastica mit Bluteosinophilic. *Schweiz Med. Wochenschr.* **17**: 817–820, 1936.

13. Chew, C.Y.C., Ziady, G.M., Raphael, M.J., Nellen, M., and Oakley, C.M. Primary restrictive cardiomyopathy (non-tropical endomyocardial fibrosis) and hypereosinophilic heart disease. *Br. Heart J.* **39**: 399–413, 1977.

14. McKusick, A. and Cockran, T.H. Constrictive endocarditis. Report of a case. *Bull. Johns Hopkins Hosp.* **90**: 90–97, 1952.

15. Clark, G.M., Valentine, E., and Blount, S.G. Endocardial fibrosis simulating constrictive pericarditis. *New Engl. J. Med.* **254**: 349–355, 1956.

16. Bishop, M.B., Bousvaross, G., Cunningham, T.J., Jain, A.C., and Davies, J.N.P. Endomyocardial fibrosis in a North American Negro. *Lancet* **2**: 750–751, 1968.

17. Farrer-Brown, G. and Tarbitt, M.H. What is the spectrum of endomyocardial fibrosis? *Trop. Geogr. Med.* **24**: 208–212, 1972.

18. Andy, J.J., Bishara, F.F., and Soyinka, O.O. Relation of severe eosinophilia and microfilariasis to chronic African endomyocardial fibrosis. *Br. Heart J.* **45**: 672–680, 1981.

19. Andy, J.J. and Bishara, F.F. Observations on clinical features of early disease of African endomyocardial fibrosis. *Trop. Cardiol.* **8**: 23–32, 1982.

20. Bana, D.S. Cardiac murmur and endocardial fibrosis associated with methysergide therapy. *Am. Heart J.* **88**: 640–655, 1974.

21. Wilcox, R.G., James, P.D., and Toghill, P.J. Endomyocardial fibrosis associated with Daunorubicin therapy. *Br. Heart J.* **38**: 860–863, 1976.

22. Mayer, D. and Bannasch, P. Endomyocardial fibrosis in rats treated with N-nitrosomorpholine. *Virchows Arch.* (A) **401**: 129–135, 1983.

23. Brockington, I.F., Olsen, E.G.J., and Goodwin, J.F. Endomyocardial fibrosis in European residents in tropical Africa. *Lancet* **1**: 583–588, 1967.

24. Jaiyesimi, F., Salimonu, L.S., and Antia, A.U. Serum immunoglobulins in children with cardiomyopathies. *Trans. R. Soc. Trop. Med. Hyg.* **78**: 127–131, 1984.

25. Shaper, A.G., Kaplan, M.H., Foster, W.D., Macintosh, D.M., and Wilks, N.E. Immunological studies in endomyocardial fibrosis and other forms of heart disease in the tropics. *Lancet* **1**: 598–606 1967.

26. Shaper, A.G., Kaplan, M.H., Mody, N.J., and Mcintyre, P.A. Malarial antibodies and auto-antibodies to heart and other tissues in the immigrant and indigenous peoples of Uganda. *Lancet* **1**: 1342–1346, 1968.

27. Osunkoya, B.O., Carlisle, R., Dawodu, A.H., and Basile, U. Histopathology of extracardiac tissues in endomyocardial fibrosis. *Afr. J. Med. Sci.* **3**: 275–282, 1972.

28. Brockington, I.F. and Olsen, E.G.J. Loffler's endocarditis and Davies endomyocardial fibrosis. *Am. Heart J.* **85**: 305–322, 1973.

29. Roberts, W.C., Leigler, D.G., and Carbone, P.P. Endomyocardial disease and eosinophilia. *Am. J. Med.* **46**: 28–42, 1969.

30. Gardner-Thorpe, C., Harriman, D.G.F., Parsons, M., and Rudge, P. Loffler's eosinophilic endocarditis with Balint's syndrome (optic ataxia and paralysis of visual fixation). *Quart. J. Med.* **40**: 249–258, 1971.

31. Nutman, T.B., Miller, K.D., Mullingan, M., and Ottesen, E.A. *Loa loa* infection in temporary residents of endemic regions: Recognition of hyper-responsive syndrome with characteristic clinical manifestations. *J. Infect. Dis.* **154**: 10–17, 1986.

32. Patel, A.K., D'Arbela, P.G., and Somers, K. Endomyocardial fibrosis and eosinophilia. *Br. Heart J.* **39**: 238–241, 1977.

33. Libanoff, A.J. and McMahon, N.J. Eosinophilia and endomyocardial fibrosis. *Am. J. Cardiol.* **37**: 438–441, 1976.

34. Farrer-Brown, G., Tarbit, M.H., Somers, K., and Hutt, M.S.R. Microvascular study of hearts with endomyocardial fibrosis. *Br. Heart J.* **34**: 1250–1254, 1972.

35. Shaper, A.G. Endomyocardial fibrosis. In: Cardiovascular Disease in the Tropics. Shaper, A.G., Hutt, M.S.R., and Fejfar, Z. (eds.), British Medical Association, London, 1974, pp. 22–41.

36. Connors, D.H., Somers, K., Hutt, M.S.R., Manion, W.C., and D'Arbella, P.G. Endomyocardial fibrosis in Uganda. An epidemiologic, clinical and pathologic study. *Am. Heart J.* **74**: 687–709, 1967, and *Am. Heart J.* **75**: 107–124, 1968.

37. Becker, B.J.P., Chatgidakis, C.B., and Van Lingen, B. Cardiovascular collagenosis with parietal endocardial thrombosis. A clinicopathologic study of forty cases. *Circulation* **VII**: 345–355, 1953.

38. Davies, J.N.P. Some considerations regarding obscure diseases affecting the mural endocardium. *Am. Heart J.* **59**: 600–631, 1960.

39. Date, A., Parameswaran, A., and Bhaktaviziam, A. Renal lesions in the obliterative cardiomyopathies. *J. Pathol.* **140**: 113–122, 1983.

40. Andy, J.J. Helminthiasis, the hypereosinophilic syndrome and endomyocardial fibrosis: Some observations and an hypothesis. *Afr. J. Med. Sci.* **12**: 155–164, 1983.

41. Morenas, P. Un cas de filariese du a Acanthocheilonema perstans avec manifestations cliniques et grosse eosinophilie. *Bull. Soc. Path. Exot.* **5**: 325–330, 1929.

42. Gerbaux, A., Garin, J.P., and Lenegre, J. Cardiopathie et filariose. *Bull. Soc. Med. Paris* **73**: 873–887, 1957.

43. Baltzenschlarger, A., Reville, P., and Finker, L. La myoendocardite fibreuse parietale de l'adulte. *Ann. Anat. Pathol.* **6**: 111–128, 1961.

44. Giraud, G., Latour, H., Puech, P., Oliver, G., and Hertault, J. Cardiopathie filarienne, etude hemodynamique. *Montpellier Med.* **55**: 44–53, 1959.

45. Fisher, E.R. and Davies, E.R. Myocarditis with endocardial elastomyofibrosis. *Am. Heart J.* **56**: 537–552, 1957.

46. Ive, F.A., Willis, J.P., Ikeme, A.C., and Brockington, I.F. Endomyocardial fibrosis and filariasis. *Quart. J. Med.* **36**: 495–516, 1967.

47. Brockington, I.F. Endomyocardial fibrosis and eosinophilia. In: Cardiovascular Disease in the Tropics. Shaper, A.G. Hutt, M.R., and Fejfar, Z. (eds.), British Medical Association, London, 1974, pp. 42–45.

48. Andy, J.J., Bishara, F.F., Soyinka, O.O., and Odesanmi, W.O. Loiasis as a possible trigger of African endomyocardial fibrosis: A case report from Nigeria. *Acta Tropica* **38**: 179–186, 1981.

49. Zilberg, B. Unusual manifestations occurring in the early stages of Bilharziasis in children. The expanded Katayama syndrome. *Central Afr. J. Med.* **16**: 251–253, 1970.

50. Zilberg, B., Sanders, E., and Lewis, B. Cerebral and cardiac abnormalities in Katayama fever. *S.A. Med. J.* **17**: 598–602, 1967.

51. Jaiyesimi, F., Onadeko, M., and Antia, A.U. Endomyocardial fibrosis, schistosomiasis and dermatosis: A new facet of an old problem. *Trop. Cardiol.* **V**: 27–33, 1979.

52. Saraiva, L.R., Tompson, G., and Lira, V. Endomiocardiofibrose na infancia relato de tres casos, um dos quais associade a communicacao interatrial. *Arq. Bras. Cardiol.* **34**: 303–306, 1980.

53. Andy, J.J., O'Connell, J.P., Daddario, R.C., and Roberts, W.C. Trichinosis causing extensive ventricular mural endocarditis with superimposed thrombosis. Evidence that severe eosinophilia damages endomyocardium. *Am. J. Med.* **63**: 824–829, 1977.

54. Gruber, G.B. and Gamper, E. Uber gehinverenderungen bei menschlicher trichinose. *Vehr. dt. Path. Ges.* **22**: 219–221, 1927.

55. McCabe, E.S. and Zatuchni, J. Fulminating trichiniasis. *Am. J. Dig. Dis.* **18**: 205–209, 1951.

56. Terplan, K., Kraus, R., and Barnes, S. Eosinophilic meningoencephalitis with predominantly cerebellar changes caused by trichinosis infection. *J. Mount Sinai Hosp.* (N.Y.) **24**: 1293–1298, 1957.

57. Spry, C.J.F., Tai, P.C., and Ogilvie, B.M. Hyper-eosinophilia in rats with *Trichinella spiralis* infection. *Br. J. Exp. Pathol.* **61**: 1–7, 1980.

58. Gould, S.E. The pathology of trichinosis. *Am. J. Clin. Pathol.* **3**: 627–643, 1943.

59. Kilduffe, R.A., Barbash, S., and Merendino, A.G. A New Jersey outbreak of trichinosis

with report of a case complicated by femoral thrombosis. *Am. J. Med. Sci.* **186**: 794–802, 1933.

60. Covey, J.E., McMahon, J.J., and Myers, H.L. Trichinosis as a cause of major arterial thrombosis. *J. Am. Med. Assoc.* **140**: 1212–1213, 1949.

61. Gerbaux, A., Ben Naceur, M., De Brux, J., and Lenegre, J. Contribution a l'etude de l'endocardite parietale fibroplastique avec eosinophilie sanguine (endocardite de Loeffler) *Arch. Mal. Coeur* **49**: 689–715, 1956.

62. Potier, J.C., Grollier, G., Le Clerc, A., Mandard, J.C., Rousselot, P., Maiza, D., Khayat, A., Verwaerde, J.C., Valla, A., and Foucault, J.P. Insuffisance mitrale secondaire a une fibrose endocardique associee a une distomatose. *Arch. Mal. Coeur* **74**: 141–147, 1981.

63. Marsden, P.D. Eosinophilia in relation to helminthic infections. In: Cecil's Text Book of Medicine Beeson, P.B., McDermott, W.C., and Wyngarden, J.B. (eds.), W.B. Saunders, Philadelphia, London, Toronto, 1979, p. 638.

64. Spry, C.J.F. Eosinophils and endomyocardial fibrosis. A review of clinical and experimental studies, 1980–1986. In: Cardiomyopathy Update I. Pathogenesis of Myocarditis and Cardiomyopathy; Recent Experimental and Clinical Studies. Kawai, C. and Abelman, W.H. (eds.), University of Tokyo Press, Tokyo, 1986, pp. 293–310.

65. Olsen, E.G.J. and Spry, C.J. Relation between eosinophilia and endomyocardial disease. *Progr. Cardiovasc. Dis.* **27**: 241–254. 1985.

66. Davies, J., Oakley, C.M., and Spry, C.J. The cardiac effects of eosinophilia. *Pract. Cardiol.* **8**: 172–181, 1982.

67. Parrillo, J.E. and Fauci, A.S. Human eosinophils. Purification and cytotoxic capability of eosinophils from patients with the hypereosinophilic syndrome. *Blood* **51**: 457–473, 1978.

68. Tai, P.C., Hayes, D.J., Clark, J.B., and Spry, C.J. Toxic effects of human eosinophil products on isolated rat heart cells *in vitro. Biochem. J.* **204**: 75–80, 1982.

69. Tai, P.C., Spry, C.J.F., Olsen, E.G.J., Ackerman, S.J., Dunnette, S., and Gleich, G.J. Deposits of eosinophil granule proteins in cardiac tissue of patients with eosinophilic endomyocardial disease. *Lancet* **1**: 643–647, 1987.

70. Acquatella, H., Schiller, N.B., Puigbo, J.J., Gomez Mancebo, J.R., Suarez, C., and Acquatella, G. Value of two-dimensional echo-cardiography in endomyocardial disease with and without eosinophilia. A clinical and pathologic study. *Circulation* **67**: 1219–1226, 1983.

71. Van Bogaert, L., Dubois, A., Janssens, P.G., Radermecker, J., Tverdy, G., and Wanson, M. Encephalitis in *Loa loa* filariasis. *J. Neurol. Neurosurg. Psychiat.* **18**: 103–119, 1955.

72. Toussaint, D. and Dannis, P. Retinopathy in generalized *Loa loa* filariasis. *Arch. Ophthalmol* **74**: 470–467, 1965.

73. Bertrand-Fontaine, S.J., Wolfrom, R., and Cagnard, V. Un cas de filariose cerebrale (double hemiplegie) au cours d'une filariose a *Loa loa. Bull. Mem. Soc. Med. Hosp. Paris* **64**: 1092–1095, 1948.

74. Skinner, J.C. Neurologic complications of trichinosis. *N. Engl. J. Med.* **238**: 317–319, 1948.

75. Basu, S.M. Encephalopathy in association with ascariasis. *Indian J. Paediat.* **46**: 228–231, 1979.

76. Yahontov, B.V., Saripov, A.S., and Niambaev, A.N. Epileptic syndrome in ascariasis and enterobiasis. *Dgurnal. Neuropatologii. Psychiat.* **78**: 378–380, 1978.

77. Kivits, M. Quatre cas d'encephalite, mortelle avec invasion du liquide cephalo-rachiden par microfilariae loa. *Ann. Soc. Belg. Med. Trop.* **32**: 235–242, 1952.

78. Wilcocks, C. and Manson-Bahr, P.E.C. (eds). Manson's Tropical Diseases, 17th ed, p. 24, Bailliere Tindal, London.

79. Gelfand, M. A Clinical study of Intestinal Bilharziasis (*Schistosoma mansoni*) in Africa. Edward Arnold, London, 1967.

80. Ottesen, E.A. The clinical spectrum of lymphatico filariasis and its immunological determinants. W.H.O./FIL/80, 160 Geneva, 1979.

81. Ravindran, M. Tropical eosinophilia presenting with neurologic features. *Br. Med. J.* **2**: 1262–1263, 1979.
82. Vakil, R.J. Cardiovascular involvement in tropical eosinophilia. *Br. Heart J.* **23**: 578–589, 1961.
83. Fediyanina, L.V. Allergic myocarditis in guinea pigs due to superinfection with ascaris. *Meditsinskaya Parazitologiya i Parazitrnye Bolezine* **49**: 67–70, 1980.
84. Spink, W.W. Cardiovascular complications of trichinosis. *Arch. Intern. Med.* **56**: 238–249, 1935.
85. Foster, D.G. Filariasis—A rare cause of pericarditis. *J. Trop. Med. Hyg.* **59**: 212–214, 1959.
86. Fey, L.D. and Moore, M.A. Fulminating trichinosis with myocarditis. *NW Med. Seattle* **53**: 701–709, 1954.
87. Harley, J.B., McIntosh, C.L., Kirklin, J.J., Maron, B.J., Gottdiener, J., Roberts, W.C., and Fauci, A.S. Atrioventricular valve replacement in the idiopathic hypereosinophilic syndrome. *Am. J. Med.* **73**: 77–81, 1982.
88. Reimann, H.A., Price, A.H., and Herbut, P.A. Trichinosis and periarteritis nodosa. *J. Am. Med. Assoc.* **122**: 274–282, 1943.
89. Cavalle, T., Galvaner, E.G., Ward, P.A., and Von Litchtenberg, F. The nephropathy of experimental hepatosplenic schistosomiasis. *Am. J. Pathol.* **76**: 433–445, 1974.
90. Veress, B., Musa, A.R., Osman, H., Asha, A., Sadding, E.W., and El Hassan, A.M. The nephrotic syndrome in the Sudan with special reference to schistosomal nephropathy. A preliminary morphologic study. *Ann. Trop. Med. Parasitol.* **72**: 357–361, 1978.
91. Pillay, V.K.G., Kirch, E., and Kurtzman, N.A. Glomerulopathy associated with filarial loasis. *J. Am. Med. Assoc.* **225**: 175–183, 1973.
92. Date, A., Kirubakaran, M.G., Gunasekaran, V., and Shastry, J.C.M. Acute eosinophilic glomerulonephritis with Bancroftian filariasis. *Postgrad. Med. J.* **55**: 905–907, 1979.
93. Akinsola, A., Ijaware, A., Ladipo, G.O.A., Thomas, J., Odesanmi, W., and Hartley, B. Loiasis and glomerulonephritis: A report of 2 cases and a review of literature. *West Afr. J. Med.* **7**: 38–44, 1988.
94. Klei, T.R., Cromwell, W.A., and Thompson, P.E. Ultrastructural glomerular changes associated with filariasis. *Am. J. Trop Med. Hyg.* **23**: 608–618, 1974.
95. Kantor, F.S. Drug allergy. In: Cecil's Textbook of Medicine Beeson, P.B., McDermott, W., and Wyngarden, J.B. (eds.), Philadelphia, London and Toronto, pp. 154–157.
96. Wynne, J. and Braunwald, E. Hypersensitivity. In: Heart Disease. A Textbook of Cardiovascular Medicine. Braunwald, E. (ed.), W.B. Saunders, Philadelphia, London, and Toronto, pp. 1487–1489.
97. Edge, J.R. Myocardial fibrosis following arsenical therapy. *Lancet* **2**: 675–677, 1946.
98. Leach, W. Case report of gummatous myocarditis. *Br. Heart J.* **22**: 149–152, 1960.
99. Gardiol, P.D. and Pitch, E. Encephalopathie et eosinophiles a propos d'un cas de tuberculose urogenitale traite par des tuberculostatiques. *Schweiz Z. Tuberk.* **14**: 212–226, 1957.

Echocardiographic Recognition and Doppler Abnormalities in Eosinophilic Endomyocardial Disease and Endomyocardial Fibrosis

Harry Acquatella, Luis Rodriguez, Juan Jose Puigbo, Jose Ramon Gomez-Mancebo, Mayaly Casanova, Ivan Combellas, and Hugo Giordano

Hospital Universitario de Caracas, Centro de Investigaciones "J.F. Torrealba" of the Ministry of Health, and Centro Medico de Caracas, Venezuela

ABSTRACT

A spectrum of echocardiographic findings is found in the EMF syndrome. In the acute/necrotic stage, heart size can be normal or dilated with decreased ejection fraction; apical irregularities or thrombus formation lying over a dyskinetic wall can also be observed. In the chronic stage, localized areas of fibrosis giving rise to strong echoes are seen at the ventricular apex with variable extension along the inflow tract and at the posterior atrioventricular valves, which may appear fibrotic and poorly mobile due to adhesions to the basal posterior endocardium. The 2-dimensional echographic pattern of normal size or mildly dilated hyperkinetic ventricles with huge atria having a typical fibrotic distribution is highly suggestive of EMF. The severity of mitral and tricuspid regurgitant lesions can be assessed by Doppler ultrasound. Pulsed-wave examination of ventricular inflow velocities may show changes suggestive of restriction. Echocardiography is extremely useful in the diagnosis and follow-up of EMF patients.

INTRODUCTION

The introduction of echocardiography in recent years has facilitated the noninvasive diagnosis of eosinophilic endomyocardial disease and endomyocardial fibrosis (EMF),[1] initially characterized by autopsy,[2-7] clinical findings,[8-11] cardiac catheterization, and angiography.[12-14] The addition of Doppler ultrasound promises an improvement in the evaluation of functional abnormalities. In this paper, we will attempt to summarize recent contributions of cardiac ultrasound in assessing the EMF syndrome.

There are two classical forms of presentation.[1,15] One, known as eosinophilic endomyocardial disease is more commonly seen in temperate countries,[2] it presents initially with marked hypereosinophilia as part of a generalized febrile illness. The other, observed initially in tropical countries,[3,4] presents as an advanced bi/univentricular heart failure showing slight or no eosinophilia and no evidence of systemic illness, and constitutes the classical tropical EMF. Extensive pathologic studies[5-7] of both syndromes concluded that each represents one extreme of a single disease entity. Recent reviews[1] support this unitarian view. The presence of hypereosinophilia might depend on how early or late in the disease process a particular patient is examined.[15] With the exception of some regions of Africa[3] and India,[16] in general endomyocardial disease is an infrequent cause of heart failure. Nevertheless, echocardiography may have increased recognition of unsuspected noneosinophilic patients. A recent review of 14,241 consecutive echocardiograms from our laboratory included 63 subjects with "restrictive syndrome" (0.44%), 26 of whom had endomyocardial disease (0.18%). Half of them were diagnosed in the last 4 years. The ratio of eosinophilic/noneosinophilic patients was 1 to 5.

Three progressive pathologic stages of cardiac involvement are described at autopsy.[7,10] Initially, acute necrosis of the endocardium lasting for some weeks is followed by a thrombotic stage in the ensuing months. A further fibrotic process of the thrombus and underlying endocardium require from several months to 2 or more years to develop. As each stage shows different morphological and functional abnormalities within the heart, different echocardiographic manifestations are also to be expected.

ACUTE/NECROTIC AND THROMBOTIC STAGES

There are not many echographic reports on EMF patients during the acute/necrotic stage. Most patients display a normal heart size and function.[17] The development of acute eosinophilic myocarditis may be suspected on clinical grounds when tachycardia and cardiomegaly with systemic and pulmonary venous congestion are present.[18] Two-dimensional echograms may show nonspecific ventricular dilatation with diminished cardiac contractility.[18-20] Cardiac hemodynamics may disclose a nonspecific profile of congestive heart failure,[18,19] with no evidence of restriction. Degranulated eosinophils in peripheral blood smears might indicate eosinophilic myocarditis[10] and endocardial biopsy is indicated for confirmation.[1,10,15] During this early stage echocardiography is not as sensitive as biopsy in diagnosing eosinophilic heart disease,[1] but it is of great help for future evaluation. In our patients with secondary (reactive) hypereosinophilia, echographic follow-up has demonstrated the absence of cardiac damage for up to 15 months.[21]

In the subsequent thrombotic phase, 2-dimensional echocardiography allows a thorough apical exploration. It is particularly useful in discovering thrombus formation over a diskinetic left or right ventricular apex, as occurred with the patient shown in Fig. 1. In the majority of patients only subtle echographic apical irregularities have been detected.[17] Because a variety of cardiac manifestations other than endocardial restriction have been described in patients with hypereosinophilia, including dilated congestive heart failure, arrhythmia-conduction disturbances, and myopericarditis, the term "eosinophilic heart disease" has been proposed.[19]

FIBROTIC STAGE

The majority of echographic reports in the literature deals with the late fibrotic stage of EMF.[13,17,21-38] The 2-dimensional echographic appearance is striking, consisting of a combination of normal or slightly dilated ventricles with severely dilated or even huge atria and, most importantly, a peculiar distribution of fibrotic patches on the ventricular endocardial surface.[21]

In a large series of autopsies from Uganda[39] distribution patterns of localized areas of ventricular endocardial fibrosis were described: type 1 affects the apex only with variable extension along the inflow tract; type 2 extends from the apex to the respective atrioventricular posterior valve along the inflow tract; type 3 comprises valvular lesions only; type 4 shows lesions in the apex and valvular regions (not affecting the intervening myocardium); and type 5 shows fibrotic patches in areas other than the apex or valves. Two-dimensional echographic studies have also shown this distribution. A greatly

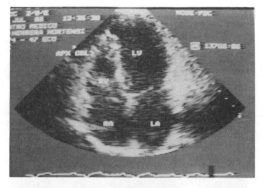

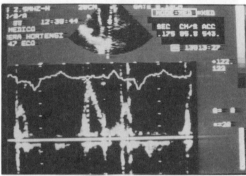

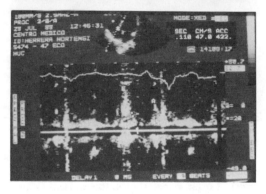

Fig. 1. Echocardiographic and Doppler study obtained 9 years after successful steroid treatment in a patient who had acute multiorgan idiopathic hypereosinophilic syndrome in 1979. A left ventricular angiogram performed during the acute stage showed a large apical thrombus and dyskinetic apex. Serial 2-dimensional echocardiograms in the ensuing months and years showed resolution of the left apical thrombus, but the apical dyskinesis persisted and enlarged (upper panel). A right ventricular apical thrombus observed in several echograms became fibrotic and finally obliterated the right ventricular apex (APX OBL). RV and RA: right ventricle and atria; LV and LA: left ventricle and atria. Middle panel shows a normal Doppler mitral inflow: early inflow peak velocity was 85.8 cm/s, deceleration time was 0.175 s. Lower panel shows the tricuspid Doppler tracing: early inflow peak velocity (E) was 47 cm/s, but deceleration time was moderately shortened, 0.110 s. This, and an increased reversal of presystolic flow at inspiration of suprahepatic vein Doppler tracing (not shown), were suggestive of mild restriction. Abbreviations are the same in subsequent figures.

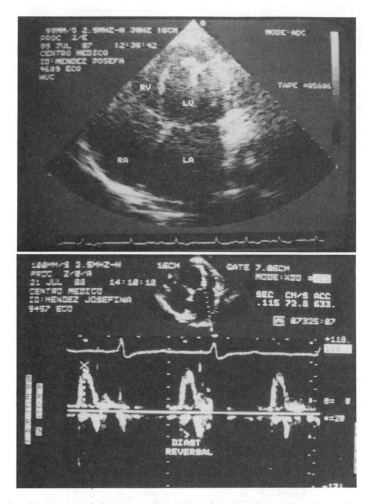

Fig. 2.   Upper panel shows a 2-dimensional 4-chamber apical view of a woman
with LV EMF. Bright echorefractile apical endocardium extending to the LV
inflow tract is apparent. Ventricular dimensions are normal while the atria are
moderately enlarged. Lower panel shows the pulsed Doppler mitral inflow
velocity tracing: peak early inflow velocity (X) is normal, 72.8 cm/s, but deceleration time is decreased to 0.115 s. In mid to late diastole reversal flow to the
atria is present.

thickened apical endocardium (type 1) is found in the left (Fig. 2) and in the right (Fig.
3) ventricles, respectively. Figure 2 also shows fibrotic extension along the inflow tract.
Echogenic fibrotic patches filling the left ventricular cavity immediately below the mitral
valve on M-mode tracings have been described,[25,31] as shown in Fig. 4 (type 3). The
posterobasal wall may only show diminished motion[31] as a subtle abnormality. Mild
to severe mitral and/or tricuspid regurgitation is frequently present, and may in part
be due to retraction and scarring of the posterior valve leaflet into the adjacent posterior
ventricular wall.[21,31] In those patients with left ventricular apical obliteration, strong
echoes of the endocardial surface are frequently seen moving forcefully inward in
systole[21] in the 4- and 2-chamber apical views. The forceful systolic contraction is quite

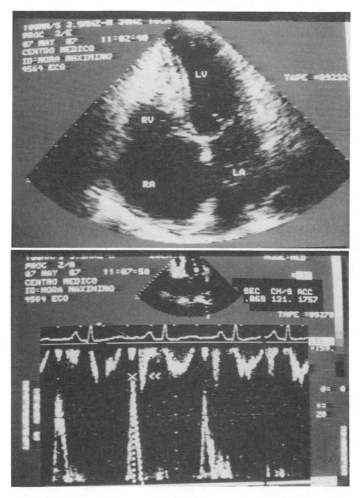

Fig. 3. Upper panel shows an almost totally obliterated RV in a severely symptomatic patient. The LV apex was spared but in real time it had an outward dyskinetic motion. Both ventricles were hyperdynamic. The interatrial septum protrudes to the left. Lower panel displays the mitral Doppler tracing showing a high peak (X) early inflow velocity of 121 cm/s, an extremely short deceleration time of 0.069 s, mid-diastolic flow reversal (<), and a very low atrial flow. Tricuspid Doppler tracing (not shown) disclosed the same abnormalities. Both valves were regurgitant.

distinct from other conditions also displaying apical thrombosis, such as myocardial infarction or chronic Chagas' disease.[21] The apical motion reflects different pathologic mechanisms: in EMF systolic function is preserved, allowing the apex to retract inwardly to the ventricular cavity, whereas in the other two conditions the underlying myocardium is ischemic or fibrotic and will display an outward dyskinetic motion. Apical obliteration is found in most[21] but not all patients.[17,31] Demonstration of the apical and submitral areas of fibrosis may explain the embolic source presented by these patients.[31]

The distribution of fibrotic areas has been clearly demonstrated by amplitude-processed, color-coded imaging depicting regions of relative intensity endomyocardial echoes, even when standard 2-dimensional imaging appeared normal.[17] Unfortunately this

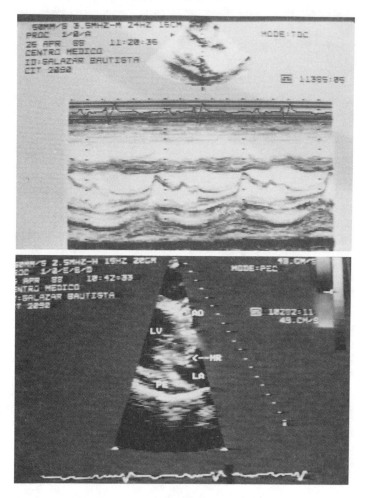

Fig. 4. Upper panel is an M-mode echocardiographic tracing from a patient whose only abnormality was a fibrotic endocardial patch posterior to the mitral valve. A mitral "b" notch is present. In the lower panel a parasternal long-axis color-flow mapping view shows in light blue a jet of mitral regurgitation (MR). In real time the posterior mitral valve was fibrotic and poorly mobile. PE: pericardial effusion.

technique is not widely available. It has been observed that biventricular involvement is present in almost all cases seen in nontropical countries,[1,13-15,17,23] and in about three-quarters of patients studied in tropical countries.[1,15,32,40] Univentricular involvement (mostly right-sided), as shown in Fig. 3, is reported frequently from equatorial Africa, predominantly from the Ivory Coast,[24] Nigeria,[28] and also in Brazil.[40] Dilatation of the right ventricular infundibulum, greatly thickened and easily seen tricuspid valves, severe tricuspid regurgitation, right ventricular volume overload, and paradoxical septal motion are common echographic findings in this last setting.

M-mode echocardiographic studies have shown increased left ventricular wall thickness and mass.[9] Echocardiographic follow-up has been suggested to estimate beneficial or detrimental changes during therapy.[4] Finally, slight to large pericardial effusion is observed in some patients.[9,13,21,34]

ECHOCARDIOGRAPHIC AND DOPPLER ASSESSMENT OF SYSTOLIC AND DIASTOLIC FUNCTION

In the chronic fibrotic stage the combination of preserved or increased systolic function associated with restrictive diastolic dysfunction is frequent. Fractional shortening (or ejection fraction) was normal or increased in 8 of 10 patients from our initial series,[21] as well as in the majority of subjects studied by other groups.[9,13,14,19,25]

Endocardial thickening affects diastolic filling of the ventricles, giving origin to non-specific M-mode echocardiographic findings which are common to other restrictive/constrictive conditions. Early in diastole, an abrupt increased filling occurs, and endocardial constraint impedes further filling in mid- to late diastole. Mitral and tricuspid regurgitation with increased regurgitant volume further contributes to the predominant early diastolic filling (see Doppler findings). Intraventricular pressure tracings show a typical dip and plateau pattern with unequal diastolic pressures in the 2 ventricles.[13] The rapid early diastolic filling gives origin on M-mode echo to a rapid early diastolic posterior motion of the posterior left ventricular posterior wall.[13,34] Similarly, the interventricular septum may also show a rapid protodiastolic anterior motion,[41] looking on M-mode like an inverted "dip-plateau."[24] This abrupt septal motion is also observed in pericardial constriction.[42] These findings depend on the complex interplay between right and left ventricular pressures which might in one instant be greater in one chamber than another,[13] probably reflecting different chamber fibrotic stiffness and respective volume overload. On M-mode[24] and on 2-dimensional 4-chamber apical view[21] an abrupt protodiastolic septal "sail" motion to the right and to the left may be seen.

Digitized M-mode echocardiograms disclosed two patterns of abnormal filling. When mitral regurgitation exists there is a decreased duration of rapid filling and increased peak rate of filling. When no mitral incompetence is present, filling is normal or tracings show a reduced peak rate and prolonged duration of filling. Digitized M-mode apparently shows no specific changes in eosinophilic myocardial disease.[17]

Doppler echocardiographic studies in EMF are lacking. Recently, abnormalities in ventricular diastolic filling have been shown by pulsed Doppler examination obtained at the tip of either the mitral or tricuspid valve, showing restrictive physiology as in other cardiac conditions.[13] In restriction, most filling occurs abruptly in very early diastole, originating an increase in peak velocity and shortening of deceleration time of the early ("E") filling wave with an associated decrease in peak velocity of atrial ("A") filling wave. Therefore, the ratio E/A is significantly greater than in normal controls. Figure 3 shows similar findings in one of our patients with a severe form of EMF: an extreme short deceleration time and greatly increased E/A ratio were present in both mitral and tricuspid valves. Diastolic regurgitation can also be present[43] (Fig. 2). Other less severe Doppler abnormalities are shown in Figs. 1 and 2, obtained from other subjects. Some of the factors contributing to an increase in early abrupt diastolic filling[44] may exist in EMF, such as increased left atrial pressure (or increased wedge pressure)[12,13,40] and normal end-systolic ventricular volume.[12,14] Nevertheless, these findings are not specific for restriction, but can also be observed in dilated congestive cardiomyopathy with mitral regurgitation[44] or can be due to very high atrial (pulmonary capillary wedge) pressure.[45] Pulmonary artery Doppler biphasic forward flow, with the majority oc-

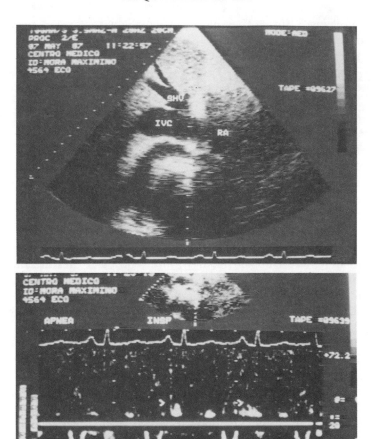

Fig. 5.   Vein abnormalities in severe RV EMF (same patient as in Fig. 3). Upper panel displays the echocardiographic aspect from a subxyphoid window, showing a severely engorged inferior vena cava (IVC), and suprahepatic veins (SHV). Lower panel depicts a pulsed-wave Doppler tracing obtained with the sample volume positioned about 2 cm into the suprahepatic vein. It shows absent forward systolic flow, and a sharp, abrupt early forward diastolic flow (Y). Inspiration (INSP) increased slightly forward flow (second Y from left) and reversal of presystolic flow (denoted as >). These findings suggest severe restriction because flow to the heart occurs only in early diastole.

curring in late diastole in an almost totally occluded right ventricle, was recently reported.[46]

Pulsed-wave Doppler investigation of peripheral veins such as the suprahepatic vein and superior vena cava have also disclosed abnormalities in filling suggestive of restriction.[43] These consists of reverse systolic flow, increased and rapid flow during early diastole, and increased reversal of presystolic flow during inspiration. Preliminary experience has disclosed similar findings (Fig. 5). Further work is necessary to estimate the sensitivity and specificity of the observed Doppler abnormalities in a larger group of patients.

Finally, color-flow mapping[47] (Fig. 4), and pulsed and continuous wave Doppler techniques widely used in estimating the severity of regurgitant lesions could also be useful in assessing these patients.

DIFFERENTIAL DIAGNOSIS

The most striking echographic finding in the acute hypereosinophilic stage of EMF is the demonstration of apical thrombus superimposed on an akinetic or dyskinetic apex. This is not specific, as up to 27% of patients with acute viral myocarditis may also present apical thrombosis[48] of similar appearance. Electrocardiographic evidence of necrosis (QS wave) simulating myocardial infarction may be found[19] which may prompt a coronary angiographic study to exclude coronary heart disease. Two of our acute hypereosinophilic patients disclosed such findings.

In the chronic stage the 2-dimensional echocardiographic combination of normal or near-normal ventricle size, dilated or huge atria, apical obliteration with bright endocardial echoes with preserved systolic inward motion, fibrotic involvement of sub-mitral/tricuspid valves, and inflow tracts constitutes a hallmark image of EMF distinct from other restrictive/constrictive conditions.[21] Absence of the particular fibrotic distribution makes the echographic diagnosis of EMF more difficult.

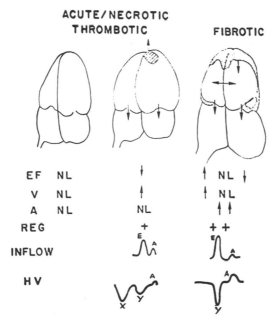

Fig. 6. Schematic diagram summarizing the spectrum of 2-dimensional echocardiographic and Doppler findings observed in EMF. In the upper drawings the heart is positioned with the apex pointing upward; the hatching denotes thrombus or endocardial scarring; the arrows point in the direction of wall motion, or mitral/tricuspid regurgitation. EF: ejection fraction; NL: normal; V and A: ventricular and atrial size, repectively; REG: mitral and or tricuspid regurgitation; INFLOW: diagram of the pulsed Doppler inflow velocities of mitral/tricuspid valves; HV: same as suprahepatic vein.

Other restrictive conditions disclosing "normal ventricles with large atria" include idiopathic restrictive cardiomyopathy due to nonspecific myocardial fibrosis,[49] nonspecific hypertrophy, Fabry's disease, cardiac transplantation, and amyloidosis.[43] Amyloid heart disease can easily be distinguished from EMF. Typical findings include normal ventricle size, a peculiar "granular sparkling" appearance of the myocardium,[50,51] thickened ventricular septal, left ventricular and right ventricular walls, decreased systolic wall thickening and left ventricular global systolic function, and thickening of the atrioventricular valves, papillary muscles, and interatrial septum. Restrictive cardiac irradiation and heart transplant are easily recognized by history. On the other hand, pericardial constriction[52] continues to be an elusive diagnosis even after cardiac catheterization; demonstration of a thickened pericardium is valuable but echocardiography has proved to be nonspecific. Furthermore, pericardial thickening in EMF can also be observed. While in EMF the atria tend to be huge, in pericardial constriction the heart looks like "a tube" with nearly normal atria. Based on M-echo appearance, one of our earlier patients was submitted to open pericardial exploration, with a negative result.[21]

Local fibrotic patches below the posterior mitral valve leaflet and inflow tract should be differentiated from submitral annular calcification. Finally, in countries where rheumatic heart disease is prevalent,[39] both situations may coexist but echocardiography is helpful in demonstrating typical rheumatic deformation of both mitral valve leaflets.

CONCLUSIONS

A thorough echocardiographic and Doppler examination should be included in the routine work-up of EMF. In countries with insufficient economic resources, the relatively low cost of cardiac ultrasound relative to cardiac catheterization should prove of great help in diagnosis and improved care of EMF patients.

REFERENCES

1. Spry, C.J.F. Eosinophils and endomyocardial fibrosis: A review of clinical and experimental studies, 1980–86. In: Pathogenesis of Myocarditis and Cardiomyopathy. Recent Experimental and Clinical Studies, Kawai, C. and Abelmann, W.M. (eds.), University of Tokyo Press, Tokyo, 1987, pp. 293–310.
2. Loffler, W. Endocarditis parietalis fibroplastica mit Bluteosinophilie. Ein eigenartiges Krankheitsbild. *Schweiz Med. Wochenschr.* **18**: 817–820, 1936.
3. Davies, J.N.P. Endomyocardial fibrosis in Africans. *East Afr. Med. J.* **25**: 10–14, 1948.
4. Davies, J.N.P. and Ball, J.D. The pathology of endomyocardial fibrosis in Uganda. *Br. Heart J.* **17**: 337–359, 1955.
5. Roberts, W.C., Liegler, D.G., and Carbone, P.P. Endomyocardial disease and eosinophilia. A clinical and pathologic spectrum. *Am. J. Med.* **46**: 28–42, 1969.
6. Roberts, W.C., Buja, L.M., and Ferrans, V.J. Loffler's fibroplastic parietal endocarditis, eosinophilic leukemia, and Davies' endomyocardial fibrosis: The same disease at different stages? *Pathol. Microbiol.* **35**: 90–95, 1970.
7. Brockington, I.F. and Olsen, E.G.J. Loffler's endocarditis and Davies' endomyocardial fibrosis. *Am. Heart J.* **85**: 308–322, 1973.
8. Chusid, M.J., Dale, D.C., West, B.C., and Wolff, S.M. The hypereosinophilic syndrome: Analysis of fourteen cases with review of the literature. *Medicine* **54**: 1–27, 1975.
9. Parrillo, J.E., Borer, J.S., Henry, W.L., Wolff, S.M., and Fauci, A.S. The cardiovascular

manifestations of the hypereosinophilic syndrome. Prospective study of 26 patients, with review of the literature. *Am. J. Med.* **67**: 572–582, 1979.

10. Olsen, E.G.J. and Spry, C.J.F. The pathogenesis of Loffler's endomyocardial disease, and its relationship to endomyocardial fibrosis. In: Progress in Cardiology, Vol. 8, Yu, P.N. and Goodwin, J.F. (eds.), Philadelphia, Lea & Febiger, 1979, pp. 281–303.

11. World Health Organization. Cardiomyopathies. Report of a WHO expert committee. *WHO Tech. Rep. Ser.* **697**: 7–64, 1984.

12. Bell, J.A., Jenkins, B.S., and Webb-Peploe, M.M. Clinical, haemodynamic, and angiographic findings in Loffler's eosinophilic endocarditis. *Br. Heart J.* **38**: 541–548, 1976.

13. Chew, C.Y.C., Ziady, G.M., Raphael, M.J., Nellen, M., and Oakley, C.M. Primary restrictive cardiomyopathy. Non-tropical endomyocardial fibrosis and hypereosinophilic heart disease. *Br. Heart J.* **39**: 399–413, 1977.

14. Hess, O.M., Turina, M., Senning, A., Goebel, N.H., Scholer, Y., and Krayenbuehl, H.P. Pre- and postoperative findings in patients with endomyocardial fibrosis. *Br. Heart J.* **40**: 406–415, 1978.

15. Olsen, E.G.J. and Spry, C.J.F. Relation between eosinophilia and endomyocardial disease. *Prog. Cardiovasc. Dis.* **27**: 241–254, 1985.

16. Kartha, C.C. and Sandhyamani, S. An autopsy study of tropical endomyocardial fibrosis in Kerala. *Indian J. Med. Res.* **82**: 439–446, 1985.

17. Davies, J., Gibson, D.G., Foale, R., Herr, K., Spry, C.J.F., Oakley, C.M., and Goodwin, J.F. Echocardiographic features of eosinophilic endomyocardial disease. *Br. Heart J.* **48**: 434–440, 1982.

18. Case records of the Massachusetts General Hospital (Case no. 18). *N. Engl. J. Med.* **302**: 1077–1083, 1980.

19. Take, M., Sekiguchi, M., Hiroe, M., Hirosawa, K., Mizoguchi, H., Kijima, M., Shirai, T., Ishide, T., and Okubo, S. Clinical spectrum and endomyocardial biopsy findings in eosinophilic heart disease. In: Myocarditis and Related Disorders, Sekiguchi, M., Olsen, E.G.J., and Goodwin, J.F. (eds.), Springer-Verlag, Tokyo, Berlin, Heidelberg, New York, 1985, pp. 243–249.

20. DePace, N.L., Nestico, P.F., Morganroth, J., Ross, J., Fox, R., Kotler, M.N., Mintz G.S., and Vassallo, R. Dilated cardiomyopathy in the idiopathic hypereosinophilic syndrome. *Am. J. Cardiol.* **52**: 1359–1360, 1983.

21. Acquatella, H., Schiller, N.B., Puigbo, J.J., Gomez Mancebo, J.R., Suarez, C., and Acquatella, G. Value of two-dimensional echocardiography in endomyocardial disease with and without eosinophilia. A clinical and pathologic study. *Circulation* **67**: 1219–1226, 1983.

22. Hernandez Pieretti, O. Echocardiographic diagnosis and evaluation of cardiomyopathies: Idiopathic hypertrophic subaortic stenosis, Chagas' heart disease and endomyocardial fibrosis. *Postgrad. Med. J.* **53**: 533–539, 1977.

23. Hall, S.W., Theologides, A., From, A.H.L., Gobel, F.L., Fortuny I.E., Lawrence, C.J., and Edwards, J.E. Hypereosinophilic syndrome with biventricular involvement. *Circulation* **55**: 217–222, 1977.

24. Dienot, B., Ekra, A., and Bertrand, E. L'echocardiographie dans 23 cas de fibroses endomyocardiques constrictives droites ou bilaterales. *Arch. Mal. Coeur* **72**: 1101–1107, 1979.

25. Pernod, J., Gerbaux, A., Vernin, P., Terdjman, M., Lelguen, C., and Droniou, J. Apport de l'echocardiographie dans le diagnostic des fibroses endomyocardiques. *Arch. Mal. Coeur* **73**: 139–146, 1980.

26. Haertel, J.C. and Castro, I. Avaliacao ecocardiografica da fibrose endomiocardica. *Arq. Bras. Cardiol.* **35**: 475–480, 1980.

27. Rodger, J.C., Irvine, K.G., and Lerski, R.A. Echocardiography in Loffler's endocarditis. *Br. Heart J.* **46**: 110–112, 1981.

28. George, B.O., Gaba, F.E., and Talabi, A.I. M-mode echocardiographic features of endomyocardial fibrosis. *Br. Heart J.* **48**: 222–228, 1982.

29. Candell Riera, J., Permanyer Miralda, G., and Soler Soler, J. Echocardiographic findings in endomyocardial fibrosis. *Chest* **82**: 88–90, 1982.

30. Lengyel, M. and Dekov, E. Two-dimensional echocardiographic features of Loffler's endocarditis. *Acta Cardiol. Brussels* **37**: 59–69, 1982.

31. Gottdiener, J.S., Maron, B.J., Schooley, R.T., Harley, J.B., Roberts, W.C., and Fauci, A.S. Two-dimensional echocardiographic assessment of the idiopathic hypereosinophilic syndrome. Anatomical basis of mitral regurgitation and peripheral embolization. *Circulation* **67**: 572–578, 1983.

32. Vijayaraghavan, G., Davies, J., Sadanandan, S., Spry, C.J., Gibson, D.H., and Goodwin, J.F. Echocardiographic features of tropical endomyocardial disease in South India. *Br. Heart J.* **50**: 450–459, 1983.

33. Rios, A. Aspectos clinicos y ecocardiograficos de la fibrosis endomiocardica. *Acta Med. Colomb.* **8**: 157–167, 1983.

34. Puigbo, J.J., Combellas, I., Acquatella, H., Marsiglia, I., Tortoledo, F., Casal, H., and Suarez, J.A. Endomyocardial disease in South America: Report on 23 cases in Venezuela. *Postgrad. Med. J.* **59**: 162–168, 1983.

35. Couto, A.A., Victer, H.J., Martins, J.C., Cunha, L.R., Golebiovski, P., Almeida, C.S. de, Pareto Junior, R.C., and Carneiro, R.D. O ecocardiograma na endomiocardiofibrose. Diagnostico diferencial. *Arch. Bras, Med.* **58**: 217–220, 1984.

36. Bletry, O., Scheuble, C., Cereze, P., Masquet, P., Priollet, P., Balafrej, M., and Godeau, P. Cardiac manifestations of the hypereosinophilic syndrome. The value of 2-dimensional echography (12 cases). *Arch. Mal. Coeur* **77**: 633–641, 1984.

37. Fawsy, M.E., Ziady, G., Halim, M., Guindy, R., Mercer, E.N., and Feteih, N. Endomyocardial fibrosis: report of eight cases. *J. Am. Coll. Cardiol.* **5**: 983–988, 1985.

38. Barria, M.A. and Carabantes, J. Fibrosis endomiocardica. *Bol. Hosp. San Juan de Dios (Chile)* **32**: 156–161, 1985.

39. Shaper, A.G., Hutt, M.S.R., and Coles, R.M. Necropsy study of endomyocardial fibrosis and rheumatic heart disease in Uganda 1950–65. *Br. Heart J.* **30**: 391–401, 1968.

40. Moraes, C.R., Buffolo, E., Lima, R., Victor, E., Lira, V., Escobar, M., Rodrigues, J., Saraiva, L., and Andrade J.C. Surgical treatment of endomyocardial fibrosis. *J. Thorac. Cardiovas. Surg.* **85**: 738–745, 1983.

41. Acquatella, H., Puigbo, J.J., Suarez, C., and Mendoza, J. Sudden early diastolic anterior movement of the septum in endomyocardial fibrosis. *Circulation* (letter) **59**: 847–848, 1979.

42. Candell Riera, J., Garcia del Castillo, H., Permanyer Miralda, G., and Soler Soler, J. Echocardiographic features of the interventricular septum in chronic constrictive pericarditis. *Circulation* **57**: 1154–1158, 1978.

43. Appleton, C.P., Hatle, L.V., and Popp, R.L. Demonstration of restrictive ventricular physiology by Doppler echocardiography. *J. Am. Coll. Cardiol.* **11**: 757–768, 1988.

44. Takenaka, K., Dabestani, A., Gardin, J.M., Russell, D., Clark, S., Allfie, A., and Henry, W.L. Pulsed Doppler echocardiographic study of left ventricular filling in dilated cardiomyopathy. *Am. J. Cardiol.* **58**: 143–147, 1986.

45. Appleton, C.P., Hatle, L.K., and Popp, R.L. Relation of transmitral flow velocity patterns to left ventricular diastolic function: New insights from a combined hemodynamic and Doppler echocardiographic study. *J. Am. Coll. Cardiol.* **12**: 426–440, 1988.

46. Presti, C., Ryan, T., and Armstrong, W.F. Two-dimensional and Doppler echocardiographic findings in hypereosinophilic syndrome. *Am. Heart J.* **114**: 172–175, 1987.

47. Helmcke, F., Nanda, N.C., Hsiung, M.C., Soto, B., Adey, C.K., Goyal, R.G., and Gatewood Jr., R.P. Color Doppler assessment of mitral regurgitation with orthogonal planes. *Circulation* **75**: 175–183, 1987.

48. Richardson, P.J., Daly, K., and Gishen P. Hemodynamic findings in biopsy proven acute myocarditis. In: Viral Heart Disease, Bolte, H.D. (ed.), Springer-Verlag, Berlin, Heidelberg, New York, Tokyo, 1984, pp. 165–172.

49. Siegel, R.J., Shah, P.K., and Fishbein, M.C. Idiopathic restrictive cardiomyopathy. *Circulation* **70**: 165–169, 1984.
50. Siqueira Filho, A.G., Cunha, C.L.P., Tajik, A.J., Seward, J.B., Schattenberg, T.T., and Giuliani, E.R. M-mode and two-dimensional echographic features in cardiac amyloidosis. *Circulation* **63**: 188–196, 1981.
51. Falk, R.H., Plehn, J.F., Deering, T., Schick Jr., E.C., Bionay, P., Rubinow, A., Skinner, M., and Cohen, A.S. Sensitivity and specificity of echocardiographic features of cardiac amyloidosis. *Am. J. Cardiol.* **59**: 418–422, 1987.
52. Engel, P.J., Fowler, N.O., Tei, C.W., Shah, P.M., Driedger, H.J., Shabetai, R., Harbin, A.D., and Franch, R.H. M-mode echocardiography in constrictive pericarditis. *J. Am. Coll. Cardiol.* **6**: 471–474, 1985.

Early and Late Results of Surgery for Endomyocardial Fibrosis

Carlos R. Moraes

Division of Thoracic Surgery, Department of Surgery, Federal University of Pernambuco Medical School and Heart Institute of Pernambuco, Hospital Portugues, Recife, Brazil

ABSTRACT

Fifty-seven patients with endomyocardial fibrosis (EMF) underwent endocardial decortication and atrioventricular valve replacement or repair between December 1977 and May 1988. There were 44 female and 13 male patients, ranging in age from 4 to 59 years (mean 31). Twenty-six patients had biventricular disease, 24 had the right-sided form, and 7 had EMF confined to the left ventricle. All were in functional class III or IV (New York Heart Association classification). The hospital mortality was 19.2% (11 patients). The causes of early death were low cardiac output syndrome (6), arrhythmia cerebral embolism, renal failure, pulmonary embolism, and sepsis. There were 11 (19.2%) late deaths but 5 had noncardiac causes. Among the 35 survivors (mean follow-up 47 months), 25 (43.8%) are in functional class I or II. The 5-year probability of survival, according to the life table analysis, is 72%, which is clearly superior to the outlook for patients medically treated. Despite the high early and late mortality, and the fact that only 43.8% of the operated patients had good late clinical results, it is concluded that, at present, surgical treatment is the only hope for patients with advanced EMF.

INTRODUCTION

Since the introduction of endocardial decortication and atrioventricular valve replacement for endomyocardial fibrosis (EMF) by Dubost[1] in France, the procedure has been performed with increasing frequency in several other countries, especially in those where the disease is more common.[2-5] This article reviews experience with 57 operated patients in Recife, Brazil, and the surgical literature.

PATIENTS

From December 1977 to May 1988, 57 patients with EMF were operated on in our institutions. There were 44 female and 13 male patients, ranging in age from 4 to 59 years (mean 31).

The time of onset of symptoms ranged from 6 months to 16 years prior to admission (mean 3.4 years). Most patients were in poor general condition and a low nutritional state. All patients had been born and spent their entire lives in Brazil. The majority (52) were classed as belonging to low socioeconomic groups, whereas 4 were considered middle class and only one patient could be regarded as belonging to the upper middle class. At the time of admission only 7 (12.3%) had increased eosinophilia.

According to the New York Association Functional Classification, 36 patients were in class III and 21 in class IV. The patients were divided into 3 groups: group I consisted of 26 (45.6%) patients with biventricular disease; group II included 24 (42.1%) patients with involvement of the right ventricle alone; and group III comprised 7 (12.3%) patients with EMF confined to the left ventricle.

Those classed as having bilateral or right-sided forms (groups I and II) had a very similar clinical picture dominated by raised venous pressure, massive hepatomegaly, and ascites with unremarkable auscultatory findings. On the other hand, patients of group III showed a clinical picture characterized by dyspnea on exertion, signs of mitral insufficiency, and pulmonary hypertension.

The chest X-ray films showed enlargement of the heart, the mean cardiothoracic ratio being 0.66 (from 0.47 to 0.83). In patients in groups I and II cardiomegaly was mainly the result of a huge right atrium. Cardiomegaly was less pronounced in patients in group III, but marked pulmonary congestion was always present.

Electrocardiograms disclosed no specific abnormalities, with multiphasic low QRS complexes or QS/QR patterns. The majority (37 patients) were in atrial fibrillation. Multiple patterns of conduction disturbances such as first degree or branch blocks were common.

M-mode echocardiography (21 patients) showed abnormalities corresponding to the cavities involved. In every patient with right-sided involvement, dilatation and hyperkinesis of the infundibulum of the right ventricle and paradoxical motion of the septum were noted. Left ventricular involvement was characterized by an abnormal posterior wall motion and the occurrence of anomalous echoes on the posterior wall, near the mitral valve. Bidimensional echocardiography (10 patients) demonstrated abnormal filling of the apex of the affected ventricle by the fibrous mass.

Cardiac catheterization was carried out in all patients and was the base of diagnosis. Right ventricular disease was manifested by a high end-diastolic pressure in this cavity and an increase in right atrial pressure. The right ventricular pressure tracings either were of the dip-plateau type or were grossly distorted, resembling those obtained from the right atrium. Left ventricular involvement was characterized hemodynamically by increased left ventricular end-diastolic pressure and the subsequent elevation of the pulmonary wedge and arterial pressures. In patients with biventricular disease, the low output of the right ventricle and tricuspid insufficiency usually prevented the development of pulmonary hypertension.

Definitive diagnosis was established in every case by selective cineangiocardiography. On the right side there was atrial dilatation, tricuspid regurgitation, and amputation of the ventricular inflow tract with a typical tunnel-like formation that allowed direct passage of the dye from the dilated atrium to the pulmonary artery. Left ventricular cineangiography revealed a globular configuration of this chamber with obliteration of the apex. Twenty-six of 33 patients with left ventricular involvement (groups I and III) had moderate to severe mitral regurgitation.

SURGICAL TECHNIQUE

All patients were operated on by means of median sternotomy with conventional hypothermic (30°C) cardiopulmonary bypass by cannulating the ascending aorta and both venae cavae. The bypass was discontinued in one patient, and both venous cannulae, blocked by thrombi from the right atrium, were replaced. The duration of cardiopulmonary bypass ranged from 38 to 165 min (mean 79). Myocardial protection was achieved by means of cold potassium cardioplegic solution, infused into the aortic root, and topical hypothermia of the heart. The intracardiac procedure was performed in one period of ischemic arrest, which lasted from 18 to 115 min (mean 48).

Endocardium decortication of the right ventricle was accomplished in 50 patients, of whom 26 had biventricular disease (group I) and 24 had the right-sided form (group II). A large right atriotomy was performed in all cases, and thrombi, when present, were removed. The tricuspid valve was resected in 45 patients. Fibrous tissue was incised below the tricuspid annulus, leaving a plane of cleavage between the fibrosis and the underlying myocardium. The dissection was directed toward the ventricular apex into the posterior wall, allowing the excision of an entire fibrous shell. After the decortication had been completed, a valve prosthesis was inserted in the tricuspid position. Five patients with biventricular disease showed limited right-side involvement, with an area of fibrosis confined to the apex of the right ventricle, and no significant tricuspid incompetence. In those cases, the endocardiectomy was carried out, but the tricuspid valve was preserved.

Left ventricular endocardiectomy was performed in 33 patients, of whom 26 had biventricular disease (group I) and 7 had the left-sided form (group III). The fibrosis of the left ventricular endocardium was resected by the same guidelines as those used for the right side. However, the approach to the left ventricular cavity varied according to the size of the left atrium. In 18 patients who had a dilated left atrium, a good exposure was obtained by a large vertical atriotomy. The remaining 15 patients, all with biventricular disease, had a normally sized left atrium and the operation was carried out either by an incision in the atrial septum after decortication of the right ventricle (6 patients) or by a limited apical left ventriculotomy (9). The latter approach was electively performed in patients with minor or no mitral regurgitation, in whom only the decortication of the left ventricle was planned. In only 7 patients was it possible to preserve the mitral valve; it was replaced in the other 26.

In this series of 57 operated patients, 54 received a bioprosthesis and only 3 received a disk-tilting valve.

OPERATIVE AND PATHOLOGICAL FINDINGS

The 50 patients with right-side involvement (groups I and II) always showed dilatation and thickening of the right atrium. Organized thrombus was found in the area of the atrial appendage in 15 (26.3%) patients and in the apex of the right ventricle in one (1.7%). The fibrous thickening obliterated the apex of the right ventricle in all cases but was limited to this area in 5 (8.7%) with biventricular disease. In the other 45 (91.3%), the fibrosis extended toward the outflow tract and to the tricuspid annulus involving the papillary muscles and retracting the valve leaflets, particularly the septal cusp, causing severe tricuspid insufficiency. A moderate pericardial effusion was present in 12 (21%) patients in groups I and II.

Lesions found in the left ventricle of 33 patients (groups I and III) were classed as limited in 7 (12.2%) with biventricular disease. In those patients, fibrosis was located at the apex with minor involvement of the papillary muscles. In the remaining 26 patients there was extensive involvement of the left ventricle, with the fibrosis extending from the apex toward the papillary muscles and the free wall of the ventricle, encroaching upon the posterior aspect of the mitral valve and thus causing severe insufficiency. The posterior papillary muscle was more often involved than the anterior. Three (5.2%) patients had thrombus in the left ventricular cavity.

Histologically, the diagnosis of EMF was confirmed in all cases. The endocardial fibrous tissue consisted essentially of collagenous connective tissue with sparse elastic fibers and without infiltration of inflammatory cells. Areas of granulation were usually seen, and more rarely calcium deposits.

RESULTS

Early Mortality

The operative mortality (up to 1 month after operation) was 19.2% (11/57). Mortality according to patient groups is given in Table 1. The causes of early deaths included low cardiac output syndrome ($n=6$), arrhythmia ($n=1$), renal failure ($n=1$), pulmonary embolism ($n=1$) sepsis ($n=1$), and cerebral embolism ($n=1$).

Postoperative Complications

Twenty-one (36.8%) of 46 survivors had a total of 36 nonfatal but severe postoperative complications (Table 2). Apart from a variable degree of low cardiac output, the main sources of morbidity were arrhythmias and complete heart block. Four of 7 patients who presented A-V block warranted permanent pacing.

Reoperation

Only one patient with biventricular disease required reoperation 2 years later to replace the mitral valve which had been preserved during the first intervention. No recurrence of fibrosis in the left ventricle was noted.

Late Mortality

Eleven (19.2%) late deaths occurred in periods of time ranging from 2 months to 7 years after operation. The causes of late death were intractable heart failure ($n=3$), cerebral embolism ($n=2$), sepsis ($n=2$), hepatic cirrhosis ($n=1$), gastrointestinal infec-

TABLE 1. Operative Mortality

Group	No.	Deaths	%
I	26	7	26.9
II	24	4	16.6
III	7	–	–
Total	57	11	19.2

p > 0.05

TABLE 2. Postoperative Complications

Type	No. patients
Low cardiac output	12
A-V heart block	7
Ventricular arrhythmias	7
Renal failure	3
Hemorrhage	3
Infection	3
Pulmonary embolism	1

TABLE 3. Late Mortality

Group	No.	Deaths	%
I	26	4	15.3
II	24	7	29.1
III	7	–	–
Total	57	11	19.2

P > 0.05.

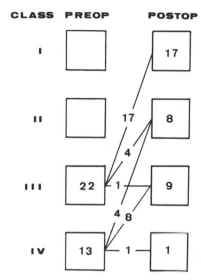

Fig. 1. New York Heart Association functional classification of 35 survivors (mean follow-up 47 months).

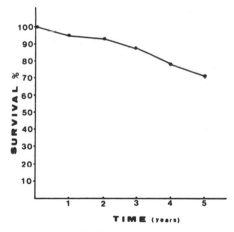

Fig. 2. Five-year actuarial survival curve.

tion ($n = 1$), pulmonary embolism ($n = 1$), and unknown ($n = 1$). Late mortality according to patient group is given in Table 3.

Survivors

Thirty-five (61.4%) patients are alive at the time of writing. The total follow-up for the 35 surviving patients was 1,628 patient/months (mean 47 months). Twenty-five (43.8%) patients are in functional class I or II (Fig. 1). Five-year actuarial probability of survival, including operative mortality, was 72% (Fig. 2).

DISCUSSION

The diagnosis of EMF, and its surgical treatment, is being made with increasing frequency in Brazil, where the disease seems to be relatively common among persons from the lower strata of the population.[5-10]

In recent years there has been a considerable increase in knowledge about the clinical features and pathophisiology of EMF. Clinical and morphologic characteristics of the disease are now well established. At present there is also strong evidence to support the theory that Loffler's endocarditis and EMF have a common pathogenesis, possibly due to a toxic effect of eosinophils on the endocardium.[11] Brockington and Olsen[12] have shown that the fibrous stages of both entities are histologically indistinguishable. In 1984, a WHO committee[13] recommended the use of the terms "eosinophilic endomyocardial disease" for the heart disease associated with a marked eosinophilia, which is usually found in temperate climates, and "tropical endomyocardial disease" for the condition commonly seen in tropical regions. The latter clinical picture was present in all our patients in whom the hypereosinophilic syndrome has not been recognized. Only 7 patients (12.3%) of our series had hematologic eosinophilia at the time of admission.

The downhill course of patients with EMF and the irreversible nature of the disease are well known.[14,15] Most patients die within 3 years of symptom onset. Medical therapy with digitalis and diuretics is often unsatisfactory, and, at present, endocardiectomy and atrioventricular valve replacement constitute the preferred form of treatment. The rationale for surgical treatment is mainly based on the fact that the systolic function of the myocardium is preserved or only slightly depressed in most patients with EMF.

The operative technique has been previously reported in detail[16] and differs little from the original method of Dubost.[17] During endocardial resection, it is important to avoid injury to the myocardium by remaining on the side of fibrosis. This is facilitated by a clear plane of cleavage between the thick endocardium and the underlying myocardium. The fibrosis tends to be thicker near the apex of the ventricles and at the bases of the papillary muscles. Most fibrous tissue should be removed because incomplete decortication can result in unsatisfactory postoperative improvement. However, we have followed the suggestion of Metras[3] to leave a thin strip of endocardium at the level of the septal leaflet and anterolateral commissure of the tricuspid valve with the aim of avoiding complete heart block. In fact, only one instance of this complication has occurred in our series since we adopted that technique. Another important technical modification that we have made is to approach the left ventricle through a limited apical ventriculotomy in patients with minor mitral incompetence, in whom only endocardiectomy is planned.

We have favored low-profile bioprosthesis for mitral and tricuspid valve replacement in patients with EMF because they are less prone to thromboembolic complications. This is particularly important with the type of patients in this series, with large atria, frequent atrial fibrillation, and social conditions that preclude anticoagulation.

The high operative mortality (19.2%) in our series indicates the severity of the cardiac condition of most patients at the time of operation. This figure is similar to that reported by other groups in Brazil,[8,9] India,[4] Ivory Coast,[18] and France.[17] A review of the literature shows that surgical treatment for EMF has been reported in 287 patients, with 54 (18.8%) operative deaths (Table 4). This experience supports the view that the operation can be carried out with an acceptable risk in patients with EMF, although the majority are in the late stage of cardiac failure. On the other hand, we think that the operative mortality is likely to improve if the operation in undertaken at an earlier stage of the disease.

Like others,[4,18] we have observed different mortality rates in patients with biventricular (26.9%), right-sided (16.6%), and left-sided (0%) forms of the disease, but the difference was not statistically significant. The difficult postoperative course with a high incidence of postoperative complications observed in our series is also a reflection of the poor preoperative conditions that have been referred to by others.[3,4]

Follow-up studies have shown no recurrence of the fibrosis to date and good clinical improvement in the majority of the reported cases. However, 32 (11.1%) late deaths have been described (Table 4). We have documented 11 late deaths, but 5 had noncardiac causes and 2 were due to cerebral embolism in patients not receiving anticoagulants.

We have followed 35 surviving patients for a total period of 1,628 patient/months (mean 47 months). Twenty-five (43.8%) are in functional class I or II, and this figure is encouraging, in contrast to the poor prognosis for nonoperative patients.[15] The 5-year probability of survival, according to the life table analysis, was 72%, and it is also clearly superior to the outlook for medically treated patients.[14,15]

TABLE 4.   Reports of Patients Operated Upon for EMF

Authors	No. of Patients	Location		Operative deaths	Late deaths
		Biventricular	Monoventricular		
Binet et al.[19]	1	0	1 (LV)	0	0
Bjorck et al.[20]	1	0	1 (RV)	0	0
Blake et al.[21]	1	0	1 (LV)	0	0
Cachera et al.[22]	6	3	3 (LV)	0	1
Costa et al.[8]	14	9	5 (LV, 3; RV, 2)	4	0
Davies et al.[23]	2	1	1 (LV)	0	0
Dubost et al.[17]	20	6	14 (LV, 5; RV, 9)	3	4
Galbut et al.[24]	1	1	0	0	0
Graham et al.[25]	1	1	0	0	0
Hess et al.[26]	4	1	3 (LV)	0	0
Ikahelmo et al.[27]	1	0	1 (LV)	0	1
John et al.[28]	1	0	1 (RV)	0	0
Laing et al.[29]	1	0	1 (RV)	0	0
Lepley et al.[30]	1	0	1 (LV)	0	0
Mady et al.[9]	39	25	14 (LV, 7; RV, 7)	11	0
Mendonca et al.[10]	15	9	6 (LV, 2; RV, 4)	1	3
Métras et al.[18]	55	20	35 (LV, 18; RV, 17)	9	6
Nair et al.[31]	1	0	1 (LV)	0	0
San Juan[32]	1	0	1 (LV)	0	0
Sheikhzadeh et al.[33]	1	1	0	0	0
Wood et al.[34]	1	0	1 (LV)	0	0
Valiathan et al.[4]	62	34	28 (LV, 9; RV, 19)	15	6
This report	57	26	31 (LV, 7; RV, 24)	11	11
TOTAL	287	137	150 (LV, 65; RV, 85)	54	32

LV: left ventricle, RV: right ventricle.

In conclusion, this study, like other reports,[4,8-10,17,18] demonstrates that surgery can be lifesaving in patients with EMF. The quality of life can be greatly improved for many patients although the long-term outlook is uncertain. The need for a valve prosthesis is a possible limitation of the operation. Moreover, the possibility of recurrence of the fibrosis still exists. However, at present, endocardiectomy and atrioventricular valve replacement or repair is the treatment of choice for patients with EMF because of the inherent grave prognosis of this condition and the ineffectiveness of medical therapy.

REFERENCES

1. Dubost, C. L'endocardectomie: Traitement chirurgical de la fibrose endocardique constrictive. *C.R. Acad. Sci.* **281**: 855–857, 1975.
2. Moraes, C.R., Buffolo, E., Victor, E., Saraiva, L., Gomes, J.M.P., Lira, V., Lima, R., Escobar, M., and Andrade, J.C.S. Endomyocardial fibrosis: Report of six patients and review of the surgical literature. *Ann. Thorac. Surg.* **29**: 243–248, 1980.
3. Metras, D., Quezzin-Colibaly, N., Quattara, K., Chauvet, J., Ekra, A., Lougechaud, A., and Bertrand, E. Endomyocardial fibrosis: Early and late results of surgery in 20 patients. *J. Thorac. Cardiovasc. Surg.* **83**: 52–64, 1982.
4. Valiathan, M.S., Balakrishnan, K.G., Sankarkumar, R., and Kartha, C.C. Surgical treatment of endomyocardial fibrosis. *Ann. Thorac. Surg.* **43**: 68–73, 1987.
5. Costa, F.D.A., Moraes, C.R., Rodrigues, J.V., Mendonca, J.T., Andrade, J.C., Buffolo, E., Succi, J.E., Carvalho, R.G., Faraco, D.L., and Costa, I.A. Early surgical results in the treatment of endomyocardial fibrosis. A Brazilian cooperative study. *Eur. J. Cardiothorac. Surg.* (in press).
6. Moraes, C.R., Buffolo, E., Lima, R., Victor, E., Lira, V., Escobar, M., Rodrigues, J., Saraiva, L., and Andrade, J.C. Surgical treatment of endomyocardial fibrosis. *J. Thorac. Cardiovasc. Surg.* **85**: 738–745, 1983.
7. Moraes, C.R., Rodrigues, J.V., Gomes, C.A., Marinucci, L., Coelho, T.C., Santos, C.L., Victor, E., and Cavalcanti, I. Dez anos de cirurgia da endomiocardiofibrose: O que aprendemos. *Rev. Bras. Cir. Cardiovasc.* **2**: 42–52, 1987.
8. Costa, F.D.A., Soeiro, A.B., Sallum, F.S., Faraco, D.L., Carvalho, R.G., Brofmann, P.R., Loures, D.R.R., and Costa, I.A. Tratamento cirurgico da endomicardiofibrose. Estudo cooperativo. *Arq. Bras. Cardiol.* **49**: 139–146, 1987.
9. Mady, C., Barretto, A.C.P., Stolf, N.A.G., Oliveira, S.A., Arteaga-Fernandez, E., Bellotti, G., Jatene, A.D., and Pileggi, F. Resultados imediatos do tratamento cirurgico da endomiocardiofibrose. *Arq. Bras. Cardiol.* **50**: 93–95, 1988.
10. Mendonça, J.T., Carvalho, M.R., Kakuda, R., Franco Filho, E., Araujo, J.A., Barros, M.L., Costa, G.B., Almeida, M.L.D., Garcia, M.H., Taqueda, M.S.S., Souza, A.O., Menezes, R.S., and Paixão, E.L.R. Endomiocardiofibrose: Tratamento cirurgico. *Rev. Circ. Cardiovasc.* **1**: 23–27, 1988.
11. Spry, C.J. Eosinophils in eosinophilic endomyocardial disease. *Postgrad. Med. J.* **62**: 609–613, 1986.
12. Brockington, I.F. and Olsen, E.G.L. Loffler's endocarditis and Davies endocardial fibrosis. *Am. Heart J.* **85**: 308, 1973.
13. Cardiomyopathies. Report of a WHO Expert Committee. *WHO Tech. Rep. Ser.* **697**: 7–64, 1984.
14. D'Arbela, P.G., Mutazindwa, T., Patel, A.K., and Somers, K. Survival after first presentation with endomyocardial fibrosis. *Br. Heart J.* **34**: 403, 1972.
15. Bertrand, E., Chauvet, J.O.D., Assamoi, M., N.Dori, R., Ekra, A., Ravinet, L., Longechaud, A., and Métras, C. Evaluation des resultats du traitement chirurgical de la fibrose endomyocardique: Etude de 31 malades opérées et 30 malades non opérées. *Bull. Acad. Natl. Med.* **166**: 1170–1186, 1982.

16. Moraes, C.R., Escobar, M., Lima, R., and Rodrigues, J.V. Technical aspects in surgery for endomyocardial fibrosis: Experience with 37 patients. *Texas Heart Inst. J.* **10**: 115–118, 1983.

17. Dubost, C., Prigent, C., Gerbaux, A., Maurice, P., Pesselecq, J., Rulliere, R., Carpentier, A., and Deloche, A. Surgical treatment of constrictive fibrous endocarditis. *J. Thorac. Cardiovasc. Surg.* **82**: 585–591, 1981.

18. Métras, D., Caulibaly, A., and Quattara, K. The surgical treatment of endomyocardial fibrosis: Results in 55 patients. *Circulation* **72** (suppl. II): 274, 1985.

19. Binet, J.P., Pcrnod, J., Kermarec, J., Colette, J., Weiler, M., Bouhey, J., and Bouvier, M. Endocardite constrictive fibroplastique: A propos d'une forme localisée au ventric gauche. *Arch. Mal. Coeur* **70**: 163–168, 1977.

20. Bjorck, V.O., Szamosi, A., and Tornell, G. Parietal fibroplastic endocarditis (Loeffler's disease): Radiological and surgical aspects in connection with a case report. *Scand. J. Thorac. Cardiovasc. Surg.* **8**: 23–26, 1974.

21. Blake, D.P., Palmer, T.E., and Olinger, G.N. Mitral valve replacement in idiopathic hyper-eosinophilic syndrome. *J. Thorac. Cardiovasc. Surg.* **89**: 630–638, 1985.

22. Cachera, J.P., Poulain, H., Menaske, P., Laurent, F., Loisance, D., and Chiche, P. Endocardite fibreuse d'origine filarienne: Traitement chirurgical. *Trop. Cardiol.* **2**: 79, 1976.

23. Davies, J., Sapsford, R., Brooksky, I., Olsen, B.G.J., Spry, C.J.F., Oakley, C.M., and Goodwin, J.F. Successful surgical treatment of two patients with eosinophilic endomyocardial disease. *Br. Heart J.* **46**: 438–445, 1981.

24. Galbut, D.L., Benson, J., Blankstein, R.L., Vignola, P.A., and Gentsch, T.O. Endomyocardial fibrosis. Preoperative diagnosis and surgical therapy. *Chest* **84**: 779–782, 1983.

25. Graham, J.M., Lawrie, G.M., Feteih, N.M., and DeBakey, M.E. Management of endomyocardial fibrosis: Successful surgical treatment of biventricular involvement and considerations of the superiority of operative treatment. *Am. Heart J.* **102**: 771–782, 1981.

26. Hess, O.M., Turina, M., Senning, A., Goebel, N.H., Scholer, Y., and Krayenbuchl, H.P. Pre- and postoperative findings in patients with endomyocardial fibrosis. *Br. Heart J.* **40**: 406–415, 1978.

27. Ikahelmo, M.J., Karkola, P.J., and Takkunen, J.T. Surgical treatment of Loeffler's eosinophilic endocarditis. *Br. Heart J.* **45**: 729–732, 1981.

28. John, S., Mani, G.K., Muralidharan, S., Krishnaswami, S., and Cherian, G. Endomyocardial fibrosis from a surgical standpoint. *J. Thorac. Cardiovasc. Surg.* **80**: 437–440, 1980.

29. Laing, H.C., Sharratt, G.P., Johnson, A.M., Davies, M.J., and Monro, J.L. Endomyocardial fibrosis in a European woman and its successful surgical treatment. *J. Thorac. Cardiovasc. Surg.* **74**: 803–807, 1977.

30. Lepley, D., Jr., Aris, A., Korns, M.E., Walker, J., and DeCunha, R.M. Endomyocardial fibrosis: A surgical approach. *Ann. Thorac. Surg.* **18**: 626–633, 1974.

31. Nair, U., Evans, T., and Oakley, D. Surgical treatment of endomyocardial fibrosis with preservation of mitral valve. *Br. Heart J.* **43**: 357–359, 1980.

32. San Juan, E. Discussion. In: Moraes, C.R. *et al.* (eds.), Tratamento cirurgico da endomiocardiofibrose. *Arq. Bras. Cardiol.* **33** (suppl. 1): 257, 1979.

33. Sheikhzadeh, A.H., Tarbiat, A., Nazarian, I., Aryanpur, I., and Senning, A. Constrictive endocarditis: Report of a case with successful surgery. *Br. Heart J.* **42**: 224–228, 1979.

34. Wood, A.E., Boyle, D., O'Hara, M.D., and Cleland, J. Mitral annuloplasty in endomyocardial fibrosis: An alternative to valve replacement. *Ann. Thorac. Surg.* **34**: 446–451, 1982.

Allergy and Eosinophils: Roles of Eosinophils in Airway Allergic Responses in Bronchial Asthma

Sohei Makino, Takeshi Fukuda, Shinji Motojima, Goro Yamada, Tatsuo Yukawa, and Yoshinori Terashi

Department of Medicine and Clinical Immunology, Dokkyo University School of Medicine, Tochigi, Japan

ABSTRACT

Peripheral blood and organ eosinophilia is a hallmark of IgE-mediated allergic diseases.[1] This almost constant association had been established by the early part of this century and has been of practical use in the diagnosis of allergic diseases including asthma. However, its role in allergy had long remained unknown. In the past 2 decades new information regarding eosinophil granule proteins, surface receptors, production of chemical mediators, kinetics of migration and T- cell factor dependency of its proliferation has been obtained. Most of this information suggests that eosinophils are effector and proinflammatory cells in IgE-mediated allergic reaction.

INTRODUCTION

This review is intended to show the role of eosinophils in the IgE-mediated allergic response by taking allergic asthma as a model of local allergic response.

STRUCTURAL AND FUNCTIONAL CHARACTERISTICS OF EOSINOPHILS[2,4]

Figure 1 shows a transmission electron micrograph of a mature human eosinophil in peripheral blood. The nucleus is mostly bilobed, and one eosinophil has around 200 characteristic specific granules which are stained red by eosin with hematoxylin and eosin (HE) staining and are made up of an electron-dense, quadrangular crystalloid core surrounded by a less dense matrix.

Currently, at least 4 cationic proteins are recognized in the granule: major basic protein (MBP), eosinophil cationic protein (ECP), eosinophil peroxidase (EPO), and eosinophil-derived neurotoxin (EDN).[5,6] The crystalloid core is composed of MBP, which is quantitatively predominant among these cationic proteins. ECP, EPO, and EDN are located in the matrix of the granule.[7,8,9] *In vitro*, MBP, ECP, and the EPO $+ H_2O_2 +$ halide system can kill helminthic parasites, especially in the larval stage. In addition, these 3 proteins are toxic for tumor cells and/or many mammalian cells, including guinea pig respiratory epithelium.[10,11] Furthermore, it has been shown that human MBP produces damage in human bronchial epithelium consisting of desquamation and destruction of ciliated cells,[12] mimickingthe epithelial damage characteristic of asthma. Other evidence for the participation of eosinophils in the allergic process is provided by the stimulation of mediator release by eosinophil granule proteins[13]: MBP, ECP,[14] and EPO $+ H_2O_2 +$ halide[15] cause calcium-, energy-, and temperature-dependent histamine release from mast cells and/or basophils.

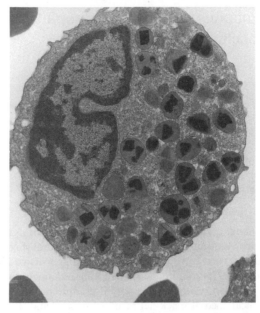

Fig. 1.   Transmission electron micrograph of a mature human eosinophil in peripheral blood.

HETEROGENEITY OF EOSINOPHILS[16]

Eosinophils can be divided into 2 groups, normodense and hypodense eosinophils. Hypodense eosinophils in blood are found in increased frequency in patients with allergic asthma,[17,18,19] allergic rhinitis,[20] peripheral eosinophilia, and parasitic infection. Functionally, hypodense eosinophils are active, showing increased production of LTC_4,[18] increased density of complement receptors,[21] the expression of IgE-Fc receptor-2,[22,23] increased density of IgG-Fc receptor,[24,25] and increased cytotoxicity.[26,27] Eosinophils in tissue such as in bronchoalveolar lavage are mainly hypodense, suggesting that eosinophils in tissue are of a stimulated form.

EOSINOPHILS IN LATE-PHASE RESPONSE OF IgE-MEDIATED ALLERGIC REACTION

In IgE-mediated allergic reaction, peripheral eosinophilia and accumulation of eosinophils at the site of allergic reaction[1] are characteristic findings. In allergic asthma the inhalation of a specific allergen causes immediate bronchoconstriction, and then late-phase airway narrowing accompanied by eosinophil infiltration in the bronchial mucosa, followed by the post-late-phase inflammatory response in the bronchi.[3,4] During these late-phase responses intense eosinophil infiltration is observed in the airway. Such findings raise the possibility that eosinophils infiltrating in the airway may cause inflammation and result in these airway responses. Other than allergic diseases, in hypereosinophilic syndrome eosinophils are considered to cause damage to the endomyocardium.[28,29]

The following description is intended to show the role of eosinophils in the late-phase

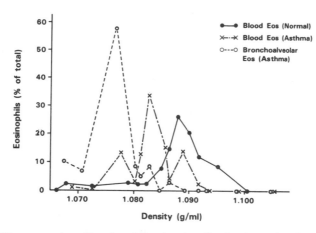

Fig. 2. Heterogeneity of eosinophils: density distribution of eosinophils from peripheral blood of a normal subject (•) and an asthmatic subject (×) and from bronchoalveolar lavage of an asthmatic subject (○).

reactions of IgE-mediated allergic response by taking allergic asthma as a model of local allergic response.

EARLY AND LATE PHASES OF IgE-MEDIATED ALLERGIC REACTION

IgE-mediated allergic response consists of 2 phases, early and late. A combination of an antigen molecule and IgE antibodies which are fixed on the surface of a mast cell causes the release of chemical mediators.[30]

Chemical mediators can be functionally categorized into 2 groups: spasmogenic and vasoactive; and chemotactic mediators. Histamine, sulfidepeptide leukotrienes (LTC_4, D_4, E_4), platelet-activating factor (PAF), and prostaglandin D_2 are spasmogenic and vasoactive mediators,[31,32] and LTB_4,[33,34] PAF,[35] HETE,[36] ECF-A,[37,38] and NCF-A[39] are chemotactic mediators.

In the early-phase response spasmogenic and/or vasoactive chemical mediators cause spasms of smooth muscle and increase vascular permeability, which result in broncho-constriction in asthma, wheal and flare response in skin testing, and nasal secretion and constipation in allergic rhinitis. This response occurs immediately after an antigen challenge and subsides within about 60 min.

In this phase no apparent infiltration of eosinophils in the tissue is observed, although eosinophils in the peripheral blood accumulate in and around the vasculatures at the site of the allergic reaction.[40] Peripheral eosinopenia develops, if antigenic challenge is great enough to collect a number of circulating eosinophils.[1,41] In the late-response period that occurs 5–8 hr after the antigen challenge, an inflammatory response is frequently observed at the site of the immediate response. In skin testing diffuse swelling and redness are observed during this period.[42] Inflammatory cells including eosinophils accumulate in the tissue.[40,43,44] In bronchial challenge with a specific antigen, late-phase narrowing of the airway is frequently associated with eosinophilia in bronchoalveolar lavage fluid.[45–47]

After the late-phase response, not infrequently inflammation and tissue destruction are observed at the site of immediate and late responses. Signs of post-late-phase inflammation become most apparently manifested in the bronchial allergic response.

THREE-PHASE RESPONSES OF ALLERGEN-INDUCED ASTHMATIC RESPONSE (Fig. 3)

Allergic response of the airway in bronchial asthma is unique, since after the immediate- and late-phase response, a post-late-phase response, which was called the subacute/chronic inflammation phase by Kay,[48] is observed.

Immediately after the antigen challenge, immediate bronchospasm occurs, and then 3–8 hr after antigen challenge, late-phase airway narrowing occurs. Following the late-phase response, the post-late response, which is characterized by bronchial hypersensitivity without narrowing of airway, is observed for 1 to 2 weeks.[49] These responses are called immediate asthmatic response (IAR), late asthmatic response (LAR), and post-late asthmatic response (PLAR), respectively.

Eosinophils in the peripheral blood diminish during IAR, and then the cells increase gradually and return to the baseline value 24 hr after.[41]

In the bronchial tissue or bronchial lumen, eosinophils start to increase 2 to 3 hr after the challenge and reach the maximum 6 hr later,[40,45,46] which seems to remain for several days or longer. LAR is not observed in all patients with IAR. Its occurrence seems to depend on a greater accumulation of eosinophils in the bronchi. DeMonchy[45] carried out bronchoalveolar lavage 6 hr after allergen inhalation and found that the number of eosinophils was higher in LAR-positive patients than in those with IAR only.[45] Nanba *et al.* also carried out bronchoalveolar lavage in LAR-positive patients 2 hr after the therapeutic termination of the LAR airway narrowing, and found an increased number of eosinophils in LAR-positive patients, while they did not find any increase in eosinophils in bronchoalveolar lavage fluid (BALF) in patients with IAR only.[47]

Post-late-phase asthmatic response, which is characterized by enhancement of bron-

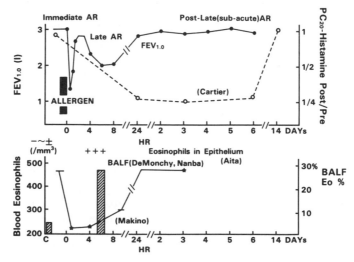

Fig. 3. Three phases of asthmatic response (AR) after a specific allergen inhalation.

chial responsiveness, is also not found in all IAR-positive patients. Again, its occurrence seems to be dependent on a greater accumulation of eosinophils in the bronchi.

Cartier et al. found an increase in bronchial responsiveness to inhaled histamine in LAR-positive patients more frequently than in IAR only.[49]

The mechanism of the bronchial hyperresponsiveness in LAR-positive patients is considered to be as follows: eosinophils infiltrate massively into the bronchial mucosa and release their granule proteins, such as MBP[50,51] and EPO,[52] and these proteins cause damage to the bronchial mucosa. The damage to the bronchial epithelium results in the exposure of the irritant receptor which enhances nonspecific bronchial responsiveness. In fact, Wardlaw et al. have observed increases in nonspecific bronchial responsiveness to inhaled methacholine in patients whose bronchoalveolar lavage fluids contained increased amounts of eosinophil-derived major basic protein.[53]

TIME COURSE OF AIRWAY NARROWING, BRONCHIAL HYPERRESPON-SIVENESS, AND EOSINOPHIL INFILTRATION IN THE BRONCHIAL MUCOSA AFTER AN ALLERGEN CHALLENGE IN SENSITIZED GUINEA PIGS: ANIMAL MODEL

In order to investigate the relationship between the eosinophil infiltration to the bronchi and airway responses after allergen-induced bronchoconstriction, measurements of respiratory resistance and bronchial responsiveness to inhaled histamine and histologic examination of the bronchi were carried out in sensitized guinea pigs before and after antigen inhalation challenge.

1) Model of Passively Sensitized Guinea Pigs[54]

Male Hartley guinea pigs were passively sensitized by injecting homologous anti-

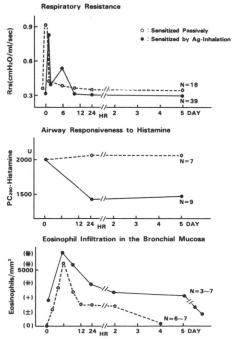

Fig. 4. Three antigen-induced airway responses and eosinophil infiltration response in guinea pigs sensitized passively or by antigen inhalation.

ovalbumin (OA) serum, which showed high titer of 48-hr PCA with reaginic activity of IgE. Forty-eight hours after sensitization, the sensitized animals were challenged by inhalations of 1% OA solution. Respiratory resistance was measured by the modified oscillation method of Mead without anesthesia and tracheotomy.

Immediately after the antigen challenge a significant increase in respiratory resistance was confirmed in all animals, but no late-phase airway narrowing was observed.

Animals were sacrificed before and 15 min, 1, 2, 4, 6, 9, 12, and 24 hr, and 2 and 4 days after challenge, and the lungs were used for histologic examination. Eosinophil infiltration started 2 hr after the antigen challenge and reached a maximum 6 hr after, then decreased gradually but remained for at least 48 hr.

Nonspecific responsiveness of the bronchi was expressed by PC_{200} (RR)-histamine which is the lowest concentration of histamine solution which induces a 200% increase in respiratory resistance. No significant decrease in PC_{200}-histamine was observed. Lellouch-Tubiana and others challenged passively sensitized guinea pigs with intravenous OA antigen, and 6 hr later observed the infiltration of eosinophils in the bronchial mucosa,[55] conforming to our inhalation challenge study.

Our observations in normal, passively sensitized guinea pigs were: the animals developed IAR but no LAR; post-late-phase bronchial hypersensitivity was not observed. Eosinophil infiltration had one peak, which reached a maximum 6 hr after the antigen challenge.

2) *Model of Actively Sensitized Guinea Pigs by Repeated Antigen Inhalations*[56-58]

Asthmatic patients are considered to be sensitized to environmental allergens and then exposed to such allergens repeatedly, resulting in persistent allergic inflammation in the airway. In order to reproduce this situation, we sensitized guinea pigs by repeated inhalations of an antigen solution and then challenged them.

Male Hartley guinea pigs were placed in an air-tight box and exposed to the aerosols of 1% OA solution for 2 hr once a week 4–10 times. The exposure was stopped when the animals showed apparent signs of dyspnea. One week later, the animals were challenged by inhalation of the antigen solution, and showed an immediate bronchoconstriction response. About half of the animals showed late-phase airway narrowing, in contrast to the passively sensitized animals.

PC_{200}-histamine was measured 24 hr and 5 days after the antigen challenge. Half of the animals showed a decrease in PC_{200}-histamine, showing the enhancement of airway responsiveness. Counting of infiltrated eosinophils in the bronchial mucosa revealed significant infiltration before the antigen challenge, and 2 hr after the challenge the infiltration started to increase and reached the first peak 6 hr later. This remained but gradually decreased for 5 days thereafter. Desquamation of the bronchial epithelium was also observed 1 and 5 days after the challenge.

Hutson *et al.* similarly sensitized guinea pigs by inhalation of OA antigen and observed immediate and late bronchial responses after intravenous antigen challenge.[59] In those inhalation-sensitized guinea pigs, the animals showed immediate- and late-phase airway narrowing and post-late-phase airway hyperresponsiveness, along with intense and prolonged infiltration of eosinophils into the bronchial mucosa.

3) *Summary of the Time Course Study*

Table 1 summarizes the differences in physiologic and histologic observations of the airway between actively and passively sensitized guinea pigs. In passively sensitized guinea pigs, eosinophil infiltration develops only one peak around 6 hr after antigen

TABLE 1. Comparison of Allergen-Induced Airway Responses between Passively Sensitized and Guinea Pigs Actively Sensitized by Inhalation

Airway response		Airway narrowing	Eosinophil infiltration	Bronchial responsiveness
Immediate	Passive	+ +	−	ND
	Active	+ +	+	ND
Late	Passive	−	+ +	ND
	Active	+ +	+ + +	ND
Postlate	Passive	−	+ −	± (24hr)
	Active	−	+ +	+ + (24hr, 5days)

challenge, while in animals actively sensitized by inhalation eosinophil infiltration develop the first peak around 6 hr after challenge and it remains for longer period.

POSSIBLE MECHANISM OF LATE-PHASE ASTHMATIC RESPONSE

We observed that half of the inhalation-sensitized animals showed LAR, while no LAR was observed in passively sensitized animals. Hutson et al. also observed LAR in inhalation-sensitized guinea pigs.[59] Increased eosinophil infiltration seems to favor the occurrence of LAR, as seen in this study and in human and experimental asthma.[45,47,60]

The possible mechanisms of LAR in inhalation-sensitized animals are as follows: 1) Eosinophils can release LTC_4[61,62] and PAF, and their increased accumulation is thought to supply more of these chemical mediators and cause edema of the bronchial mucosa and spasm of the bronchial smooth muscle. 2) MBP and EPO also enhance histamine release from basophils and/or mast cells.[13-15]

POSSIBLE MECHANISM OF POST-LATE-PHASE ASTHMATIC RESPONSE

Half of the inhalation-sensitized animals showed enhancement of bronchial responsiveness to inhaled histamine, while no such enhancement was observed in passively sensitized animals. Again, increased eosinophil infiltration seems to lead to the occurrence of this post-late asthmatic response, as seen in the present study. In human asthma, LAR is accompanied by increased accumulation of eosinophils and is frequently followed by post-LAR.[45,47,49]

The possible mechanisms are as follows: 1) infiltrating eosinophils can cause damage to the bronchial mucosa by releasing their toxic granule proteins.[10,44] 2) Destruction of the bronchial epithelium causes the sensitization of the irritant receptor, sensory nerve ending of the Vagus nerve, and results in the enhancement of vaso-vagal reflex bronchoconstriction. 3) A decrease in epithelium-derived relaxation factor, EpDRF,[63] due to the desquamation of the bronchial epithelium occurs. 4) Eosinophil-derived MBP causes the destruction of epithelial ciliary movement and induces retention of bronchial secretion.[64]

CHEMICAL MEDIATORS CHEMOTACTIC TO EOSINOPHILS

PAF and LTB_4 are major chemotactic chemical mediators in allergic reaction, and HETE and ECF-A tetrapeptides have much less chemotactic activity.[65-67] These

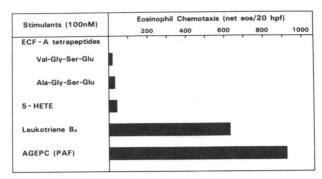

Fig. 5. Human eosinophil chemotactic activity of ECF-A tetrapeptides, leukotriene B_4 and PAF. Each bar is the mean ($N=3$) of a single experiment.

chemical mediators are released from mast cells and basophils by specific antigen exposure. In addition to these cells, PAF and/or LTB_4 is released from alveolar macrophages,[68,69] eosinophils,[70-72] neutrophils,[73,74] and monocytes/lymphocytes,[75] and platelets by IgE-mediated or other mechanisms. *In vitro* PAF and LTB_4 are significantly potent in chemotactic activity to human eosinophils.[65-67]

In our study of Boyden's chamber,[65] the upper chamber was filled with human eosinophil suspension of 98 % purity, and the lower chamber was filled with the solutions of various chemical mediators. Cells were incubated for 2 hr for migration. PAF and LTB4 demonstrated eosinophil-chemotactic activity in a dose-dependent manner. Figure 5 shows the number of eosinophils that migrated through filters to the chemical mediators, all in a concentration of 100 nM. PAF and LTB_4 attracted about 900 and 600 eosinophils per 20 fields, respectively, while HETE and ECF-A were about 1/20th as potent.

The specificity of chemotactant receptors can be shown by either the inhibition of receptor-specific blockers or desensitization of cellular receptors by exposure to ahigh concentration of chemotactants. PAF receptor antagonist CV3988, 1 to 10 μM, suppressed the eosinophil migration to PAF solution, $3 \times 10-8\mu$M, dose-dependently. Pretreatment of eosinophils with 1 μM LTB_4 made the cells unresponsive to LTB_4, but those cells showed normal chemotactic activity to PAF and zymosan-activated serum. These observations shows the specificity of the PAF or LTB_4 receptor of eosinophils.[65] Similarly, intrabronchially or intravenously introduced PAF causes eosinophilia in the bronchial mucosa in rabbits and baboons.[76,77]

In order to evaluate the *in vivo* chemotactic roles of PAF and other chemical mediators, we pretreated sensitized guinea pigs with PAF blocker CV6029 or ketotifen, an inhibitor of chemical mediator release, and challenged them with OA solution inhalation. After the animals showed definite bronchoconstriction, they were sacrificed 6 hr after the antigen challenge. CV6029 and ketotifen significantly suppressed eosinophil accumulation in the bronchial mucosa.[78,79]

Similarly, Lellouch-Tubiana *et al.* have reported that PAF blockers, WEB 2086 and BN, significantly suppressed eosinophil infiltration in guinea pigs challenged with an intravenous antigen.[55] These observations suggest that PAF and possibly LTB_4 can be major chemoattractants to induce eosinophil infiltration in the bronchial mucosa in airway allergy.

ROLES OF T-CELL-DERIVED FACTORS ON EOSINOPHIL ACCUMULATION

In addition to eosinophil chemotactic factors, T-cell-derived factors have been shown to play critical roles of antigen-induced eosinophil accumulation in the airway.

Akutsu and others[79] immunized male Hartley guinea pigs by intraperitoneal injection of OA with aluminum hydroxide and challenged by the inhalation of OA solution. Eosinophil accumulation in the airway showed 2-peaked time course. The first peak was around 6 hours and the second peak was around 24 hours after the antigen challenge. As described in the preceding chapter, the pretreatment with PAF antagonist, CV6029, suppressed the first peak but did not suppress the second peak, suggesting that the first peak was induced in part by PAF.

On the other hand the pretreatment with cyclosporine A, a suppressor of T-cell function, did not suppress the first peak but it did suppress the second peak, suggesting that the second peak is dependent on T-cell function.

These results suggest that in actively sensitized guinea pigs the first peak of eosinophil accumulation during late-phase response is dependent on PAF and the second peak

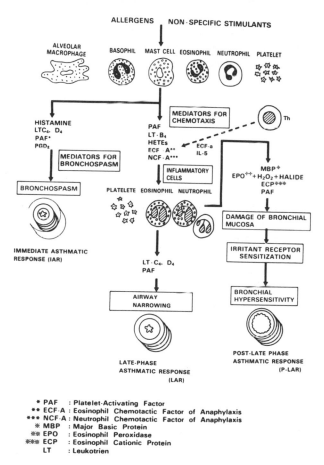

Fig. 6. Possible roles of eosinophils in 3 phases of asthmatic response after a specific allergen exposure.

during post-late-phase response is dependent on T-cell-derived factor(s). In fact, Hirotsu, Hirashima and others[43] isolated T-cell-derived ECF from the the delayed phase (24 hours old) of eosinophil-rich inflammatory sites by an antigen challenge in sensitized guinea pigs. There is a possibility that such T-cell factor may attract eosinophil to the antigen-induced inflammatory sites of the airway, too.

IL-5 is one of eosinophil colony stimulating factor and produced by T-cells. IL-5 enhances the effect of PAF on eosinophils. In chemotaxis, Numao and others[80] showed pretreatment of eosinophil with IL-5 enhanced PAF-induced chemotaxis in Boyden chamber. IL-5 itself did not show any chemotactic activity.

In summary, T-cell-derived factors cause or enhance eosionophil accumulation by antigen challenge in the site of allergic reaction, by (1) chemotaxis of eosinophils by possible ECF released by antigen-stimulated T-cells, (2) enhancement of PAF-induced eosinophil chemotaxis by IL-5, and (3) prolonged survival of eosinophil migrated to the site of allergic reaction by IL-5.[81]

SUMMARY: EOSINOPHILS AS EFFECTOR AND PROINFLAMMATORY CELLS IN THE LATE PHASE OF IgE-MEDIATED ALLERGIC REACTION

Clinical and experimental observation in IgE-mediated allergic response suggest that eosinophils play critical roles in the induction of late-phase and postlate-phase reaction. In late-phase reaction accumulated eosinophils release LTC_4 and PAF and cause local inflammation. In post-late-phase reaction eosinophil granule proteins, major basic protein and eosinophil peroxidase, cause damage to the tissue and induce functional disturbances specific to the organs. In the airway the enhancement of responsiveness is observed in the post-late phase. In airway allergic response, accumulation of eosinophils in the bronchi seems to induce the development of late-phase airway narrowing and post-late-phase bronchial hyperresponsiveness as seen in guinea pigs sensitized by repeated antigen inhalations.

Eosinophils accumulation at sites of allergic reaction is considered mostly to be hypodense and activated, and to expose IgE-Fc receptor-2 and IgG-Fc receptor. It is thought that antigen can stimulate these eosinophils and cause the release of their granule proteins and chemical mediators like mast cells. Such sequences can amplify the allergic inflammation.

From the clinical point of view, control of eosinophil migration and activation are critical to control allergic diseases.

ACKNOWLEDGMENT

A part of this study was supported by a grant from the Ministry of Education (No. 62440038).

REFERENCES

1. Cohen, S.G. and Ottesen, E.A. The eosinophil, eosinophilia and eosinophil-related disorders, In: Allergy. 2nd ed., Middleton, E., Jr., Reed, C.E., and Ellis, E.F. (eds.), Mosby, St. Louis, 1983, pp. 701–770.
2. Fukuda, T., Akutsu, I., Numao, T., Motojima, S., and Makino, S. The eosinophil in asthma. *Triangle* (Sandoz. Basel) **273**: 103–112, 1988.
3. Makino, S. Bronchial hyperreactivity, eosinophils in brochial asthma, and their relation

to prophylactic therapy. In: PAF (Platelet-activation factor) and Airway Hyperreactivity in Asthma. Makino, S. (ed.), Excerpta Medica, Asian Pacific Series No. 77, 1987, pp. 12 –20.

4. Frigas, E. and Gleich, G.J. The eosinophil and the pathophysiology of asthma. *J. Allergy Clin. Immunol.* **77**: 527–537, 1986.

5. Peters, M.S., Rodriguez, M., and Gleich, G.J. Localization of human eosinophil granule major basic protein, eosinophil cationic protein, and eosinophil-derived neurotoxin by immunoelectron microscopy. *Lab. Immunol.* **54**: 656–662, 1986.

6. Venge, P., Dahl, R., Hallgern, R., and Olsson, I. Cationic proteins of human eosinophils and their role in the inflammatory reaction in the eosinophil. In: Health and Disease. Mahmoud, A.A.F. and Austen, K.F. (ed.) Grune & Stratton, New York, 1980, pp. 131 –144.

7. Butterworth, A.E., Wasson, D.L., Gleich, G.J., Loegering, D.A., and David, J.R. Damage to schistosomula of *Shistosoma mansoni* mansoni induced directly by eosinophil major basic protein. *J. Immunol.* **122**: 221–229, 1979.

8. Jong, E.C., Mahmoud, A.A.F., and Klebanoff, S.J. Peroxidase-mediated toxicity to schistosomula of *Schisotosoma mansoni. J. Immunol.* **126**: 468–471, 1981.

9. Ackerman, S.J., Gleich, G.J., Loegering, D.A., Richarson, B.A., and Butterworth, A.E. Comparative toxicity of purified human eosinophil granule cationic proteins for schistosomula of *Schistosoma mansoni. Am. J. Trop. Med. Hyg.* **34** (4): 735–745, 1985.

10. Motojima, S., Frigas, E., Loegering, D.A., and Gleich, G.I. Toxicity of eosinophil cationic proteins for guinea pig tracheal epithelium *in vitro. Am. Rev. Respir. Dis.* **139**: 801–805, 1989.

11. Frigas, E., Loegering, D.A., and Gleich, G.J. Cytotoxic effect of the guinea pig eosinophil major basic protein on tracheal epithelium. *Lab. Immunol.* **42**: 35–43, 1980.

12. Frigas, E., Loegering, D.A., Solley, G.O., Farrow, G.M., and Gleich, G.J. Elevated levels of the eosinophil granule major basic protein in the sputum of patients with bronchial asthma. *Mayo Clin. Proc.* **56**: 345, 1981.

13. O'Donnell, M.C., Ackerman, S.J., Gleich, G.J., and Thomas, L.L. Activation of basophil and mast cell histamine release by eosinophil granule major basic protein. *J. Exp. Med.* **157**: 1981–1991, 1983.

14. Zheutlin, L.M., Ackerman, S.J., Gleich, G.J., and Thomas, L.L. Stimulation of basophil and rat mast cell histamine release by eosinophil-derived cationic proteins. *J. Immunol.* **133**: 2180–2185, 1984.

15. Henderson, W.R., Chi, E.V., and Klebanoff, S.J. Eosinophil peroxydase-induced mast cell secretion. *J. Exp. Med.* **152**: 265–279, 1980.

16. Fukuda, T., Numao, T., Akutsu, I., and Makino, S. Heterogeneity of eosinophils. *J. Allergy Clin. Immunol.* **83**: 369–373, 1989.

17. Schult, P.A., Lega, M., Jadidi, S., Vertis, R., Waner, T., Graziano, F.M., and Busse, W.W. The presence of hypodense eosinophils and diminished chemiluminescence response in asthma. *J. Allergy Clin. Immunol.* **81**: 429–437, 1988.

18. Kauffman, K.F., Belt, B., Monchy, J.R.D., Boelens, H., and Vries, K. Leukotriene C4 production by normal-density and low-density eosinophils of atopic individuals and other patients with eosinophilia. *J. Allergy Clin. Immunol.* **79**: 611–619, 1987.

19. Fukuda, T., Donnette, S.L., Reed, C.E., Ackerman, S.J., Peters, M.S., and Gleich, G.J. Increased numbers of hypodense eosinophils in the blood of patients with bronchial asthma. *Am. Rev. Respir. Dis.* **132**: 981–985, 1985.

20. Frick, W.E., Sedgwick, J.B., and Busse, W.W. Hypodense eosinophils in allergic rhinitis. *J. Allergy Clin. Immunol.* **82**: 119–125, 1988.

21. Capron, M., Kazatchkine, M.D., Fischer, E., Joseph, M., Butterworth, A.E., Kusnierz, J.P., Prin, L., Papin, J.P., and Capron, A. Functional role of the α-chain of complement receptor type 3 in human eosinophil-dependent antibody-mediated cytotoxicity against schistosomes. *J. Immunol.* **139**: 2059–2065, 1987.

22. Jouault, T., Capron, M., Balloul, J.M., Ameisen, J.C., and Capron, A. Quantitative and

qualitative analysis of the Fc receptor for IgE (Fc & RII) on human eosinophils. *Eur. J. Immunol.* **18**: 237–241, 1988.

23. Capron, M., Jouault, T., Prin, L., Joseph, M., Ameisen, J.C., Butterworth, A.E., Papin, J.P., Kusnierz. J.P., and Capron, A. Functional study of a monoclonal antibody to IgE Fc receptor (Fc & R2) of eosinophils, platelets, and macrophages. *J. Exp. Med.* **164**: 72–89, 1986.

24. Winvist, I., Olofsson, T., Olsson, I., Persson, A., and Hallberg, T. Altered density, metabolism and surface receptors of eosinophils in eosinophilia. *Immunology* **47**: 531–539, 1982.

25. Shaw, R.J., Walsh, G.M., Cromwell, O., Moqbel, R., Spry, C.J.F., and Kay, A.B. Activated human eosinophils generate SRS-A leukotriens following IgG-dependent stimulation. *Nature* **316**: 150–152, 1985.

26. Prin, L., Capron, M., Tonnel, A., Bletry, O., and Capron, A. Heterogeneity of human peripheral eosinophils: Variability in cell density and cytotoxic ability in relation to the level and the origin of hypereosinophilia. *Int. Archs. Allergy Appl. Immunol.* **72**: 336–346, 1983.

27. De Simone, C., Donnelli, G., Meli, D., Rosati, F., and Sorice, F. Human eosinophils and parasite diseases, II. Characterization of two cell fractions isolated at different densities. *Clin. Exp. Immunol.* **48**: 249–255, 1982.

28. Spry, C.J.F. Eosinophils in endomyocardial disease. *Postgrad. Med. J.* **62**: 609–613, 1986.

29. Tai. P.C., Ackerman, S.J., Spry, C.J.F., Dunnette, S., Olsen, E.G. J., and Gleich, G.J. Deposits of eosinophil granule proteins in cardiac tissues of patients with eosinophilic endomyocardial disease. *Lancet.* **1**: 643–647, 1987.

30. Schleimer, R.P., MacGlashan, D.W.J.R., Peters, S.P., Pinkard, R.N., Adkinson, N.F. Jr., and Lichtenstein, L.M. Characterization of inflammatory mediator release from purified human lung mast cells. *Am. Rev. Respir. Dis.* **133**: 614–617, 1986.

31. Drazen, J.M. and Austen, K.F. Leukotrienes and airway responses. *Am. Rev. Respir. Dis.* **136**: 985–998, 1987.

32. Henderson, W.R. Jr. Eicosanoids and lung inflammation. *Am. Rev. Respir. Dis.* **135**: 1175–1185, 1987.

33. Fukuda, T., Numao, T., Yamada, G., and Makino, S. Immunopharmacological study of PAF-induced eosinophil chemotaxis, 4th Immunopharmacology Symposium (Tokyo), Miyamoto, T. (ed.), DMB Japan, 1986, pp. 43–53. (in Japanese)

34. Nagy, L., Lee, T.H., Goetzl, E.J., Pickett, W.C., and Kay, A.B. Complement receptor enhancement and chemotaxis of human neutrophils and eosinophils by leukotriens and other lipoxygenase products. *Clin. Exp. Immunol.* **47**: 541–547, 1982.

35. Wardlaw, A.J. and Kay, A.B. PAF-acether is a potent chemotactic factor from human eosinophils. *J. Allergy Clin. Immunol.* **77** (suppl.): 1986 (abstract).

36. Goetzl, E.J. and Pickett, W.C. The human PMN leukocyte chemotactic activity of complex hydroxyeicosatetrainoic acids (HETEs). *J. Immunol.* **125**: 1789, 1980.

37. Goetzl, E.J. and Austen, K.F. Natural eosinophiltactic peptides: Evidence of heterogeneity and studies of structure and function. In: The Eosinophils in Health and Disease. Mahmoud, A.A.F. and Austen, K.F. (eds.), Grune & Stratton, New York, 1980, pp. 149–165.

38. Kay, B., Stechshulte, D.J., and Austen, K.F., An eosinophil leukocyte chemotactic factor of anphylaxis. *J. Exp. Med.* **133**: 602–619, 1971.

39. Buchanan, D.R., Cromwell, O., and Kay, A.B. Neutrophil chemotactic acitivity in acute severe asthma (status asthmaticus). *Am. Rev. Respir. Dis.* **136**: 1397–1402, 1987.

40. Aita, S., Ikeda, C., Narimatsu, H., Noguchi, H., Yokokawa, H., Idei, H., Sugisaki, T., and Takahashi, T. Endoscopic and histological studies on bronchi in patients with brochial-asthma by fibrooptic brochoscopic challenge with house dust allergens. *Jpn. J. Allergology* **32**: 274–281, 1983. (in Japanese)

41. Dahl, R., Venge, P., and Olsson, I. Variations blood eosinophils and eosinophil cationic protein in serum in patients with bronchial asthma. *Allergy* **33**: 211–215, 1978.

42. Frew, A.J. and Kay, A.B. The pattern of human late-phase skin reactions to extracts of

aeroallergens. *J. Allergy Clin. Immunol.* **81**: 1117–1121, 1988.

43. Hirotsu, Y., Hirashima, M., and Hayashi, H. The mediation of tissue eosinophilia in hyper-sensitivity reaction, III, Separation of two different eosinophil chemotactic factors and transfer of those factors by serum or cells from sensitized guinea-pigs. *Immunology* **48**: 59–67, 1983.

44. Ishizaki, M. Experimental histological study on allergic conjunctivities due to Japanese cedar pollen. *Allergy* Vol. 35, No. 12, 1986.

45. De Monchy, J.G.R., Kauffman, H.F., Venge, P., Koeeter, G.H., Jansen, H.M., Sluiterm, H.J., and Vrie, S.K. Bronchoalaveolar eosinophilia during allergen-induced late asthmatic reaction. *Am. Rev. Respir. Dis.* **131**: 373–376, 1985.

46. Bruijnzeel, P.L.B., de Monchy, J.G.R., Verhagen, J., and Kauffman, H.F. The eosinophilic granulocyte, an active participant in the late phase asthmatic reaction. *Bull. Eur. Physio-pathol Respir. Clin. Resp. Physiol.* **22** (suppl. 7): 54–61, 1986.

47. Nanba, K., Tanizaki, K., and Kimura, I., Studies on mechanism of late asthmatic response using bronchoalveolar lavage. *Jpn. J. Allergology* **37**: 67–74, 1988. (in Japanese)

48. Kay, A.B. Mediators and inflammatory cells in asthma. In: Asthma. Kay, A.B. (ed.), Black-well, Oxford, 1986, pp. 1–10.

49. Cartier, A., Thompson, N.C., Frith, P.A., *et al.* Allergen-induced increase of bronchial responsiveness to histamine: Relationship to the late asthmatic response and change in airway caliber. *J. Allergy Clin. Immunol.* **70**: 170–177, 1982.

50. Filley, W.V., Holley, K.E., Kephart, G.M., and Gleich, G.J. Identification of immuno-fluorescence of eosinophil granule major basic protein in lung tissues of patients with bronchial asthma. *Lancet* **ii**: 11–16, 1982.

51. Frigas, E., Loegering, D.A., Solley, G.O., Farrow, G.M., and Gleich, G.J. Elevated levels of the eosinophil granule major basic protein in the sputum of patients with bronchial asthma. *Mayo Clin. Proc.* **56**: 345–353, 1981.

52. Khalife, J., Capron, M., Cesbron, J., Tai, P., Tealman, H., Prin, L., and Capron, A. Role of specific IgE antibodies in peroxidase (EPO) release from human eosinophils. *J. Immunol.* **137**: 1659–1664, 1986.

53. Wardlaw, A.J., Dunnette, S., Gleich, G.J., Colling, J.V., and Kay, A.B. Eosinophils and mast cells in bronchoalveolar lavage in subjects with mild asthma. Relationship to bron-chial hyperreactivity. *Am. Rev. Respir. Dis.* **137**: 62–69, 1988.

54. Yukawa, T., Terasshi, Y., Fukuda, Y.T., Makino, S., Hosono, K., and Soejima, K. His-tological studies of guinea-pig bronchi following inhaled antigen exposure, 1. Single an-tigen challenge-induced eosinophil infiltration and epithelial damage in passively sensitized models. *Jpn. J. Allergology* **36**: 227–237, 1987. (in Japanese)

55. Lellouch-Tubiana, A., Lefort, J., Simon, M., Pfister, A., and Vargaftig, B.B. Eosinophil recruitment into guinea-pig lungs after PAF-acether and allergen administration: Modula-tion by prostacyclin, platelet depletion and selective antagonists. *Am. Rev. Respir. Dis.* **137**: 948–954, 1988.

56. Terashi, Y., Yukawa, T., Fukuda, T., and Makino, S. Late phase response in the guinea-pig airway caliber following inhaled antigen exposure1:1. comparative studies between passively and actively sensitized models. *Jpn. J. Allergol* **37**: 980–991, 1988. (in Japanese)

57. Terashi, Y., Yukawa, T., Terashi, K., Motojima, S., Fukuda, T., and Makino, S. Allergen-induced late asthmatic response (LAR) occurs in actively sensitized guinea-pigs (PGs), but not in passively sensitized guinea-pigs. *J. Allergy Clin. Immunol.* **81**: 194, 1988. (sum-mary)

58. Yukawa, T., Fukuda, T., and Makino, S. Experimental asthma in guinea pigs. *Jpn. J. Allergy* **35**: 627, 1986. (in Japanese)

59. Hutson, P.A., Church, M.K., Clay, T.P., Miller, P., and Holgate, S.T. Early and late-phase bronchoconstriction after allergen challenge of nonanesthetized guinea pigs. *Am. Rev. Respir. Dis.* **137**: 548–557, 1988.

60. Iijima, H., Ishii, M., Yamauchi, K., Chao, C., Kimura, K., Shimura, S., Shindoh, Y., Inoue,

H., Mue, S., and Takishima, T. Bronchoalveolar lavage and histologic characterization of late asthmatic response in guinea pigs. *Am. Rev. Respir. Dis.* **136**: 922–929, 1987.

61. Kajita, T., Yui, Y., Mita, H., Taniguchi, N., Saito, H., Mishima, T., and Shida, T. Release of leukotriene C4 from human eosinophils and its relation to the cell density. *Int. Srchs. Allergy Immun.* **78**: 406–410, 1985.

62. Mahauthaman, R., Howell, C.J., Spur, M.B.W., Youlten, L.J.F., Clark, T.J.H., and Lessof, M.H., and Lee, T.H. The generation and cellular distribution of leukotriene C_4 in human eosinophils stimulated by unopsonized zymosan and glucan particles. *J. Allergy Clin. Immunol.* **81**: 696–705, 1988.

63. Flavahan, N.A., Slifman, N.R., Gleich, G.J., and Vanhoutte, P.M. Human eosinophil major basic protein causes hyperreactivity of respiratory smooth muscle. *Am. Rev. Respir. Dis.* **138**: 685–688, 1988.

64. Hastie, A.T., Loegering, D.A., Gleich, G.J., and Keuppers, F. The effect of purified major basic protein on mammalian ciliary acitivity. *Am. Rev. Respir. Dis.* **135**: 848–853, 1987.

65. Fukuda, T., Numao, T., Akutsu, I., Motojima, S., and Makino, S. *In vitro* model of eosinophil migration into the site of acute allergic reactions. *J. Allergy Clin. Immunol.* **81**: 206, 1988. (summary)

66. Tamura, N., Agurawal, D.K., Suliaman, F.A., and Townley, R.G. Effect of platelet activating factor on the chemotaxis of normodense eosinophils from normal subjects. *Biochem. Biophys. Commun.* **142**: No. 3, 1987.

67. Wardlaw, A.J., Moqbel, R., Cromwell, O., and Kay, A.B. Platelet-activating factor—A potent chemotactic and chemokinetic factor for human eosinophils. *J. Clin. Invest.* **78**: 1701–1706, 1986.

68. Gosset, P., Tonnel, A.B., Joseph, M., Prin, L., Mallart, A., Charon, J., and Capron, A. Secretion of a chemotactic factor for neutrophils and eosinophils by alveolar macrophage from asthmatic patients. *J. Allergy Clin. Immunol.* **74**: 827–834, 1984.

69. Arnoux, B., Joseph, M., Sinoes, M.H., Tonnel, A.B., Duroux, P., Capron, A., and Benveniste, J. Antigenic release of PAF-acether and β-glucuronidase from alveolar macrophages of asthmatics. *Bull. Eur. Physiopathol. Respir.* **23**: 119–124, 1987.

70. Lee, T., Lenihan, D.J., Malone, B., Roddy, L.L., and Wasserman, S.I. Increased biosynthesis of platelet-activating factor in activated human eosinophils. *J. Biol. Chem.* **259**: 5526–5530, 1984.

71. Weller, P.F., Lee, C.W., Foster, D.W., Corey, E.J., Austen, K.F., and Lewis, R.A. Generation and metabolism of 5-lipoxygenase pathway leukotrienes by human eosinophils: Predominant production of leukotriene C_4. *Proc. Natl. Acad. Sci. USA* **80**: 7626–7630, 1983.

72. Bruijnzeel, P.L.B., de Monchy, J.G.R., Verhagen, J., and Kauffman, H.F., The eosinophilic granulocyte, an active participant in the late phase asthmatic reaction. *Bull. Eur. Physiopathol. Respir. Coin. Resp. Physiol.* **22** (suppl 7): 54–61, 1986.

73. Lotner, G.Z., Lynch, J.M., Betz, S.J., and Henson, P.M. Human neutrophil-derived platelet activating factor. *J. Immunol.* **124**: 676–684, 1980.

74. Ludwig, J.C., Hoppen, C.L., McManus, L.M., Mott, G.E., and Pinckard, R.N. Modu lation of platelet-activating factor (PAF) synthesis and release from human polymorphonuclear leukocytes (PMN): Role of extracellular albumin. *Arch. Biochem. Biophys.* **241**: 337–347, 1985.

75. Rosenbach, T. and Czarnetzki, B.M. Comparison of the generation *in vitro* of chemotactically active LTB-4 and its omega-metabolites by human neutrophils and lymphocytes-monocytes. *Clin. Exp. Immunol.* **69** (1): 221–228, 1987.

76. Yamada, G. Effects of platelet-activating factor on normal subjects and rabbits. 4th Immunopharmacology Symposium (Tokyo), Tomioka, H. (ed.), DMB Japan, Tokyo, 1986, pp. 99–114.

77. Arnoux, B., Denjean, A., Page, C.P., Nolibe, D., Morley, J., and Benveniste, J. Accumulation of platelets and eosinophils in baboon lung after PAF-acether challenge. *Am. Rev. Respir. Dis.* **137**: 855–860, 1988.

78. Yukawa, T., Fukuda, T., Amagai, M., Ikemori, R. Makino, S., Yamaguchi, K., Hosono, K., and Soejima, K. Histological study of late-phase response of airway allergy in guinea-pigs. In: Proceedings of the 3rd Symposium of Immunopharmacology, Tokyo. Tomika, H. (ed.). DMB Japan, Tokyo, 1985, pp. 117–137.
79. Akutsu, I., Fukuda, T., Amagai, M., Numao, T., and Makino, S., Contribution of PAF to early-phase but not delayed-phase infiltration of eosinophils in a guinea pig model of asthma. *J. Allergy Clin. Immunol.*, **83**: 273, 1989.
80. Numao, T, Fukuda, T., Akutsu, I., Makino, S., Enokihara, H., and Honjo, T. Selective enhancement of eosinophil chemotaxis by recombinant human interleukin 5. *J. Allergy. Clin. Immunol.* **83**: 299, 1989. (abstract).
81. Austen, K.F. Regulation of the chemical phenotypes of eosinophils and mast cells by factors in the microenvironment. In: Proceeding of the XIII International Congress of Allergology and Clinical Imunology, 1988 in Montreux, Switzland.

The Japanese Survey of Eosinophilic Heart Disease

Machiko Take,* Morie Sekiguchi,** and Minoru Shibuya*

* Institute of Geriatrics, Tokyo Women's Medical College, Tokyo, Japan
** The Heart Institute of Japan, Tokyo Women's Medical College, Tokyo, Japan

ABSTRACT

Eosinophilic heart disease in Japan has been surveyed. Sixty-one cases were collected from the literature and in addition our experiences have been included from 1961 to 1988. Eighty percent of patients were thought to have the idiopathic hypereosinophilic syndrome. Eighty-nine percent had other organ involvement. The patients presented with various nonspecific signs and symptoms, and cardiac injury was found incidentally in some cases. From cardiac examinations and histopathologic studies, not only endomyocardial but also pericardial, myocardial, and pancardiac injury was found. It is concluded that a wide range of cardiac abnormalities can be present in patients with eosinophilia.

Since Löffler[1] reported endocarditis parietalis fibroplastica with blood eosinophilia in 1936, various diseases associated with peripheral blood eosinophilia have been reported to involve the heart. It is known that eosinophil granule proteins are toxic to tissue cells and eosinophils themselves can contribute to cardiac injury to some degree.[2-4]

A survey of eosinophilic heart disease in Japan was undertaken from the literature and our own patients from 1961 to 1988. A profile of eosinophilic heart disease in Japan is introduced in this paper, based on 61 patients with eosinophilic heart disease (Table 1). Eleven of them were admitted to our hospital and examined by us.[5,6] The male to female ratio was 2.2:1, and the age range was from 1 year and 4 months to 83 years (mean 43.8 years).

The diseases which caused the eosinophilia were the idiophathic hypereosinophilic syndrome (HES)[7] in 49 patients (80%), leukemia and lymphoma in 5, carcinoma in 2, antituberculosis drugs in 2, suspected parasitosis in 2, and allergic condition to an unknown allergen in one. The maximum blood eosinophil count and mortality rate are shown in Table 2. Fewer than 1,000 eosinophils/mm³ was mostly found in endomyocardial fibrosis (EMF). HES patients with more than 50,000 eosinophils/mm³ had a high mortality rate.

The patients presented with a variety of nonspecific symptoms and signs including dyspnea, fever, cough, general malaise, skin lesions, and edema (Table 3). Organ involvement is summarized in Table 4. Cardiac injury was found incidentally in some patients. By definition, all patients had cardiovascular and hematologic involvement, except for 2 who had EMF. All other organs can be involved in eosinophilic heart disease, and 89% in this survey had other organ involvement.

TABLE 1. Breakdown of Patients ($n=61$)

	No. of patients	
Male	42	2.2
Female	19	1

Age range: 1 y 4 M–83 y (m±S.D.) 43.8±18.2 y

TABLE 2. Eosinophil Counts

/mm³	No. of patients (%)	Died (%)
0— 100	0 (0)	0 (0)
101— 1,000	4 (6.7)	3 (75)
1,001—10,000	25 (41.7)	5 (20)
10,001—50,000	28 (46.7)	12 (42.9)
50,001—	3 (5.0)	3 (100)
Total	60	22 (37.3)

TABLE 3. Signs and Symptoms ($n=61$)

Symptom	No. of patients	(%)
Dyspnea	36	(59)
Fever	30	(49)
Cough	26	(43)
General malaise	20	(33)
Skin eruption	18	(30)
Edema	17	(28)
Chest pain, oppression	16	(26)
Palpitation	13	(21)
Sputum	13	(21)
Stridor, bronchial asthma	12	(20)
Abdominal pain, fullness	10	(16)
Gastrointestinal disorder	10	(16)
Pruritus	9	(15)
Syncope, unconsciousness	7	(11)
Short breath	7	(11)
Hypoesthesia, paraesthesia	6	(10)
Muscle weakness	5	(8)
Rhinitis	5	(8)

Cardiac injury was examined by physical examination, electrocardiogram, echocardiography, and endomyocardial biopsy. Upon auscultation, mitral regurgitation was the most frequent finding (20% of patients). Aortic regurgitation and mitral stenosis were found in one case each. A friction rub, suggestive of pericarditis, was found in 8% of patients (Table 5). Electrocardiograms most commonly showed ST-T changes, and 9 patients with such changes had left ventricular hypertrophy. In several cases, abnormal Q waves and ST-T changes similar to those of acute myocardial infarction were present, suggesting the existence of acute endomyocarditis.

Various conduction disturbances and arrhythmias were also found (Table 6). Echocardiography (Table 7) revealed pericardial effusion in half of the patients. Abnormal

TABLE 4.   Organ Involvement ($n=61$)

Organ	No. of patients	(%)
Cardiovascular	61	(100)
Hematologic	59	(97)
Pulmonary	33	(54)
Skin	26	(43)
Nerve system	15	(25)
Lymph node	15	(25)
Liver	14	(23)
Gastrointestinal	9	(15)
Spleen	8	(13)
Muscle	7	(11)
Nasosinuses	6	(10)
Kidney	3	(5)
Joint	2	(3)
Gallbladder	1	(2)

TABLE 5.   Auscultation ($n=61$)

Finding	No. of patients	(%)
Mitral regurgitation	12	(20)
S3	10	(16)
S4	9	(15)
Apical systolic murmur	6	(10)
Friction rub	5	(8)
Tricuspid regurgitation	3	(5)
Summation gallop	3	(5)
Aortic regurgitation	1	(2)
Ejection click	1	(2)
Opening snap	1	(2)

TABLE 6.   ECG Changes ($n=61$)

Change	Cases	(%)		No. of patients	(%)
Negative T	29	(48)	I A-V block	3	(5)
ST depression	26	(43)	II A-V block	2	(3)
ST elevation	12	(20)	III A-V block	2	(3)
Sinus tachycardia	12	(20)	PAC—atrial tachycardia	3	(5)
LVH	9	(15)	RAD	3	(5)
Abnormal Q	8	(13)	LAD	2	(3)
Low voltage	7	(11)	RBBB+LAD	1	(2)
P-sinistrocardiale	6	(10)	VT	2	(3)
Af—AF	6	(10)	P-dextrocardiale	1	(2)
Poor R wave	6	(10)	Sinus arrest	1	(2)
PVC	5	(8)	IVCD	1	(2)
CRBBB—iRBBB	5	(8)	Junctional rhythm	1	(2)

echos in the left ventricle (in 19%) and the right ventricle (6%) were found, suggesting thrombi. Enlargement of ventricles and atria and asymmetrical left ventricular hypertrophy were also found.

TABLE 7.   Echocardiographic Findings ($n=31$)

Finding	No. of patients	(%)
Pericardial effusion	15	(48)
Enlargement of LV	7	(23)
RV	4	(13)
LA	6	(19)
RA	1	(3)
Abnormal echo in LV	6	(19)
RV	2	(6)
Asymmetrical LVH	3	(10)

TABLE 8.   Endomyocardial Biopsy Findings

	Literature $n=10$	Authors' $n=11$	Total $n=21$	(%)
Myocardial fibrosis	5	10	15	(71)
Myocardial degeneration	6	9	15	(71)
Myocardial disarrangement	0	10	10	(48)
Endocardial thickening	3	6	9	(43)
Cell infiltration	2	7	9	(43)
Eosinophilic infiltration	4	1	5	(24)
Mural thrombus	2	1	3	(14)

TABLE 9.   Macroscopical Findings in Autopsied Hearts ($n=21$)

Finding	No. of patients	(%)
Thrombus in RV	10	(48)
LV	9	(43)
RA	2	(10)
LA	2	(10)
PML	1	(5)
Hypertrophy of LV	9	(43)
RV	7	(33)
Dilatation of LV	4	(19)
RV	1	(5)
Valvular deformity of MV	3	(14)
TV	3	(14)
AV	1	(5)

Cardiac weight: 310–780 g
(m ± S.D.)   (459.3 ± 135.5)
$n=18$ adults

Endomyocardial biopsy was performed in 21 of 61 patients. Eleven cases were examined by us and 10 in other hospitals (Table 8). The incidence of pathologic findings was different according to the observer. Eosinophil infiltration was found only in 5 patients (24%). EMF was the nonspecific type in some cases.

Twenty-three of 61 patients (37.7%) died and 21 were autopsied. The gross anatomic findings are presented in Table 9. Fourteen (67%) had thrombi: 10 (48%) in the right ventricle, 9 (43%) in the left ventricle, 2 (10%) in the right atrium, 2 (10%) in the left atrium, and one on the posterior mitral valve leaflet. Hypertrophy and dilatation of

TABLE 10. Histopathological Findings in Autopsied Hearts ($n=21$)

Finding	No. of patients	(%)
Mural thrombus	15	(71)
Endocardial thickening	15	(71)
cell infiltration	6	(29)
eosinophilic infiltration	3	(14)
Myocardial fibrosis	14	(67)
cell infiltration	7	(33)
eosinophilic infiltration	6	(29)
degeneration	4	(19)
Pericardial thickening	4	(19)
cell infiltration	3	(14)

both ventricles were observed. Valvular deformities were found in the mitral, tricuspid, and aortic valves. In 2 patients large aortic emboli were found. In 10 (48%), lesions on both sides of the heart were found, 4 on the left side, 4 on the right side, and 2 undetermined.

The histopathologic findings of autopsied hearts are presented in Table 10. These findings and the biopsy findings shown in Table 8 are comparable except for the lower incidence of mural thrombi in biopsy specimens. From cardiac examination and histopathologic studies not only endomyocardial but perimyocardial and pancardiac injury was found. The clinical features of cardiac failure developed in the end-stage of eosinophilic heart disease were divided into 2 types, the restrictive or constrictive type and the dilated type.[5,8]

It is concluded that a wide range of cardiac abnormalities can be present in patients with eosinophilia.

REFERENCES

1. Löffler, W. Endocarditis parietalis fibroplastica mit Bluteosinophilie. Ein eigenartiges Krankheitsbild. *Schweiz. Med. Wochenschr.* **17**: 817–820, 1936.
2. Olsen, E.G.J. and Spry, C.J.F. The pathogenesis of Löffler's endomyocardial disease and its relationship to endomyocardial fibrosis. *Prog. Cardiol.* **8**: 281–303, 1979.
3. Tai, P.-C., Hayes, D.J., Clark J.B., and Spry, C.J.F. Toxic effects of human eosinophil secretion products on isolated rat heart cells *in vitro. Biochem. J.* **204**: 75–80, 1982.
4. Tai, P.-C., Ackerman, S.J., Spry C.J.F. Dunnette, S., Olsen, E.G., and Gleich, G.J. Deposits of eosinophil granule proteins in cardiac tissues of patients with eosinophilic endomyocardial disease. *Lancet* 643–647, 1987.
5. Take, M., Sekiguchi, M., Hiroe, M., Hirosawa, K., Mizoguchi, H., Kijima, M., Shirai, T., Ishida, T., and Okubo, S. Clinical spectrum and endomyocardial biopsy findings. *Heart Vessels* (Suppl. 1): 243–249, 1985.
6. Sekiguchi, M., Yu, Z.-X., Take, M., Hiroe, M., Hirosawa, K., Shirai, T., Ishide, T., and Takahashi, T. Ultrastructural features of the endomyocardium in patients with eosinophilic heart disease. An endomyocardial biopsy study. *Jpn. Circul. J.* **48**: 1375–1382, 1984.
7. Fauci, A.S., Harley, J.B., Roberts, W.C., Ferrans, V.J., Gralnick, H.R., and Bjournson, B.H. NIH conference; the idiopathic hypereosinophilic syndrome: Clinical, pathophysiologic, and therapeutic considerations. *Ann. Int. Med.* **97**: 78–92, 1982.
8. De Pace, N.L., Nestice, P.F., Morganroth, J., Ross, J., Fox, R., Kotler, M.N., Mintz, G.S., and Vassallo, R. Dilated cardiomyopathy in the hypereosinophilic syndrome. *Am. J. Cardiol.* **52**: 1359–1360, 1983.

Clinical Studies on Endomyocardial Fibrosis in Patients with Hypereosinophilia: An Historical Review

C.J.F. Spry and Po-Chun Tai

St. George's Hospital Medical School, London, U.K.

ABSTRACT

Eosinophilic endomyocardial fibrosis (E-EMF) is a disease that is now well recognized in patients with many different forms of eosinophilia, especially the idiopathic hypereosinophilic syndrome. The development of knowledge about the disease, and its relationship with eosinophils, is documented historically. The main clinical and cardiologic features of the disease are described, including its occurrence in children. The importance of recent work on the toxic properties of eosinophils and the presence of the eosinophil granule proteins in the areas of damage in the heart are emphasized. Current medical and surgical treatment of the heart disease is outlined, and possible areas of further work on E-EMF are suggested.

INTRODUCTION

Eosinophilic endomyocardial fibrosis (E-EMF) was probably first seen in 1893 in a 31-year-old woman who had a tumor in the neck, with a blood eosinophil count of $57.6 \times 10^9/l$. At postmortem the right ventricular endocardium was found to be covered with a grayish-white mural thrombus.[1] In 1936 Professor W. Löffler published detailed clinical descriptions of 2 patients in Basel, Switzerland, who had E-EMF. His first patient was a woman of 45 who died one year after presentation, with severe right- and left-sided eosinophilic endomyocardial disease. The second was a 37-year-old man who died after 21 months, with similar complications. In one patient the heart disease was associated with a severe illness, whereas the second patient presented with heart failure without a systemic illness. Another difference was that eosinophilia increased in one patient whereas it disappeared shortly before death in the other.[2] An English translation of Löffler's seminal paper was published in 1948,[3] and the disease was reviewed in a German paper published that year.[4]

A second form of this disease, called tropical endomyocardial fibrosis (T-EMF), as it is mainly confined to tropical regions, has been known since 1946.[5] For several years these diseases were considered to be distinct, although the possibility that there was a disease spectrum ranging from T-EMF to Löffler's endomyocardial fibrosis was suggested by Davies and Ball, as early as 1955.[6] However, histologic studies in the 1970s demonstrated that they were pathologically indistinguishable, despite the different clinical settings in which they were found. In the first of these papers, published in 1970, detailed postmortems were carried out on 3 men aged 25, 26, and 35 who had died with idiopathic hypereosinophilic syndrome (HES). The findings supported the possibility that T-EMF might be a later stage, or an inactive form, of E-EMF.[7]

The second, more detailed report was published in 1973. This was a comparative pathologic and clinical review of 90 patients with E-EMF. The eosinophilia was of unknown cause in 50%, reactive in 25% (polyarteritis, asthma, drug sensitivity, Hodgkin's disease, and carcinomas), and due to eosinophilic leukemia (or HES) in 25%. Among 30 hearts examined, 10 were in the acute necrotic stage, with an illness lasting a mean of 5.5 weeks; 8 were in the later thrombotic stage, with an illness of 10 months; and 12 were in the fibrotic stage, with an illness lasting 24.5 months. Samples from 16 patients in the thrombotic and fibrotic stages of E-EMF were compared with 32 specimens from patients with T-EMF, and no significant pathologic differences were found. It was concluded that T-EMF and E-EMF had a similar pathogenesis, such as a toxic effect of eosinophils on the myocardium.[8]

By 1972 the frequent occurrence (20% or more) of E-EMF in patients with "eosinophilic leukemia" (2 rare disorders occurring together with high frequency) led to the suggestion that there might be an intimate cause-effect relationship between the 2 disorders, similar to that of the cardiopulmonary lesions in the metastatic carcinoid syndrome: "Forceful cardiac contractions might cause excessive destruction of eosinophils, and a continued high concentration of their chemicals, and hydrolytic enzymes within the heart. This in turn may cause endocardial inflammation, and injury. In prolonged eosinophilia, regardless of etiology, this sort of change is likely to occur more frequently, and to be more severe. It would appear that the endocardial lesion is the result of the eosinophilia. . . ."[9]

Twenty-six patients with E-EMF were described during the period 1936–1957 and reviewed by Weiss-Carmine. Several patients had arteritic lesions, and thromboemboli were also noted to be an important feature of the disease.[10] Another review was published in 1955.[11]

A second major review of E-EMF was carried out in 1963 with details of 14 further patients, including 3 more of their own, by Brink and Weber (1963). This paper suggested that high blood neutrophil counts might be associated with EMF, although this has not been substantiated subsequently.[12]

By 1980, over 100 patients with E-EMF had been described.[13] Because an underlying eosinophilic disorder, which was often HES, dominated the clinical picture, the heart disease was usually described in less detail. However, the general awareness that cardiac complications were the main presentation in at least half of the patients with HES, and that over 80% would finally develop heart disease,[14] stimulated detailed cardiologic studies on those patients. Two series of patients with HES, who have a high incidence of E-EMF, have been studied over more than a decade in the U.S.A.,[15] and by us.[16] T-EMF, with or without eosinophilia, was initially described in African patients.[17]

There have been detailed reports from a number of other countries in the last few years, including South India in 1983[18,19] and 1986,[20] the Ivory Coast in 1985,[21] Venezuela in 1983,[22] Brazil in 1984,[23] Japan in 1985,[24] Thailand in 1984,[25] Spain in 1982,[26] the Middle East in 1985,[27] and France in 1983.[28] In French-speaking regions, no attempt was made to distinguish the tropical forms of the disease from the eosinophilic form. In other countries, they are often described separately. In 1979, an analysis of the cardiological features of E-EMF was reported from the National Institutes of Health (NIH), Bethesda, Maryland, U.S.A.[15] That paper reviewed 65 previous case reports, in which 57% had histologic features of E-EMF, combined with descriptions of a further 26 patients. M-mode echocardiograms were thought to show an increased left ventricular wall thickness and raised left ventricle mass in 18 of 22 patients (82%). It was suggested that this was an early feature of cardiac involvement in HES, and might be helpful in following the progression of the disease. In 7 of 8 patients who did not show a good response to treatment with prednisolone, with or without hydroxyurea, there appeared to be a progression of echocardiographic abnormalities, whereas in 8 of 10 patients adequately treated, this did not occur. Although this was one of the first detailed descriptions of the disease, using a combination of echocardiography and ventricular angiocardiograms, cardiac biopsies were not done in any of the 26 patients. Three of the 26 patients died: one following busulphan treatment, one with a possible arrhythmia, and one with the Budd-Chiari syndrome. Although only one patient had emboli, because of the likely presence of thrombi in the left ventricle of some patients, it was recommended that anticoagulation should be carried out. Several patients had angiographic evidence of coronary artery disease, but this was not a clinical problem in any of those patients.

The cardiologic features of E-EMF seen in outpatients range from apparent normality in patients in the earliest stage to gross heart failure in patients in the late fibrotic stage of the disease. In 1974, a review of the cardiovascular complications which occurred in NIH patients with HES and eosinophilic leukemia showed that they were the same, and that the endocardial lesions were indistinguishable from those seen in T-EMF.[29] A further report from the same center was made in 1983.[30]

The awareness of the high incidence of eosinophilic heart disease in patients with persistent eosinophilia has made many clinicians more alert to the earlier signs of cardiac involvement: asymptomatic murmurs and microembolic disease, especially splinter hemorrhages, minor strokes, and nonspecific ECG abnormalities.[31] Today, eosinophilic heart disease can be recognized when it gives rise to a number of different abnormalities, besides a restrictive cardiomyopathy. In a series of 14 patients, which was published in 1985 by Take and colleagues in Japan,[24] 5 patients had acute carditis, 3 had electrical disturbances, 3 had ventricular dilatation, and 3 had a restrictive cardiomyopathy.

DISEASE ASSOCIATIONS

Introduction

An additional reason for believing that E-EMF was caused by eosinophils, besides those mentioned above, was the occurrence of this type of heart disease in many of the diseases which produce an eosinophilia. The only common features in these different diseases were the presence of a marked increase in blood eosinophils and endocardial lesions.[32–35] By definition, E-EMF always occurs in patients who have had, or who continue to have, eosinophilia. In some patients the clinical features of the underlying eosinophilic disorders, such as leukemia, may mask or affect the clinical presentation of the heart disease, which used to be only diagnosed at a late stage in the development of the cardiac pathology, although methods are now available for recognizing it at an early stage.

It can occur in patients with any of the principal causes of a chronic eosinophilia. For example, a 52-year-old man was described in 1959, who had tuberculosis, treated with isoniazid and PAS. He developed an eosinophil count of $14 \times 10^9/l$, and died later with E-EMF. Other early works, describing patients with infections, an eosinophilia, and endomyocardial disease, were also reviewed in this report. Those included patients with syphilis, malaria, tonsillitis, amoebiasis, dengue fever, and allergic reactions to parasites, including *Loa loa*.[36] In Western countries the most common disease association is HES, but it also includes parasitic diseases, chronic drug reactions, and tumor-induced eosinophilia.

Parasitic Diseases

Although it is unusual for patients in Western countries with E-EMF to have a parasitic infection, in 1972 a 40-year-old woman was described who died with E-EMF, and an eosinophilia of 60–70%, and who was found to have a 10-m long *Taenia saginata* worm in her intestines.[37] Patients with E-EMF and fascioliasis have also been reported from France in 1975[38] and 1978.[39]

Solid Tumors

There are several case reports of carcinoma of lung-induced E-EMF, in which the onset of the heart disease could be correlated with the eosinophilia. We reviewed those reports in 1985, and added details of a patient of our own in 1985.[40] One of the first descriptions of this association was reported from London in 1975. The patient was a 51-year-old man with a large cell carcinoma of the lung, who was studied over a 2-year period before he died of heart failure, and was found to have biventricular E-EMF at postmortem. He also had alcohol-induced flushing attacks, violent headaches, and eosinophil counts which rose as the tumor mass increased and fell after excision of the main tumor mass and subsequent radiotherapy. It was suggested that E-EMF was the result of an allergic response to the tumor, involving eosinophils.[41] Other reports of a similar disease process were published in the U.S.A. in 1982[42] and 1983.[43]

Eosinophilic Leukemia

E-EMF is an important complication of eosinophilic leukemia. A review in 1961 showed that, among 9 patients with acute eosinophilic leukemia with blast cells, 5 had cardiovascular abnormalities. Seven of the 11 patients who only had mature blood eosinophils (which might today be called HES) also had heart involvement. This is a total of 12 cases of heart disease in 20 patients (60%).[44] In 1978 E-EMF was described in a patient with Philadelphia chromosome-positive chronic myeloid leukemia and a hypoplastic right ventricle.[45] In 1965 a patient was described who had marked blood eosinophilia with blast cells in the circulation, and who developed EMF.[46]

Lymphocytic Leukemia

E-EMF has also been seen in patients with lymphocytic leukemia-associated hypereosinophilia.[47,48]

Eosinophilic Pneumonia

An unusual clinical story of a woman with chronic eosinophilic pneumonia, who developed hypereosinophilia and E-EMF, was given in a clinicopathologic conference in 1980. When she was 31, she developed pulmonary infiltrates, with an eosinophil count of 6.4×10^9/l. She improved on treatment with 13 mg/day prednisolone. At age 35, after the steroids had been stopped and the eosinophilia had recurred, she developed chest pain, severe heart failure with an enlarged heart, and a pericardial effusion. A right ventricular biopsy showed E-EMF in the acute necrotic stage. Treatment with steroids, warfarin, and digoxin resulted in an improvement.[49]

Hypersensitivity Reactions

Patients with a drug-induced hypersensitivity disease may develop E-EMF. In 1946 a 41-year-old man was described who had been treated with neoarsphenamine for syphilis, and developed an eosinophilia of 2.5×10^9/l, with heart failure which was found to be due to E-EMF.[50] In 1959, E-EMF was described as a complication of eosinophilia due to streptomycin hypersensitivity.[51] Vasculitic diseases with eosinophilia are also known to be able to lead to the development of E-EMF, including the Churg-Strauss syndrome.[52]

Negative Associations

Several diseases that give rise to persistent eosinophilia are very rarely associated with eosinophilic heart disease, even though they may result in a high blood eosinophil count for long periods. These include bronchial asthma, crytogenic eosinophilic pneumonia[53] (but see above), hayfever, and other allergic disorders. This implies that there may be a protective factor(s) in the blood of those individuals, or that the stimuli that cause eosinophil degranulation in these diseases are different, and only affect eosinophils which are distant from the heart. One possibility is that α-2 macroglobulin may act as an inhibitor in these diseases, as this protein has been shown to bind to eosinophil cationic protein in serum.[54]

CLINICAL FEATURES

Introduction

As the majority of patients with E-EMF have HES, the most extensive studies have been carried out in this group of patients, and most is known about the clinical features of the disease in this setting. About half the patients present with late-stage disease, and half develop it during the subsequent several years. The age and sex incidence of patients reflect that of HES: a mean age of 37 years. We reviewed the clinical features and pathophysiology of E-EMF in 1983,[56] 1985,[57] and 1987.[58,59] In 1988 we published a book on the properties of eosinophils, including their involvement in cardiovascular diseases, and this account is based on one of the chapters, with permission.[60] The main features at the bedside are signs of chronic heart failure, with wasting and edema, and heart murmurs which are most marked in patients with mitral incompetence.

Differential Diagnosis

In the late stage of the disease it has many features in common with other forms of restrictive cardiomyopathy, and it can be confused with pericardial constriction. The difficulty in distinguishing constrictive pericarditis and E-EMF was well illustrated by a case report from the Johns Hopkins Hospital in 1952. The correct diagnosis was only made when surgery was carried out to remove what was thought to be a constricting pericardium.[61] Löffler himself described the ways in which E-EMF is now known to affect cardiac function: "Endocardial thickening prevents normal diastolic relaxation of the ventricles, and thrombotic masses decrease the capacity of the ventricles."[62] Unlike T-EMF, ascites is uncommon, and edema of the face and upper extremities is not often seen, even when the patients are in gross heart failure, with persistently high right atrial pressures and pulmonary edema.

E-EMF IN INFANCY AND CHILDHOOD

E-EMF complicating HES can occur in infancy and childhood. Examples include:
—a girl aged 5 years, who died within a month of presenting with HES. At postmortem, there were thrombi in the left ventricle and right atrium, and emboli in a pulmonary artery, but there was no EMF, probably because the illness was of such short duration.[63]
—a child aged 7 years, who developed HES. She died after a 10-month illness, and

was found to have bilateral E-EMF, with peripheral emboli originating from the left ventricle.[64]

—a 9-year-old boy died after a 10-month illness due to HES, and showed the features of E-EMF at postmortem.[65]

—a boy aged 12, who was found to have an eosinophil count of $170 \times 10^9/l$. Three years after the onset of his illness, he died with congestive cardiac failure due to bilateral E-EMF.[66]

INVESTIGATIONS

Radiology

The cardiac silhouette is generally normal in patients with the early or later stages of E-EMF, until heart failure supervenes. In occasional patients calcification can be seen in lateral chest radiographs, although this is much more common in T-EMF. Marked calcification was reported in one patient.[67] When pulmonary edema occurs this has no special features. Pleural effusions and pericardial effusions are sometimes seen.

Electrocardiography

Electrocardiograms are normal until the later thrombotic and fibrotic stages of the disease have developed, when there are repolarization changes characteristic of endocardial lesions. Following the development of heart failure, a number of other abnormalities in the ECG can develop, but none of these has diagnostic value.

Holter monitoring has generally not been of great help, except in defining the types of arrythmias that often develop sporadically in patients who have the late stage of the disease, and who may be improved by antiarrythmic therapy. However, as arrythmias usually respond to successful cardiac surgery (valve replacement with or without endocardectomy), arrythmias seem to be more related to heart failure than to involvement of conducting system, or other sites by the fibrotic process.[68]

Conduction defects have been reported on several occasions.[69] Arrythmias were a problem in a 48-year-old man with E-EMF, who had conduction defects, a wandering atrial pacemaker, and intermittent 2:1 dissociation, which required treatment with a pacemaker.[70] Another example was in a 79-year-old man who developed complete heart block.[71] This study also reviewed 65 other cases of E-EMF, and found that 19 (29%) had conduction disturbances. A His-bundle electrogram has been carried out on a patient with E-EMF. Right atrial pacing showed an increased Pl-A interval from 25 msec to 100 msec, followed by Mobitz type 1 block. This suggested that there was a conduction delay in the atrium and AV node, possibly due to fibrous tissue. Details of the catheterization and angiocardiography findings in this patient were also published.[72] It may be very difficult to place a transvenous pacing electrode into the right ventricle, due to the presence of thrombus and fibrosis in the cavity,[73] and an open procedure may be preferable. Ventricular fibrillation has been documented in a few patients.

Echocardiography

Echocardiography is the most useful technique for defining the structural changes within the heart and the abnormalities in the ventricular wall characteristic of EMF. M-mode echocardiograms are most useful in defining the mitral valve defect that occurs in the late stage of the disease. M-mode echocardiography findings were described in 1977 in 10 patients with HES studied at the NIH. Symmetrical thickening of the left ventricle of greater than 11 mm, with increased left ventricular mass (greater than 275 g), was reported in all the patients. These observations have not been confirmed in other series of patients with E-EMF, and they remain puzzling[74]

Two-dimensional (2-D) echocardiography, which can be combined with color-coded enhancement of the images, has provided clear evidence during life of the sites of involvement of the heart in endocardial fibrosis, the abnormalities in the septal wall, and the presence of thrombi within the heart. It has become the technique of choice in first-line investigations of patients suspected of having endomyocardial disease.[75,76] Unfortunately, only patients in the late stage of the disease show abnormalities that can be considered characteristic of this disorder. These include enhanced echos from the endocardium in either ventricle, the septum, and the base of the posterior papillary muscle. In 1980 the findings were published of 2-D echocardiography in 21 patients at the NIH.[15] In 9 patients who had clinical evidence of mitral regurgitation, the 2-D echo features were correlated with the gross features seen at operation or at postmortem. In 6 patients who had peripheral emboli, the presence of thrombus or thickening of the posterobasal wall of the left ventricle was detected, and it was suggested that this was the site of origin of these emboli.[55] Three patients with HES were described from Philadelphia, U.S.A., in 1983, with cardiac dilatation on echocardiography.[77] Mural thrombi have also been clearly shown by echocardiography[78] and computed tomography.[79] In 1987, pulsed-Doppler echocardiography showed the marked contribution of right atrial systole to pulmonary flow in a woman with HES and a large right ventricular thrombus.[80]

Patients with a marked eosinophilia and E-EMF appear to be forming thrombi continually, as judged by high serum levels of platelet factor 4, β-thromboglobulin, and high fibrinogen (Davies et al., 1986, unpublished). The possible importance of this mechanism in the induction of E-EMF has been outlined in an echocardiographic study in which thrombi were considered to precede and/or augment the fibrotic process, leading to atrioventricular valve dysfunction. It was suggested that scar formation in the ventricles in patients with E-EMF was the result of the organization and incorporation of thrombus into the ventricular cavity wall,[55] although this has not been seen in other studies.

A detailed report on echocardiographic studies on E-EMF was reported from Hungary in 1982,[81] and this led to a correct diagnosis in 6 of 8 patients.[82]

In London, M-mode and 2-D echocardiography were done on 9 patients with E-EMF, among our series of patients with HES at Hammersmith Hospital. The value of this series, which was also published in 1982, was that all the patients had undergone full cardiologic investigations, and the extent and staging of their heart disease was known. Amplitude-processed 2-D echocardiography appeared to be more sensitive than conventional 2-D echocardiography in detecting areas of increased relative echo intensity. M-mode echocardiography only showed nonspecific abnormalities, but was particularly useful in assessing the functional defects in myocardial function and mitral valve disease. It was also clear from that study that echocardiography was not as sensitive as endocardial biopsy in detecting the earlier stages of the disease. This limitation may be important if echocardiography is to be used to monitor the effects of treatment on the progression of endocardial fibrosis, as it may not be sensitive enough in some patients to detect small but functionally significant deterioration in cardiac performance.[83]

Cardiac Catheterization

Before the introduction of echocardiography, E-EMF was often mistaken for constrictive pericarditis, and cardiac catheterization with pressure studies was then the only technique for providing a definitive diagnosis of the disease prior to operation. One of the first patients in whom this was done was reported on in 1956.[84]

Intracardiac pressure studies are used today to help in the assessment of pulmonary hypertension, the work of each side of the heart, and to assist in functional studies of the possible effectiveness of steroids and other drugs in preventing the progression of the disease to the later thrombotic and fibrotic stages. Angiocardiography, which is usually carried out at the same time, is also helpful in defining the extent of the lesions and the effects of these lesions on ventricular function. Angiocardiography is particularly good at demonstrating intracavity thrombi.

We published the results of detailed cardiovascular assessments of 11 patients with E-EMF who were studied at Hammersmith Hospital between 1975 and 1981.[85] Other examples of the results of these studies were in 2 patients reported from St. Thomas' Hospital, London, in 1976,[86] and a 45-year-old man described in the U.S.A. in 1977. The latter patient died 14 months after the onset of heart failure due to biventricular E-EMF complicating HES. He underwent a variety of cardiac investigations, including catheterization, with pressure studies and cardiac biopsy, and although his blood eosinophil counts were reduced with hydroxyurea and vincristine, his disease appeared to progress.[87] An earlier report in 1974 of right-sided catheterization showed almost complete obliteration of the ventricle.[88]

Pressure studies during left ventricular catheterization of a woman in 1987 with an eosinophilia of $6.068 \times 10^9/l$ showed a 90 mmHg subaortic gradient while the catheter was pulled back from the apex to the aortic root. This was interpreted as evidence for an obstructive cardiomyopathy, but was more likely due to thrombus which was also demonstrated in the cavity.[89]

Cardiac Biopsy

Cardiac biopsy of E-EMF has been carried out since 1972. Histologic studies on these biopsies and on postmortem material have defined the 3 stages of the disease. It has become one of the principal methods for diagnosing it in its early stages. This technique has the theoretical advantage that it samples the endocardium, which is the principal site of the lesion being studied.[90] Occasionally, the endocardium is so thickened by fibrous tissue that it may not be possible to obtain a biopsy. As the fibrotic areas are surrounded by softened areas of acute inflammation, the myocardium may also be perforated. There are also several examples of pericardial hematoma which have resulted from cardiac biopsy.

The use of endocardial biopsy to help in the diagnosis of endomyocardial fibrosis has been used in London since 1976, when the findings in 2 patients were reported,[86] and in the U.S.A. since 1980.[91,92] The experiences at the NIH were reviewed in 1982.[93] Right ventricular biopsy is most commonly carried out, because the lesions of E-EMF are always bilateral. If the tropical form of the disease is suspected, it may also be necessary to carry out left ventricular biopsy, because the lesions can occasionally be restricted to the left side of the heart. In the earlier stages of the disease, biopsy of the septal wall can usually provide diagnostic material. Generally 4 to 7 biopsies are taken. In the late stage of the disease, fibrotic lesions may not be easily sampled, and the catheter may move to unaffected endocardium from which normal samples may be obtained.

The histologic appearance of E-EMF shows involvement of the endocardium, underlying areas of the myocardium, small vessels, and interstitial tissues in the granulation tissue layer of the heart. These lesions are confined to the inflow tract and part of the outflow tract of the heart, where a rolled edge is often seen in postmortem samples. Occasionally, thrombi can be found attached to the mitral or tricuspid valve leaflets, and less commonly to the walls of the atria. Results of histologic studies of E-EMF, using both light and electron microscopy, were reported from the U.K. in 1981 and 1982,[94,95] Denmark in 1977,[96] and Japan in 1984[97] and 1985.[98] Electron microscopy of eosinophilic heart disease has shown the presence of degranulated cells within the heart.

Histopathology

One of the most striking demonstrations of the interaction between eosinophils and the heart is in an ultrastructural study from Japan, where degranulating eosinophils were seen adjacent to a cardiac myocyte in a cardiac biopsy from a patient with eosinophilic endomyocardial disease.[98] A monoclonal antibody that only binds to activated eosinophils[99] can be used to ascertain the presence of these cells in the blood, but no formal study has yet been carried out to determine whether the number of activated cells in the circulation can be used to define or monitor patients most likely to develop E-EMF.

In 1987, we reported the results of an immunopathologic study on cardiac tissues taken at necropsy or at cardiac biopsy from 18 patients with E-EMF, to look for the presence of the toxic eosinophil granule proteins within the heart. Serial sections were stained for eosinophil major basic protein by indirect immunofluorescence, and for eosinophil cationic protein (ECP), the eosinophil neurotoxin (EDN/EPX), and activated eosinophils with alkaline-phosphatase-linked monoclonal antibodies. Activated eosinophils and secreted eosinophil granule proteins were mainly detected within the necrotic and later-stage thrombotic lesions in areas of acute tissue damage in the endocardium and in the walls of small blood vessels. These findings suggested that eosinophil granule proteins could cause the cardiac muscle damage and vascular injury that lead to the development of EMF.[100]

TREATMENT

The treatment of E-EMF depends on the stage at which it is diagnosed. In the early acute necrotic stage, the aim is to prevent progression of the disease. In the later thrombotic phase, the goal is to prevent emboli and further disease progression. In the final stage it becomes necessary to treat heart failure and to consider the use of surgery. As yet there is no medical treatment that will prevent the progression of E-EMF, although there is preliminary evidence that prednisolone 5–15ng/d slows the progression of the disease. The insensitivity of echocardiography in following the disease progression, except in the later stages, is clearly a difficulty here, and cardiac biopsy has not been carried out routinely in treated or untreated patients to determine which form of therapy might be most effective.

The recognition that endocardial thrombi were clinically important,[101] and that thromboembolic complications were the most common cause of death in patients with E-EMF,[16] has led to the general use of anticoagulation in this disorder. However, there is no convincing evidence that this has resulted in a reduction in vascular occlusive episodes. Indeed, we have treated several patients who developed large emboli after anticoagulation was begun.

There is a growing body of evidence that eosinophils may stimulate the coagulation system, not only by effects on the clotting sequence,[102–104] but also by affecting endothelial cells and platelets.[105] Heparin may not be as effective as warfarin in controlling the formation of clots in patients with HES. This was seen in a patient who had mitral and tricuspid valve replacement with Bjork-Shiley prostheses for E-EMF, and was then treated with subcutaneous heparin every 8 hours instead of warfarin. One month later he was admitted to hospital with a thrombosed mitral valve and peripheral emboli. The mitral valve was replaced with a porcine graft. When the coagulation response to heparin was assessed, he was found to need over twice the expected amount of heparin, and it is recommended that the activated clotting time should be carefully assessed in these patients in view of their increased thrombotic tendency.[106]

Antiplatelet drugs, including aspirin and dipyridamole, have also been used, but again, their efficacy in this condition has not been proven. Anticoagulation should be continued for life after cardiac surgery for E-EMF.[107]

Medical treatment that improves the underlying eosinophilic disorder in patients with HES in turn may prevent the progression of heart disease in these patients, but no long-term reports have yet been published of their use, or of different forms of medical treatment, such as chronic steroid treatment, cytotoxic drugs, or other medication. Steroids may benefit patients by inhibiting eosinophil granule secretion and, as a result, the amount of granule toxin present within the heart. This was shown to have occurred in a 51-year-old woman in the acute necrotic stage of E-EMF complicating asthma and with radiculopathy, who was treated with prednisolone 60 mg/day for several days, followed by tapering lower doses. Cardiac biopsies were done before this and 2 months later, when the acute changes had resolved.[108]

CARDIAC SURGERY

At one time the apparently poor prognosis of the underlying eosinophilic disorder discouraged surgeons from attempting a surgical approach to E-EMF. However, the outlook for the underlying eosinophilic disorder has improved so much in the last decade that surgery has become a worthwhile form of treatment in patients with severe EMF.

There is no consensus on the stage at which surgery should be carried out, whether the mitral valve should be preserved,[109] the type of valve that should be used, or the possible danger of an increased thrombotic tendency affecting the new valve. Prior to 1980, early work in Switzerland and the U.S.A. had led some surgeons to suspect that valve replacement would not benefit EMF patients due to the high incidence of thromboembolic complications. Indeed, occasional patients have been described who developed prosthetic valve endocarditis. Three of the patients in the series at the NIH who developed heart failure complicating HES had atrioventricular valve replacements. One patient had recurrent thrombotic involvement of the valves despite anticoagulation, and after those had been replaced with porcine allografts the patient died with *Staphylococcus aureus* endocarditis. The other 2 patients, one of whom also had removal of a left ventricular thrombus, did much better postoperatively, although there was little improvement in pulmonary hypertension. That report emphasized the serious feature of the hypercoaguable state in this disease, the importance of carrying out valve replacement early, before irreversible changes have occurred in the lungs and other organs as a result of the heart failure, and the possible value of steroids.[110] This danger was seen in a 45-year-old Finnish woman with asthma, and an eosinophilia of $9.4 \times 10^9/l$ who developed intracardiac thrombi. Removal of the thrombus and replacement of the mitral valve with a Bjork-Shiley tilting disk valve only prolonged the life of the patient for 14 months, as she died after the prosthesis had become blocked with thrombus, despite treatment with anticoagulants.[111] A patient with HES in India was reported to have died from a pulmonary embolus from the right ventricle in 1985.[112] Removal of a large intracavity thrombus can be successfully carried out, as described in 1982 in a patient with an underlying malignant eosinophilic disorder.[113]

Each center has its own approach as to how surgery should be carried out. The principal points to emphasize are that the restricting fibrotic tissue can be removed successfully, and that it does not recur at the sites of surgery. The lesions may be more difficult to see at operation than in angiograms, and the extent of fibrous tissue removal should be decided preoperatively. A plain of cleavage can be found in some patients; in others a ragged surface will be left, but this does not cause any special postoperative problems. The valves should be replaced with the best known material on which thrombi will not form, in view of this high risk in EMF patients.

When mitral valve incompetence suddenly occurs in a patient with left ventricular disease, the effects are much more serious than when a similar process occurs on the right side of the heart, and surgery then becomes urgent.

By 1985, there were reports on the use of surgery in 41 patients with E-EMF. Four of these patients were operated on in Budapest, Hungary, between 1979 and 1984. Two required thrombectomy, 2 had bilateral valve replacements, and 2 died. Although eosinophilia persisted in the 2 survivors, there was no evidence for recurrence of the endocardial disease, and the patients were much improved.[82,114]

In 1980, we published details of the first 2 patients at Hammersmith Hospital with severe E-EMF who underwent open-heart surgery. One patient, with predominant right ventricular disease, was treated by right ventricular endocardectomy with tricuspid and mitral xenograft valve replacement. This patient is now in chronic heart failure again due to defective ventricular diastolic function, which is being investigated further. In the second patient, it was only necessary to replace the mitral valve. Both patients showed marked clinical improvement postoperatively, as confirmed by cardiac catheterization and angiography. Our review of the results of surgery on 22 other patients with endocardial fibrosis, some of whom had eosinophilia, showed equally encouraging results overall. In none of those patients was there any evidence of the recurrence of endocardial lesions or progression of heart damage for periods of up to 7 years.[115]

Three patients with HES and E-EMF were reported from St. Thomas' Hospital, London, in 1976. One of them, a 47-year-old man, underwent mitral annuloplasty and coronary bypass surgery, and remains well 16 years later.[86]

Probably the first patient to have surgery for E-EMF in the U.S.A. was a 16-year-old boy with HES and heart failure, who had a Hancock mitral valve replacement on April 1, 1976. However, his disease, including the heart failure, progressed, and he died 19 months later.[116] Mitral valve surgery was also successful in a 23-year-old black woman with blood eosinophil counts reaching 8.75×10^9/l, who had E-EMF causing mitral regurgitation. This responded well to mitral valve surgery.[117] A further account of the successful use of surgery for endomyocardial fibrosis was reported from Houston, Texas, in 1981,[118] but there has been no comprehensive survey of the North American experience of surgery for EMF.

RELATIONSHIP WITH T-EMF

The first suggestions that E-EMF and T-EMF might have a common pathogenesis was made in the Ivory Coast in 1956[119] and in Nigeria in 1970, where it was proposed that "the eosinophil leucocytes in susceptible persons, by some unknown mechanism, caused endo- and myocardial damage."[120] Subsequent papers have emphasized this possibility, describing the way in which eosinophils might be damaged as they hit the wall of the ventricle where they could release toxic substances, or binding to thrombotic material on the endocardium, and damaging underlying contractile tissues.

We first became interested in these possibilities in 1975, and our subsequent experimental studies have confirmed that eosinophils have a marked propensity to damage myocardial cells through a unique series of interactions with cardiac cells. This is discussed in our accompanying paper.[121]

CONCLUSIONS

Why the lesions are localized to the endocardium in this disease is still unknown. One main possibility is that the thrombus layer on the endocardium concentrates the cells and the toxic proteins, so that the underlying tissue receives the largest amounts of toxic granule constituents. The second possibility is that endocardial cells have a metabolic or structural difference from other parts of the heart and other tissues, which makes them susceptible to eosinophil-mediated damage. The peculiar blood supply to the cells in this region indicates that they might differ from other parts of the heart in their response to inflammatory cells, but this has yet to be documented.

Two of the most toxic cationic proteins in eosinophil granules, ECP and EDN/EPX, both have ribonuclease activity, and are probably evolved from a common gene.[122] Whether ribonucleases have a special capacity to damage the endocardium has not yet been studied. Other possibilities that have been considered are a special blood supply to this part of the heart and the turbulent effects of the bloodstream on the inflow tract and apex of the ventricles.

Future work on endocardial fibrosis is needed to discover the causes of the eosinophilic disorders that give rise to this disease, the nature of the stimuli that induce eosinophil secretion within the heart, and the factors within the endomyocardium which localize the lesions to these unusual anatomical sites. It is hoped that when more is known about these events effective forms of therapy and prevention of EMF may become available, and it may be possible to distinguish patients who are at risk of developing this restrictive cardiomyopathy among the many patients who have eosinophilia due to allergic and parasitic diseases but do not develop heart disease.

ACKNOWLEDGMENTS

We acknowledge the generous financial support of the British Heart Foundation and the Wellcome Trust of our work in this field during the past 13 years.

REFERENCES

1. Reinbach, G. Ueber das Verhalten der Leukocyten bei malignen Tumoren. *Arch. Klin. Chir.* **46**: 486–562, 1983.
2. Löffler, W. Endocarditis parietalis fibroplastica mit Bluteosinophilie, ineigenartiger Krankheitsbild. *Schweiz. Med. Wochenschr.* **17**: 817–820, 1936.
3. Lennox, B. Acute parietal endocarditis in a case of status asthmaticus. A possible early stage of Löffler's endocarditis parietalis fibroplastica with eosinophilia. *J. Pathol. Bacteriol.* **60**: 621–628, 1948.
4. Berblinger, W. Zur kenntnis der Endocarditis parietalis fibroplastica. *Schweiz. Med. Wochenschr.* **78**: 829–832, 1948.

5. Bedford, D.E. and Konstam, G.L.S. Heart failure of unknown aetiology in Africans. *Br. Heart J.* **8**: 236–237, 1946.

6. Davies. J.N. and Ball, J.D. The pathology of endomyocardial fibrosis in Uganda. *Br. Heart J.* **17**: 337–359, 1955.

7. Roberts, W.C., Buja, L.M., and Ferrans, V.J. Löffler's fibroplastic parietal endocarditis, eosinophilic leukemia, and Davies' endomyocardial fibrosis. The same disease at different stages? *Path. Microbiol.* (Basel) **35**: 90–95, 1970.

8. Brockington, I.F. and Olsen, E.G. Löffler's endocarditis and Davies' endomyocardial fibrosis. *Am. Heart J.* **85**: 308–322, 1973.

9. Yam, L.T., Li, C.Y., Necheles, T.F., and Katayama, I. Pseudoeosinophilia, eosinophilic endocarditis and eosinophilic leukemia. *Am. J. Med.* **53**: 193–202, 1972.

10. Weiss-Carmine, S. Die Endocarditis parietalis fibroplastica mit Bluteosinophilie (Löffler) und ihre stellung im Rahman der Parietalendokard fibrosen. *Schweiz. Med. Wochnschr.* **87**: 890–898, 1957.

11. Hoffman, F.G., Rosenbaum, D., and Genovese, P.D. Fibroplastic endocarditis with eosinophilia (Löffler's endocarditis parietalis fibroplastica). Case report and review of literature. *Ann. Intern. Med.* **42**: 668–680, 1955.

12. Brink, A.J. and Weber, H.W. Fibroplastic parietal endocarditis with eosinophilia. Loeffler's endocarditis. *Am. J. Med.* **34**: 52–70, 1963.

13. Webb-Peploe, M.M. Eosinophilic heart disease. In: Specific Heart Muscle Disease, Symons, C., Evans, T., and Mitchell, A.G. (eds.), Wright PSG, Bristol, 1983, pp. 24–32.

14. Spry, C.J. The hypereosinophilic syndrome: Clinical features, laboratory findings and treatment. *Allergy* **37**: 539–551, 1982.

15. Parrillo, J.E., Borer, J.S., Henry, W.L., Wolff, S.M., and Fauci, A.S. The cardiovascular manifestations of the hypereosinophilic syndrome. Prospective study of 26 patients, with review of the literature. *Am. J. Med.* **67**: 572–582, 1979.

16. Spry, C.J. Davies, J., Tai, P.C., Olsen, E.G., Oakley, C.M., and Goodwin, J.F. Clinical features of fifteen patients with the hypereosinophilic syndrome. *Q.J. Med.* **52**: 1–22, 1983.

17. Davies, J.N. Some considerations regarding obscure diseases affecting the mural endocardium. *Am. Heart J.* **59**: 600–631, 1960.

18. Davies, J., Spry, C.J., Vijayaraghavan, G., and De Souza, J.A. A comparison of the clinical and cardiological features of endomyocardial disease in temperate and tropical regions. *Postgrad. Med. J.* **59**: 179–185, 1983.

19. Cherian, G., Vijayaraghavan, G., Krishnaswami, S., Sukumar, I.P., John, S., Jairaj, P.S., and Bhaktaviziam, A. Endomyocardial fibrosis: Report on the hemodynamic data in 29 patients and review of the results of surgery. *Am. Heart J.* **105**: 659–666, 1983.

20. Balakrishnan, K.G., Venkitachalam, C.G., Pillai, V.R., Subramanian, R., and Valiathan, M.S. Postoperative evaluation of endomyocardial fibrosis. *Cardiology* **73**: 73–84, 1986.

21. Bertrand, E., Chauvet, J., Assamoi, M.O., et al. Results, indications and contra-indications of surgery in restrictive endomyocardial fibrosis: Comparative study on 31 operated and 30 non-operated patients. *East Afr. Med. J.* **62**: 151–160, 1985.

22. Puigbo, J.J., Combellas, I., Acquatella, H., Marsiglia, I., Tortoledo, F., Casal, H., and Suarez, J.A. Endomyocardial disease in South America—Report on 23 cases in Venezuela. *Postgrad. Med. J.* **59**: 162–169, 1983.

23. Carvalho, F.R., Matos, S., Victor, E.G., Saraiva, L., Brindeiro Filho, D., Maranhao, E., and Moraes, C.R. Phonomechanocardiographic findings in endomyocardial fibrosis. *Angiology* **35**: 63–70, 1984.

24. Take, M., Sekiguchi, M., Hiroe, M., Hirosawa, K., Mizoguchi, H., Kijima, M., Shirai, T., Ishide, T., and Okubo, S. Clinical spectrum and endomyocardial biopsy findings in eosinophilic heart disease. *Heart Vessels* (suppl.) **1**: 243–249, 1985.

25. Sueblinvong, V. and Sanpradit, M. Endomyocardial fibrosis in Thai children. *J. Med. Assoc. Thai.* **67**: 334–340, 1984.

26. Vallejo, J.L., Alvarez, E.F., Acedo, J.M., and Salem, F.M. Endomyocardial fibrosis with

aortic, mitral, and tricuspid valve involvement. *Arch. Intern. Med.* **142**: 1925–1927, 1982.

27. Fawzy, M.E., Ziady, G., Halim, M., Guindy, R., Mercer, E.N., and Feteih. N. Endomyo-cardial fibrosis: Report of eight cases. *J. Am. Coll. Cardiol.* **5**: 983–988, 1985.

28. Dubost, C., Prigent, C., Gerbaux, A., Maurice, P., Passelecq, J., Rulliere, R., Carpentier, A. and DeLoche, A. Surgical approaches in endomyocardial disease (abstract). *Postgrad. Med. J.* **59**: 160–161, 1983.

29. Roberts, W.C., Buja, L.M., Buckley, B.H., O'Connell, J.P., and Ferrans, V.J. Endomyo-cardial disease and eosinophilia (Loeffler's disease). *Am. J. Cardiol.* **133**: 166, 1974.

30. Harley, J.B., Fauci, A.S., and Gralnick, H.R. Noncardiovascular findings associated with heart disease in the idiopathic hypereosinophilic syndrome. *Am. J. Cardiol.* **52**: 321–324, 1983.

31. Cameron, J., Radford, D.J., Howell, J.O., and Brien M.F. Hypereosinophilic heart disease. *Med. J. Aust.* **143**: 408–410, 1985.

32. Olsen, E.G. and Spry, C.J. The pathogenesis of Löffler's endomyocardial disease and its relationship to endomyocardial fibrosis. *Prog. Cardiol.* **8**: 281–303, 1979.

33. Löffler's eosinophilic endocarditis (editorial). *Lancet* **ii**: 1028–1029, 1981.

34. Spry, C.J., Davies, J., and Tai, P.C. Eosinophils and endomyocardial fibrosis. *Contrib. Microbiol. Immunol.* **7**: 212–217, 1983.

35. Spry, C.J. Eosinophils in eosinophilic endomyocardial disease. *Postgrad. Med. J.* **62**: 609–613, 1986.

36. Remmele, W. and Sessner, H.H. Zur morphologischen Patholgie und Klinik der Endo-carditis parietalis fibroplastica sit Bluteosinophilie (Löffler). *Klin. Wochenschr.* **37**: 374–385, 1959.

37. Appel, J. Loeffler's endocarditis in the organism hypersensitized by *Taenia saginata. Acta. Morphol. Acad. Sci. Hung.* **20**: 133–137, 1972.

38. Dallocchio, M., Clementy, J., Mullen, P., Jacquinet, J.P., Bricaud, D.H., and Broustet, P. Fibrose endomyocardique autochtone observee au cours d'une distomatose. *Arch. Mal. Coeur* **68**: 329–2, 1975.

39. Potier, J.C., Khayat, A., and Foucault, J.P. Distomatosis and cardiac disease. Apropos of 2 new cases. Trials of classification and pathogenetic hypotheses. *Arch. Mal. Coeur* **71**: 1299–1306, 1978.

40. Spry, C.J., Weetman, A.P., Olsson, I., Tai, P.C., and Olsen, E.G. The pathogenesis of eosinophilic endomyocardial disease in patients with carcinomas of the lung. *Heart Vessels* **1**: 162–169, 1985.

41. Barrett, A.J. and Barrett, A. Bronchial carcinoma with eosinophilia and cardiomegaly. *Br. J. Dis. Chest* **69**: 287–292, 1975.

42. Slungaard, A., Vercellotti, G., Zanjani, E., Ascensao, J., and Jacob, H.S. Tumor-induced eosinophilia and endocardial fibrosis: Evidence for ectopic eosinophilopoietin production and toxic O_2 metabolite-mediated endothelial damage. *Trans. Assoc. Am. Physicians* **95**: 8–11, 1982.

43. Yakulis, R. and Bedetti, C.D. Löffler's endocarditis. Occurrence with malignant lymphoma with a high content of epithelioid histiocytes ('Lennert's lymphoma'). *Arch. Pathol. Lab. Med.* **107**: 531–534, 1983.

44. Bentley, H.P., Jr, Reardon, A.E., Knoedler, J.P., and Krivit, W. Eosinophilic leukemia. Report of a case, with review and classification. *Am. J. Med.* **30**: 310–322, 1961.

45. Smith, J.W. Hypoplastic right ventricle with eosinophilic endocarditis and patent foramen ovale. *West. J. Med.* **129**: 64–67, 1978.

46. Lohr, K., and Jahnecke, J. Ueber einer fall von Endocarditis parietalis fibroplastica mit Bluteosinophilie (Löffler) mit dem klinischer bild einer "eosinophilen leukamie." *Dtsch. Arch. Klin. Med.* **210**: 110, 1965.

47. Blatt, P.M., Rothstein, G., Miller, H.L., and Cathey, W.J. Löffler's endomyocardial fibrosis with eosinophilia in association with acute lymphoblastic leukemia. *Blood* **44**: 489–493, 1974.

48. Gaynon, P.S. and Gonzalez Crussi, F. Exaggerated eosinophilia and acute lymphoid leukemia. *Am. J. Pediatr. Hematol. Oncol.* **6**: 334–337, 1984.
49. Case records of the Massachusetts General Hospital. Weekly clinicopathological exercise. Case 18–1980. *N. Engl. J. Med.* **302**: 1077–1083, 1980.
50. Edge, J.R. Myocardial fibrosis following arsenical therapy. *Lancet* ii:[675–677, 1946.
51. Gardiol, D. and Picht, E. Encephalopathy and myocarditis with an eosinophilia. A case of urogenital tuberculosis treated with tuberculostatic drugs. *Schweiz. Zeit. Tuberk. Pneumon.* **14**: 212–226, 1959.
52. Lanham, J.G., Cooke, S., Davies, J., and Hughes, G.R. Endomyocardial complications of the Churg-Strauss syndrome. *Postgrad, Med. J.* **61**: 341–344, 1985.
53. Angelillo, V.A., Kanner, R.E., and Renzetti, A.D., Jr. Chronic eosinophilic pneumonia: A report of four cases and a review of the literature. *Am. J. Med. Sci.* **273**: 279–287, 1977.
54. Peterson, C.G. and Venge, P. Interaction and complex-formation between the eosinophil cationic protein and alpha 2-macroglobulin. *Biochem. J.* **245**: 781–787, 1987.
55. Gottdiener, J.S., Maron, B.J., Schooley, R.T., Harley, J.B., Roberts, W.C., and Fauci, A.S. Two-dimensional echocardiographic assessment of the idiopathic hypereosinophilic syndrome. Anatomic basis of mitral regurgitation and peripheral embolization. *Circulation* **67**: 572–578, 1983.
56. Olsen, E.G. and Spry, C.J. The pathophysiology of endomyocardial fibrosis. *Arq. Bras. Cardiol.* **38**: 319–323, 1982.
57. Olsen, E.G. and Spry, C.J. Relation between eosinophilia and endomyocardial disease. *Prog. Cardiovasc. Dis.* **27**: 241–254, 1985.
58. Spry, C.J. Eosinophils and endomyocardial fibrosis: A review of clinical and experimental studies 1980–86. In: Pathogenesis of Myocarditis and Cardiomyopathy: Recent Experimental and Clinical Studies. Kawai, C. and Abelmann, W.A. (eds.), Cardiomyopathy Update 1, University of Tokyo Press, Tokyo, 1987, pp. 293–310.
59. Spry, C.J. Eosinophilia and the heart. In: Immunological Aspects of Cardiovascular Diseases. Littler, W.A. (ed.), Clinical Immunology and Allergy, Bailliere Tindall, London, 1988, 1: pp. 591–606.
60. Spry, C.J. The Eosinophil. A Comprehensive Review, and Guide to the Scientific and Medical Literature, Oxford University Press, Oxford, 1988.
61. McKusick, V.A. and Cochrane, T.H. Constrictive endocarditis. Report of case. *Bull. Johns Hopkins Hosp.* **90**: 90–97, 1952.
62. Löffler, W. The pathogenetic significance of the so-called endocarditis parietalis fibroplastica. *Bull. Schweiz. Akad. Med. Wiss.* **2**: 287, 1947.
63. Rasche, R.F., Kelsch, R.D., and Weaver, D.K. Löffler's endocarditis in childhood. *Br. Heart J.* **35**: 774–776, 1973.
64. Knorr, D. and Scheppe, K.J. Löffler's fibroplastic parietal endocarditis with eosinophilia in a seven-year-old child. *Z. Kinderheilkd.* **81**: 102–112, 1958.
65. Olson, T.A., Virmani, R., Ansinelli, R.A., Lee, D.H., Mosijczuk, A.D., Marsella, R.C., and Ruymann, F.B. Cardiomyopathy in a child with hypereosinophilic syndrome. *Pediatr. Cardiol.* **3**: 161–169, 1982.
66. Libanoff, A.F. and McMahon, N.J. Eosinophilia and endomyocardial fibrosis. *Am. J. Cardiol.* **37**: 438–441, 1976.
67. Lengyel, M., Arvay, A., and Palik, I. Massive endocardial calcification associated with endomyocardial fibrosis. *Am. J. Cardiol.* **56**: 815–816, 1985.
68. Cohen, J., Davies, J., Goodwin, J.F., and Spry, C.J. Arrhythmias in patients with hypereosinophilia: a comparison of patients with and without Löffler's endomyocardial disease. *Postgrad. Med. J.* **56**: 828–832, 1980.
69. Karle, H. and Videbaek, A. Eosinophilic leukaemia or a collagen disease with eosinophilia. *Dan. Med. Bull.* **13**: 41–45, 1966.
70. Smith, L.H. Jr. and Boushey, H. Eosinophilia and eosinophilic carditis. *California Med.* **3**: 388–395, 1969.

71. Raizner, A.E., Silverman, M.E., and Waters, W.C. III. Conduction disturbances and pacemaker failure in Löffler's endomyocarditis. *Am. J. Med.* **53**: 343–347, 1972.

72. Gould, L., Reddy, C.V., Chua, W., Swamy, C.R., and Dorismond, J.C. Fibroplastic parietal endocarditis with eosinophilia. *Angiology* **28**: 779–787, 1977.

73. Scott, M.E. and Bruce, J.H. Löffler's endocarditiis. *Br. Heart J.* **37**: 534–538, 1975.

74. Borer, J.S., Henry, W.L., and Epstein, S.E. Echocardiographic observations in patients with systemic infiltrative disease involving the heart. *Am. J. Cardiol.* **39**: 184–188, 1977.

75. Bletry, O., Scheuble, C., Cereze, P., Masquet, C., Priollet, P., Balafrej, M., and Godeau, P. Cardiac manifestations of the hypereosinophilic syndrome. The value of 2-dimensional echography (12 cases). *Arch. Mal. Coeur.* **77**: 633–641, 1984.

76. Rodger, J.C., Irvine, K.G., and Lerski, R.A. Echocardiography in Löffler's endocarditis. *Br. Heart J.* **46**: 110–112, 1981.

77. DePace, N.L., Nestico, P.F., Morganroth, J., Ross, J., Fox, R., Kotler, M.N., Mintz, G.S., and Vassallo, R. Dilated cardiomyopathy in the idiopathic hypereosinophilic syndrome. *Am. J. Cardiol.* **52**: 1359–1360, 1983.

78. Kudenchuk, P.J., Hosenpud, J.D., and Fletcher, S. Eosinophilic endomyocardiopathy. *Clin. Cardiol.* **9**: 344–348, 1986.

79. Patterson, N.W., Brenbridge, A.N., and Paling, M.R. Computed tomography of mural thrombosis in the hypereosinophilic syndrome. *J. Comp. Tomogr.* **8**: 129–132, 1984.

80. Presti, C., Ryan, T., and Armstrong, W.F. Two-dimensional and Doppler echocardiographic findings in hypereosinophilic syndrome. *Am. Heart J.* **114**: 172–175, 1987.

81. Lengyel, M. and Dekov, E. Two-dimensional echocardiographic features of Loffler's endocarditis. *Acta. Cardiol.* (Brussels) **37**: 59–69, 1982.

82. Arvay, A., Lengyel, M., Meszaros, R., and Palik, I. Surgical experience with thrombotic and fibrotic forms of non-tropical eosinophilic endomyocardial disease. *Thorac. Cardiovasc. Surg.* **33**: 314–316, 1985.

83. Davies, J., Gibson, D.G., Foale, R., Heer, K., Spry, C.J., Oakley, C.M., and Goodwin, J.F. Echocardiographic features of eosinophilic endomyocardial disease. *Br. Heart J.* **48**: 434–440, 1982.

84. Clark, G.M., Valentine, E., and Blount, S.G. Endocardial fibrosis simulating constrictive pericarditis. Report of a case with determinations of pressure in the right side of the heart and eosinophilia. *N. Engl. J. Med.* **254**: 349–355, 1956.

85. Davies, J., Spry, C.J., Sapsford, R., Olsen, E.G., de Perez, G., Oakley, C.M., and Goodwin, J.F. Cardiovascular features of 11 patients with eosinophilic endomyocardial disease. *Quart. J. Med.* **52**: 23–39, 1983.

86. Bell, J.A., Jenkins, B.S., and Webb Peploe, M.M. Clinical, haemodynamic and angiography findings in Löffler's eosinophilic endocarditis. *Br. Heart J.* **38**: 541–548, 1976.

87. Hall, S.W., Jr., Theologides, A., From, A.H.,G obel, F.L., Fortuny, I.E., Lawrence, C.J., and Edwards, J.E. Hypereosinophilic syndrome with biventricular involvement. *Circulation* **55**: 217–222, 1977.

88. Blair, H.T., Chahine, R.A., Raizner, A.E., Gyorkey, F., and Luchi, R.J. Unusual hemodynamics in Löffler's endomyocarditis. *Am. J. Cardiol.* **34**: 606–609, 1974.

89. Miller, W., Walsh, R., and McCall, D. Eosinophilic heart disease presenting with features suggesting hypertrophic obstructive cardiomyopathy. *Cathet. Cardiovasc. Diagn.* **13**: 185–188, 1987.

90. Przybojewski, J.Z. Endomyocardial biopsy: A review of the literature. *Cathet. Cardiovasc. Diagn.* **11**: 287–330, 1985.

91. Galbut, D.L., Benson, J., Blankstein, R.L., Vignola, P.A., and Gentsch, T.O. Endomyocardial fibrosis. Preoperative diagnosis and surgical therapy. *Chest* **84**: 779–782, 1983.

92. Nippoldt, T.B., Edwards, W.D., Holmes, D.R., Jr., Reeder, G.S., Hartzler, G.O., and Smith, H.C. Right ventricular endomyocardial biopsy: Clinicopathologic correlates in 100 consecutive patients. *Mayo Clin. Proc.* **57**: 407–418, 1982.

93. Fauci, A.S., Harley, J.B., Roberts, W.C., Ferrans, V.J., Gralnick, H.R., and Bjornson,

B.H. NIH conference. The idiopathic hypereosinophilic syndrome. Clinical, pathophysiologic, and therapeutic considerations. *Ann. Intern. Med.* **97**: 78–92, 1982.

94. Baandrup, U. and Olsen, E.G. Critical analysis of endomyocardial biopsies from patients suspected of having cardiomyopathy. 1. Morphological and morphometric aspects. *Br. Heart J.* **45**: 475–486, 1981.

95. Olsen, E.G. The pathology of cardiomyopathy. Present state of knowledge. *Arq. Bras. Cardiol.* **38**: 325–329, 1982.

96. Baandrup, U. Löffler's endocarditis and endomyocardial fibrosis—a nosologic entity? *Acta. Pathol. Microbiol. Scand.* (A) **85**: 869–874, 1977.

97. Sekiguchi, M., Yu, Z.X., Take, M., Hiroe, M., Hirosawa, K., Shirai, T., Ishide, T., and Takahashi, T. Ultrastructural features of the endomyocardium in patients with eosinophilic heart disease. An endomyocardial biopsy study. *Jpn. Circ. J.* **48**: 1375–1382, 1984.

98. Nakayama, Y., Kohriyama, T., Yamamoto, S., Deguchi, H., Suwa, M., Kino, M., Hirota, Y., Imamura, K., Kitaura, Y., Kawamura, K., and Spry, C.J. Electron-microscopic and immunohistochemical studies on endomyocardial biopsies from a patient with eosinophilic endomyocardial disease. *Heart Vessels* (suppl.) **1**: 250–255, 1985.

99. Tai, P.C., Spry, C.J., Peterson, C., Venge, P., and Olsson, I. Monoclonal antibodies distinguish between storage and secreted forms of eosinophil cationic protein. *Nature* **309**: 182–184, 1984.

100. Tai, P.C., Ackerman, S.J., Spry, C.J., Dunnette, S., Olsen, E.G., and Gleich, G.J., Deposits of eosinophil granule proteins in cardiac tissues of patients with eosinophilic endomyocardial disease. *Lancet* i: 643–647, 1987.

101. Tanino, M., Kitamura, K., Ohta, G., Yamamoto, Y., and Sugioka, G. Hypereosinophilic syndrome with extensive myocardial involvement and mitral valve thrombus instead of mural thrombi. *Acta. Pathol. Jpn.* **33**: 1233–1242, 1983.

102. Malklewicz, B., Pajdak, W., Okulski, J., and Lisiewicz, J. Recherches sur l'activite thromboplastique des eosinophiles d'un malade atteint de leucemie eosinophilique. *Haematologica* (Pavia) **5**: 439–446, 1971.

103. Dahl, R. and Venge, P. Enhancement of urokinase-induced plasminogen activation by the cationic protein of human eosinophil granulocytes. *Thromb. Res.* **14**: 599–608, 1979.

104. Venge, P., Dahl, R., and Hallgren, R. Enhancement of factor XII dependent reactions by eosinophil cationic protein. *Thromb. Res.* **14**: 641–649, 1979.

105. Lee, T., Lenihan, D.J., Malone, B., Roddy, L.L., and Wasserman, S.I. Increased biosynthesis of platelet-activating factor in activated human eosinophils. *J. Biol. Chem.* **259**: 5526–5530, 1984.

106. Hanowell, S.T., Kim, Y.D., Rattan, V., and MacNamara, T.E. Increased heparin requirement with hypereosinophilic syndrome. *Anesthesiology* **55**: 450–452, 1981.

107. Russo, P.A., Wright, J.E., Ho, S.Y., Maneksa, J.R., and Clitsakis, D. Endocardectomy for the surgical treatment of endocardial fibrosis of the left ventricle. *Thorax* **40**: 621–625, 1985.

108. Kim, C.H., Vlietstra, R.E., Edwards, W.D., Reeder, G.S., and Gleich, G.J. Steroid-responsive eosinophilic myocarditis: Diagnosis by endomyocardial biopsy. *Am. J. Cardiol.* **53**: 1472–1473, 1984.

109. Wood, A.E., Boyle, D., O'Hara, M.D., and Cleland, J. Mitral annuloplasty in endomyocardial fibrosis: An alternative to valve replacement. *Ann. Thorac. Surg.* **34**: 446–451, 1982.

110. Harley, J.B., McIntosh, C.L., Kirklin, J.J., Maron, B.J., Gottdiener, J., Roberts, W.C., and Fauci, A.S. Atrioventricular valve replacement in the idiopathic hypereosinophilic syndrome. *Am. J. Med.* **73**: 77–81, 1982.

111. Ikaheimo, M.J., Karkola, P.J., and Takkunen, J.T. Surgical treatment of Löffler's eosinophilic endocarditis. *Br. Heart J.* **45**: 729–732, 1981.

112. Ramakrishnan, T.S., Wolfe, L.W., and Dhand, V.P. A case of acute hypereosinophilic syndrome with post-mortem findings. *Indian Heart J.* **37**: 399–401, 1985.

113. Fournial, G., Schlanger, R., Berthoumieu, F., Pris, J., Marco. J., and Eschapasse, H.

Surgery for cardiac complications caused by endocardial mural fibrin deposits in a hyper-eosinophilic syndrome. *Circulation* **65**: 1010–1014, 1982.

114. Arvay, A. and Lengyel, M. Endomyocardial fibrosis with successful surgical treatment in a Hungarian woman. *Cor. Vasa.* **25**: 191–195, 1983.

115. Davies, J., Sapsford, R., Brooksby, I., Olsen, E.G., Spry, C.J., Oakley, C.M., and Goodwin, J.F. Successful surgical treatment of two patients with eosinophilic endomyocardial disease. *Br. Heart J.* **46**: 438–445, 1981.

116. Valenzuela, R., McMahon, J.T., Glassy, F.J., Golish, J.A., and Caggiano, V. An unusual ultrastructural neutrophil abnormality of unknown function. *Cleve. Clin. J. Med.* **54**: 49–54, 1987.

117. Adams, H.W. and Mainz, D.L. Eosinophilic ascites. A case report and review of the literature. *Am. J. Dig. Dis.* **22**: 40–42, 1977.

118. Graham, J.M., Lawrie, G.M., Feteih, N.M., and Debakey, M.E. Management of endomyocardial fibrosis: Successful surgical treatment of biventricular involvement and consideration of the superiority of operative intervention. *Am. Heart J.* **102**: 771–782, 1981.

119. Gerbaux, A., Brux, J. de, Bennaceur, M., and Lenegre, J. L'endocardite parietale fibroplastique avec eosinophilie sanguine (endocardite de Löffler). *Bull. Mem. Soc. Med. Hosp. Paris* **72**: 456–465, 1956.

120. Brockington, I.F., Luzzatto, L., and Osunkoya, B.O. The heart in eosinophilic leukaemia. *Afr. J. Med. Sci.* **1**: 343–352, 1970.

121. Tai, P.C. and Spry, C.J. Eosinophil effector mechanisms: Studies on the ways in which eosinophils induce endomyocardial fibrosis. In this volume, pp. 99–107.

122. Gleich, G.J., Loegering, D.A., Bell, M.P., Checkel, J.L., Ackerman, S.J., and McKean, D.J. Biochemical and functional similarities between human eosinophil-derived neurotoxin and eosinophil cationic protein: Homology with ribonuclease. *Proc. Natl. Acad. Sci. USA* **83**: 3146–3150, 1986.

Eosinophil Effector Mechanisms: Studies on the Ways in Which Eosinophils Induce Endomyocardial Fibrosis

Po-Chun Tai and Christopher J.F. Spry

St. George's Hospital Medical School, London, U.K.

ABSTRACT

There has been a great increase in our knowledge of how eosinophils induce inflammatory responses, largely as a result of molecular studies on their granule proteins and their production of reactive oxygen species and other newly synthesized secretion products. The basic proteins with the most cytotoxic potential are the eosinophil cationic protein (ECP), the eosinophil-derived neurotoxin (EDN), eosinophil peroxidase (EPO), and eosinophil major basic protein (MBP). *In vitro* studies have shown that eosinophil secretion products damage heart cells by an initial induction of membrane lesions leading to activation of the sodium/potassium ATPase, followed by specific inhibition of mitochondrial respiration. These short-term effects now need to be related to long-term studies on eosinophils and their capacity to cause tissue injury, as eosinophils can survive for many weeks in culture and in vivo, where they continue to degranulate and produce further toxic products.

INTRODUCTION

Eosinophilic endomyocardial disease has been recognized for many years as a major complication of hypereosinophilic disorders, the most common being the idiopathic hypereosinophilic syndrome.[1,2] The finding that most, if not all, patients with heart damage had circulating eosinophils with fewer granules than normal led to the realization that eosinophil granule proteins may be involved in the development of endomyocardial fibrosis (EMF) in these disorders.[3] Evidence has accumulated from several studies which showed that eosinophils are potent proinflammatory cells capable of damaging a variety of parasites[4-6] and mammalian cells, including heart cells *in vitro*.[7] A recent multicenter study carried out in the U.K. and the U.S.A. has demonstrated localization of both eosinophil cationic protein (ECP) and eosinophil major basic protein (MBP) in acute and chronic lesions in cardiac biopsies, and postmortem material from patients with eosinophilic endomyocardial disease.[8] Taken together, these findings support a pathogenetic role for eosinophils in the development of EMF.

EOSINOPHIL GRANULE PROTEINS

Eosinophils can be distinguished from other cell types by the presence of cytoplasmic granules which contain large amounts of 3 unique highly basic proteins: ECP, eosinophil-derived neurotoxin (EDN), and eosinophil peroxidase (EPO), which can be solubilized and secreted to the outside of the cell.[9] The basic proteins with the most cytotoxic potential are ECP, EDN, EPO, and MBP. MBP is not confined to eosinophils, as it

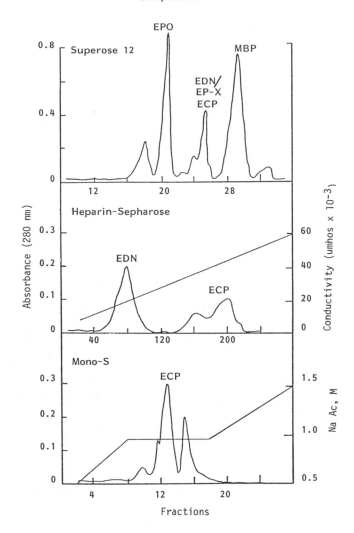

Fig. 1.   Purification of EPO, ECP, EDN, and MBP on sequential gel filtration, heparin-Sepharose and fast protein liquid chromatography. On heparin-Sepharose, EDN elutes at a lower salt concentraion than ECP. ECP can be further resolved into 3 peaks on Mono-S FPLC.

is also found in human placental X cells and basophils.[9] These cationic proteins can be purified to homogeneity by sequential chromatography on gel filtration, followed by heparin-Sepharose[9] and fast protein liquid chromatography (Fig. 1).[10]

   Unlike ECP, EDN, and EPO, which are located in the granule matrix, MBP comprises the granule crystalloid.[11] Biosynthetic studies of ECP and EPO have shown that these 2 proteins are synthesized initially as larger molecular weight precursor forms which are then cleaved into smaller molecular weight storage forms.[10,12] Studies with monoclonal antibody EG2, which only binds to the solubilized and secreted forms of ECP, have shown that ECP undergoes further antigenic changes during secretion, where it develops greater molecular weight heterogeneity.[13] Amino acid sequencing and molecular studies have shown that ECP and EDN are closely homologous and are specialized ribonucleases.[14] MBP, on the other hand, has no known enzymatic activity. The reduced and alkylated form of MBP is more toxic than native MBP, but the reason for this is unclear.[15]

ECP is the most cytotoxic of the 4 basic granule proteins. It has been found to be at least 8 times more toxic than MBP for the schistosomula of *Schistosoma mansoni*,[15] where it produces blebs followed by disruption of the parasite surface and extrusion of parasite content.[5] The mechanism of this ECP-mediated damage is unknown, but it is not related to its ribonuclease activity.[15] In addition, ECP can synergize with cytoplasts (intact cytoplasm devoid of granules which are capable of generating reactive oxygen species) in the killing of schistosomula,[16] so that *in vivo* only relatively small amounts of ECP are required to inflict damage to adjacent cells and tissues.

EDN is less cytotoxic than ECP for parasites, although it is 10 times more potent as a ribonuclease and neurotoxin.[17] Monoclonal antibodies that inhibit the ribonuclease activity of EDN had no effect on its cytotoxic capacity, but it is not known if this had any effect on its neurotoxicity. It would be interesting to see whether other ribonucleases, especially pancreatic ribonuclease (which shares homology with EDN and ECP) are also toxic to brain tissues. EPO catalyzes the formation of hypochlorite ions and hydrogen peroxide, and provides a potent cytotoxic mechanism in the presence of hydrogen peroxide and a halide for some parasites, bacteria, tumors, and various mammalian cells *in vitro*.[18] EPO is also capable of "arming" macrophages to become more effective in killing bacteria.[19]

EOSINOPHIL ACTIVATION AND SECRETION

The realization that eosinophils, like macrophages, can be activated to become more effective in damaging cells and tissues came from studies that showed that eosinophils from patients with schistosomiasis had an increased capacity to kill schistosomula of *S. mansoni* compared to normal eosinophils.[20] This finding initiated a series of studies which confirmed that, unlike normal individuals, eosinophils from patients with eosinophilia exhibit marked structural and functional heterogeneity.[21–23] On metrizamide density gradients, patients' eosinophils were found to consist of normal and light density populations.[23] The light density eosinophils have been shown by several groups to be activated, with increased expression of membrane receptors for immunoglobulins and complement components and membrane antigens detected by monoclonal antibodies.[21,23] However, there is no evidence to suggest that these light density, activated eosinophils are derived from a lineage separated from normal density eosinophils, and they probably represent normal density eosinophils at a more advanced stage in maturation.[23] Interestingly but not surprisingly, the factors responsible for increased eosinophil production were also found to be capable of activating eosinophils.[24–26] Several of these eosinopoietic/activating factors have now been purified, characterized, and cloned. These include eosinophil-activating factor (EAF),[27] granulocyte-macrophage colony-stimulating factor (GM-CSF),[28] and interleukin 5 (IL-5).[29] Of these, IL-5 is the most potent in stimulating eosinophil proliferation, maturation, and activation. EAF activates eosinophils by inducing the mobilization and solubilization of ECP, and hence increasing the propensity of the cell to secrete.[27] The mode of action of the other factors is as yet unknown.

Several research groups have been studying the membrane events that induce eosinophils to release their granule proteins, as this is clearly an important site for therapeutic intervention. A number of stimuli have been found to trigger the release of

TABLE 1.   The Binding of Monoclonal Antibody Eol to Normal and Light Density Eosinophils

Patient	% eosinophils binding Eol		125I-Eol cpm × 10⁻³	
	Normal	Light	Normal	Light
JC	95	92	18.50	22.90
AR	90	95	23.30	26.00
JR	98	96	15.23	17.89

10^6 purified eosinophils were incubated with 1/100 dilution of purified Eol, washed, and then followed by 1/40 dilution of a rabbit anti-mouse IgG. The proportion of fluorescing cells was assessed out of 200 cells scored.

In the radioactive cell binding studies, light density eosinophils were harvested from 22% metrizamide, and were greater than 95% pure, with no contaminating mononuclear cells or platelets. The 5% contaminants were neutrophils.

eosinophil granule proteins *in vitro*, including IgG, IgE, IgA, C3b, EAF, and membrane antigens detected by monoclonal antibodies.[9,30,31] We have recently studied the interaction of eosinophils with monoclonal antibody Eol, which belongs to the CD9 panel of anti-leukocyte antibodies. Eol is interesting because it has cellular specificities similar to those of IL-5, as it only binds eosinophils, pre-B cells, and platelets.[32] Unlike the other group of monoclonal antibodies to eosinophils, Eol does not bind neutrophils (Tai, unpublished). Immunofluorescence experiments have shown that Eol binds to all normal and light density eosinophils. However, light density eosinophils appear to have more Eol binding sites per cell, as shown by radioactive cell binding studies (Table 1). This observation prompted us to examine the capacity of Eol to induce eosinophil secretion. Experiments showed that Eol is a potent inducer of ECP secretion, but only after multivalent cross-linking by a second antibody has occurred (Table 2).

All of the secretory stimuli tested so far only released up to 40% of each granule protein from eosinophils.[33] This may be due partly to the short incubation times used in previous studies. As it is now possible to culture eosinophils *in vitro* for many weeks in the presence of GM-CSF or IL-5,[34–36] it should now be possible to carry out experiments to see how eosinophils become completely degranulated as seen *in vivo*.

The ability of various stimuli to induce selective secretion of granule proteins from eosinophils have been studied by 2 groups. The first group has shown that IgE induced the secretion of EPO but not of ECP, whereas stimulation with IgG induced the reverse.[31] The second group, in Sweden, has demonstrated that synthetic glycerides induced the release of as much as 40% of EDN/EPX, but little or no ECP.[33] It was suggested that this differential release of granule proteins may be due to the different compartmentalization of the granule proteins. If these observations are confirmed, they might help to explain why patients with asthma do not develop eosinophilic endomyocardial disease, and vice versa, as different granule proteins are released in the different disease settings.

EOSINOPHILS AND CARDIOVASCULAR INJURY

The major complications of the hypereosinophilic syndrome are EMF and thromboembolic disease.[2,37] Heart damage is associated with early myocardial cell necrosis and the eventual deposition of fibrous tissue.[38] There have been attempts to discover how eosinophils might induce these cardiovascular lesions. A recent study has shown that the injection of human ECP into mice produced myocarditis in 2 of 5 animals.[39]

TABLE 2. ECP Secretion Induced by Monoclonal Antibody Eol

	ECP-released ng/10^6 eosinophils mean $\pm$ S.D.
Eosinophils alone	1400 ± 327
Eosinophils[a] + Eol	1740 ± 256
Eosinophils[b] + Eol + anti-mouse IgG	14540 ± 260
Eosinophils + zymosan/C3b	4730 ± 170

[a] Light density eosinophils (10^6) were incubated with 1/100 dilution of purified Eol for 1 hr at 37°. Supernatants were removed for ECP estimations.

[b] Light density eosinophils (10^6) were incubated with 1/100 dilution of Eol at 4° for 30 min. The cells were washed and further incubated with 1/20 dilution of rabbit anti-mouse IgG at 37° for 1 hr.

Zymosan/C3b was used as a positive control for these experiments.

In vitro studies on the role of eosinophils in inflammation have centered mainly on direct cytotoxicity experiments, or on the capacity of eosinophils (or their purified granule proteins) to alter the functions of adjacent cells. We have shown that eosinophil secretion products kill rat heart cells by an initial effect on the plasma membrane, which leads to activation of sodium-potassium ATPase.[7] This membrane effect is probably similar to the pore formation induced by ECP on liposomes.[40] EDN, EPO, and MBP do not induce pore formation. It is not known at present if secretion products can enter the plasma membrane by a translocase system, but if they can, then these toxic proteins also inhibit mitochondrial respiration, especially 2-oxoglutarate dehydrogenase-dependent respiration.[7]

An interesting possibility is that rather than damaging host tissues, a more important function of eosinophils *in vivo* is to induce changes in the properties of other cellular and serum components of acute and chronic inflammation. A key event in inflammation is the emigration of eosinophils through the endothelium of blood vessels into tissue sites. Studies on eosinophil-endothelial cell interactions have shown that eosinophils are unable to kill endothelial cells, but they reduce the production of endothelial cell prostacycline, which could lead to increased thromboembolic complications.[41]

Human eosinophils, especially light density eosinophils, secrete large amounts of PAF when stimulated with the calcium ionophore A23187,[42] and this may also be related to the high incidence of thromboembolic disease in eosinophilic endomyocardial disease. In addition, ECP and MBP can both activate the coagulation system.[43,44] ECP interacts with factor XI and activates plasminogen, but the site of MBP action is unknown. Both cationic proteins are also powerful inhibitors of heparin and streptokinase by virtue of their high basicity.

Recently, two groups have described a fibrogenic factor in human eosinophil secretion products (which was absent in neutrophil secretion products) (Take, Sekiguchi, Tai, and Spry, unpublished) and in guinea pig and human eosinophil granule extracts,[45] which stimulated the proliferation of human fibroblasts in culture. This factor could account for the close association between eosinophils and fibrogenesis.

CONCLUSIONS

The *in vitro* studies, combined with clinical observations,[46] provide a strong argument for a role for eosinophils in chronic tissue injury, especially damage to the heart. As the only features that distinguish eosinophils from other cells are their highly cationic granule proteins, it seems likely that these granule proteins are responsible for the eosinophil-mediated tissue damage. However, there are many patients with hypereosinophilia who do not develop cardiac complications, and this would suggest that there are intrinsic mechanisms for inhibiting the release of granule proteins, or neutralizing their effects, once they have been released. In this context, ECP has been found to bind to α-2 macroglobulin in normal serum[47] and this interaction may represent a protective mechanism.

Several important issues remain unexplained. For instance, what is the cause of the eosinophilia in such patients? What is the nature of the stimulus that leads to eosinophil secretion *in vivo*, and why is the endocardium especially susceptible to this type of injury? At present, there are no proven therapeutic methods for preventing eosinophil-dependent tissue damage *in vivo*, but several drugs, particularly corticosteroids,[48,49] can partially inhibit eosinophil secretion *in vitro*. Further detailed studies on the unique eosinophil granule proteins and their functions are clearly required in order to find out more about how eosinophils take part in inflammation, which may lead to the development of novel strategies for treating eosinophil-induced tissue lesions.

ACKNOWLEDGMENTS

We are grateful to the many clinical and scientific colleagues who have contributed to the work discussed here, and for the financial support of the Wellcome Trust, the British Heart Foundation, and the Medical Research Council.

REFERENCES

1. Spry, C.J. The hypereosinophilic syndrome: Clinical features, laboratory findings and treatment. *Allergy* 37: 539–551, 1982.
2. Spry, C.J., Davies, J., Tai, P.C., Olsen, E.G., Oakley, C.M., and Goodwin, J.F. Clinical features of fifteen patients with the hypereosinophilic syndrome. *Quart. J. Med.* 52: 1–22, 1983.
3. Spry, C.J. and Tai, P.C. Studies on blood eosinophils. II. Patients with Loffler's cardiomyopathy. *Clin. Exp. Immunol.* 24: 423–434, 1976.
4. Ackerman, S.J., Gleich, G.J., Loegering, D.A., Richardson, B.A., and Butterworth, A.E. Comparative toxicity of purified human eosinophil granule cationic proteins for schistosomula of *Schistosoma mansoni. Am. J. Trop. Med. Hyg.* 34: 735–745, 1985.
5. McLaren, D.J., McKean, J.R., Olsson, I., Venges, P., and Kay, A.B. Morphological studies on the killing of schistosomula of *Schistosoma mansoni* by human eosinophil and neutrophil cationic proteins *in vitro. Parasitol. Immunol.* 3: 359–373, 1981.
6. Waters, L.S., Taverne, J., Tai, P.C., Spry, C.J., Targett, G.A., and Playfair, J.H. Killing of *Plasmodium falciparum* by eosinophil secretory products. *Infect. Immunol.* 55: 877–881, 1987.
7. Tai, P.C., Hayes, D.J., Clark, J.B., and Spry, C.J. Toxic effects of human eosinophil products on isolated rat heart cells *in vitro. Biochem. J.* 204: 75–80, 1982.
8. Tai, P.C., Ackerman, S.J., Spry, C.J., Dunnette, S., Olsen. E.G., and Gleich, G.J. Deposits of eosinophil granule proteins in cardiac tissues of patients with eosinophilic endomyocardial disease. *Lancet* 1: 643–647, 1987.
9. Gleich, G.J. and Adolphson, C.R. The eosinophilic leukocyte: Structure and function. *Adv. Immunol.* 39: 177–253, 1986.

10. Olsson, I., Persson, A.M., and Winqvist, I. Biochemical properties of the eosinophil cationic protein and demonstration of its biosynthesis *in vitro* in marrow cells from patients with an eosinophilia. *Blood* **67**: 498–503, 1986.

11. Egesten, A., Alumets, J., von Mecklenburg, C., Palmegren, M., and Olsson, I. Localization of eosinophil cationic protein, major basic protein, and eosinophil peroxidase in human eosinophils by immunoelectron microscopic technique. *J. Histochem. Cytochem.* **34**: 1399–1403, 1986.

12. Olsson, I., Persson, A.M., Stromberg, K., Winqvist, I., Tai, P.C., and Spry, C.J. Purification of eosinophil peroxidase and studies of biosynthesis and processing in human marrow cells. *Blood* **66**: 1143–1148, 1985.

13. Tai, P.C., Spry, C.J., Peterson, C., Venge, P., and Olsson, I. Monoclonal antibodies distinguish between storage and secreted forms of eosinophil cationic protein. *Nature* **309**: 182–184, 1984.

14. Gleich, G.J., Loegering, D.A., Bell, M.P., Checkel, J.L., Ackerman, S.J., and McKean, D.J. Biochemical and functional similarities between human eosinophil-derived neurotoxin and eosinophil cationic protein: Homology with ribonuclease. *Proc. Natl. Acad. Sci. USA* **83**: 3146–3150, 1986.

15. Hamann, K.J., Barker, R.L., Loegering, D.A., and Gleich, G.J. Comparative toxicity of purified human eosinophil granule proteins for newborn larvae of *Trichinella spiralis*. *J. Parasitol.* **73**: 523–529, 1987.

16. Yazdanbakhsh, M., Tai, P.C., Spry, C.J., Gleich, G.J., and Roos, D. Synergism between eosinophil cationic protein and oxygen metabolites in killing of schistosomula of *Schistosoma mansoni*. *J. Immunol.* **138**: 3443–3447, 1987.

17. Gullberg, U., Widegren, B., Arnason, U., Egesten, A., and Olsson, I. The cytotoxic eosinophil cationic protein (ECP) has ribonuclease activity. *Biochem. Biophys. Res. Commun.* **139**: 1239–1242, 1986.

18. Jong, E.C., Chi, E.Y., and Klebanoff, S.J. Human neutrophil-mediated killing of schistosomula of *Schistosoma mansoni*: Augmentation by schistosomal binding of eosinophil peroxidase. *Am. J. Trop. Med. Hyg.* **33**: 104–115, 1984.

19. Ramsey, P.G., Martin, T., Chi, E., and Klebanoff, S.J. Arming of mononuclear phagocytes by eosinophil peroxidase bound to *Staphylococcus aureus*. *J. Immunol.* **128**: 415–420, 1982.

20. David, J.R., Vadas, M.A., Butterworth, A.E., de Brito, P.A., Carvalho, E.M., David, R.A., Bina, J.C., and Andrade, Z.A. Enhanced helminthotoxic capacity of eosinophils from patients with eosinophilia. *N. Engl. J. Med.* **303**: 1147–1152, 1980.

21. Prin, L., Capron, M., Tonnel, A.B., Bletry, O., and Capron, A. Heterogeneity of human peripheral blood eosinophils: Variability in cell density and cytotoxic ability in relation to the level and the origin of hypereosinophilia. *Int. Arch. Allergy Appl. Immunol.* **72**: 336–346, 1983.

22. Spry, C.J. Synthesis and secretion of eosinophil granule substances. *Immunol. Today* **6**: 332–335, 1985.

23. Tai, P.C., Bakes, D.M., Barkans, J.R., and Spry, C.J. Plasma membrane antigens on light density and activated human blood eosinophils. *Clin. Exp. Immunol.* **60**: 427–436, 1985.

24. Lopez, A.F., Begley, C.G., Williamson, D.J., Warren, D.J., Vadas, M.A., and Sanderson, C.J. Murine eosinophil differentiation factor. An eosinophil-specific colony-stimulating factor with activity for human cells. *J. Exp. Med.* **163**: 1085–1099, 1986.

25. Lopez, A.F., Sanderson, C.J., Gamble, J.R., Campbell, H.D., Young, I.G., and Vadas, M.A. Recombinant human interleukin 5 is a selective activator of human eosinophil function. *J. Exp. Med.* **167**: 219–224, 1988.

26. Metcalf, D., Begley, C.G., Johnson, G.R., Nicola, N.A., Vadas, M.A., Lopez, A.F., Williamson, D.J., Wong, G.G., Clark, S.C., and Wang, E.A. Biologic properties *in vitro* of a recombinant human granulocyte-macrophage colony-stimulating factor. *Blood* **67**: 37–45, 1986.

27. Thorne, K.J., Richardson, B.A., Veith, M.C., Tai, P.C., Spry, C.J., and Butterworth, A.E. Partial purification and biological properties of an eosinophil-activating factor. *Eur. J. Immunol.* **15**: 1083–1091, 1985.

28. Lopez, A.F., Williamson, D.J., Gamble, J.R., Begley, C.G., Harlan, J.M., Klebanoff, S.J., Waltersdorph, A., Wong, G., Clark, S.C., and Vadas, M.A. Recombinant human granulocyte-macrophage colony-stimulating factor stimulates *in vitro* mature human neutrophil and eosinophil function, surface receptor expression, and survival. *J. Clin. Invest.* **78**: 1220–1228, 1986.

29. Campbell, H.D., Tucker, W.Q., Hort, Y., Martinson, M.E., Mayo, G., Clutterbuck, E.J., Sanderson, C.J., and Young, I.G. Molecular cloning, nucleotide sequence, and expression of the gene encoding human eosinophil differentiation factor (interleukin 5). *Proc. Natl. Acad. Sci. USA* **84**: 6629–6633, 1987.

30. Tai, P.C., Capron, M., Bakes, D.M., Barkans, J., and Spry, C.J. Monoclonal antibodies to human eosinophil plasma membrane antigens enhance the secretion of eosinophil cationic protein. *Clin. Exp. Immunol.* **63**: 728–737, 1986.

31. Khalife, J., Capron, M., Cesbron, J.Y., Tai, P.C., Taelman, H., Prin, L., and Capron, A. Role of specific IgE antibodies in peroxidase (EPO) release from human eosinophils. *J. Immunol.* **137**: 1659–1664, 1986.

32. Saito, H., Yamada, K., Breard, J., Yoshie, O., and Mathe, G. A monoclonal antibody reactive with human eosinophils. *Blood* **67**: 50–55, 1986.

33. Peterson, C. Eosinophil granule proteins. Biochemical and functional studies. Doctoral thesis, Uppsala University, Sweden, 1987, pp. 57.

34. Clutterbuck, E.J. and Sanderson, C.J. Human eosinophil hematopoiesis studied *in vitro* by means of murine eosinophil differentiation factor (IL5): Production of functionally active eosinophils from normal human bone marrow. *Blood* **71**: 646–651, 1988.

35. Rothenberg, M.E., Owen, W.F., Jr., Silberstein, D.S., Soberman, R.J., Austen, K.F., and Stevens, R.L. Eosinophils cocultured with endothelial cells have increased survival and functional properties. *Science* **237**: 645–647, 1987.

36. Silberstein, D.S. and David, J.R. The regulation of human eosinophil function by cytokines. *Immunol. Today* **8**: 380–385, 1987.

37. Davies, J., Spry, C.J., Sapsford, R., Olsen, E.G., de Perez, G., Oakley, C.M., and Goodwin, J.F. Cardiovascular features of 11 patients with eosinophilic endomyocardial disease. *Quart. J. Med.* **52**: 23–39, 1983.

38. Olsen, E.G. and Spry, C.J. The pathogenesis of Loffler's endomyocardial disease and its relationship to endomyocardial fibrosis. *Prog. Cardiol.* **8**: 281–303, 1979.

39. Kishimoto, C., Spry, C.J., Tai, P.C., Tomioka, N., and Kawai, C. The *in vivo* cardiotoxic effect of eosinophilic cationic protein in an animal preparation. *Jpn. Circ. J.* **50**: 1264–1267, 1986.

40. Young, J.D., Peterson, C.G., Venge, P., and Cohn, Z.A. How human eosinophil cationic protein damages target membranes. In: Inflammation: Basic Mechanisms, Tissue Injurying Principles and Clinical Models. Venge, P. and Lindblom, A. (eds.), Almqvist & Wibsell International, Stockholm, Sweden, 1985.

41. Davies, J., Powell, D., McCall, E., Hegde, G., and Spry, C.J. Thrombogenic mechanisms in the hypereosinophilic syndrome. Submitted, 1988.

42. Jouvin-Marche, E., Grzych, J.M., Boullet, C., Capron, M., and Benveniste, J. Formation of PAF-acether by human eosinophils (abstract). *Fed. Proc.* **43**: 1924, 1984.

43. Venge, P., Dahl, R., Hallgren, R., and Olsson, I. Cationic proteins of human eosinophils and their role in the inflammatory reaction. In: The Eosinophil in Health and Disease. Mahmoud, A.A., Austen, K.F., and Simon, A.S. (eds.), Grune and Stratton, New York 1980, pp. 131–142.

44. Gleich, G.J., Loegering, D.A., Kueppers, F., Bajaj, S.P., and Mann, K.G. Physicochemical and biological properties of the major basic protein from guinea pig eosinophil granules. *J. Exp. Med.* **140**: 313–331, 1974.

45. Pincus, S.H., Ramesh, K.S., and Wyler, D.J. Eosinophils stimulate fibroblast DNA synthesis. *Blood* **70**: 572–574, 1987.

46. Spry, C.J. Eosinophilia and the heart. In: Immunological Aspects of Cardiovascular Diseases. Littler, W.A. (ed.), Clinical Immunology and Allergy, Bailliere Tindall, London, 1988, 1: 591–606.

47. Peterson, C.G. and Venge, P. Interaction and complex-formation between the eosinophil cationic protein and alpha 2-macroglobulin. *Biochem. J.* **245**: 781–787, 1987.

48. Cook, R.M. and Smith, H. Ability of drugs to affect the activity of rat peritoneal eosinophils and neutrophils *in vitro* (abstract). Presented to the 6th International Congress of Immunology, Toronto, Canada, 1986.

49. Winqvist, I., Olofsson, T., and Olsson, I. Mechanisms for eosinophil degranulation; release of the eosinophil cationic protein. *Immunology* **51**: 1–8, 1984.

On the Existence of Arrhythmia-Conduction (Electric) Disturbance Type of Cardiomyopathy (ECM)

Morie Sekiguchi,* Atsuyo Hasegawa,* Motonari Hasumi,* Michiaki Hiroe,** and Shin-ichi Nunoda***

* The Heart Institute of Japan, Tokyo Women's Medical College, Tokyo 162, Japan
** Department of Radiology, Tokyo Women's Medical College, Tokyo 162, Japan
*** The First Department of Internal Medicine, Shinshu University School of Medicine, Matsumoto, Japan

ABSTRACT

There are cases of cardiomyopathy which are not easily classifiable into hypertrophic, dilated or restrictive type. They often show ventricular arrhythmia, right or left bundle branch block, intraventricular conduction disturbance, atrioventricular conduction disturbance and sinus node dysfunction (sick sinus syndrome). Endomyocardial biopsy in such cases reveals advanced myocardial degeneration or fibrosis. The description "arrhythmia-conduction disturbance type of cardiomyopathy" is appropriate for this category of myocardial disease. We propose the simpler term "electric disturbance type cardiomyopathy (ECM)." In our series of studies of cardiomyopathy employing endomyocardial biopsy in 573 cases, 264 were hypertrophic, 224 were dilated and 85 (14.8%) were classified into the ECM.

INTRODUCTION

It is a generally accepted functional concept that there are two major types of cardiomyopathy, the hypertrophic type, characterized by thickening of the interventricular septum or the free wall of the left ventricle, and the dilated type, characterized by a reduced left ventricular ejection fraction.[1,2] However, we have frequently experienced cases of myocardial disease, often associated with cardiac arrhythmias or disorders of conduction, which do not belong to either of the two major functional categories.[3-7]

In many cases of cardiomyopathy, there is neither thickening of the intraventricular septum or the ventricular wall nor is there an apparent decrease in the left ventricular ejection fraction. In our studies of endomyocardial biopsy over the past 23 years,[8-12] including right atrial biopsy, we have encountered cases where the pathologic changes are confined to the right atrial myocardium without changes in the right ventricle. Accordingly, we have termed such cases "atrial cardiomyopathy."[6,14]

In our investigation of patients with right bundle branch block as the only clinical feature, we have found advanced pathology in the right ventricular biopsy specimens.[6] Similarly in sarcoidosis,[27] where right bundle branch block and atrioventricular block are the predominant features of the cardiac disorder, it is not possible to functionally categorize such cases as either the hypertrophic or dilated type of heart muscle disease We therefore propose an addtional category of cardiomyopathy, namely "non-hypertrophic and non-dilated," characterized by cardiac arrhythmias or conduction (electric) disturbances as the predominant clinical manifestation. In this way, both clinical and pathologic features can be more easily reconciled. An analysis of this third category of cardiomyopathy is presented with our proposed term "Electric Disturbance type Cardiomyopathy (ECM)."[5,6]

FEATURES OF THE ELECTRIC DISTURBANCE TYPE CARDIOMYOPATHY (ECM)

(1) There is no evidence of hypertrophic cardiomyopathy, in that there is no thickening of the left ventricular free wall or at the apex.

(2) There are no clinical signs suggestive of dilated cardiomyopathy, and the echocardiogram, left ventriculogram and radionuclide ventriculography show left ventricular ejection fraction exceeding 50%.

(3) There are no clinical features suggestive of mitral valve prolapse.

(4) Nonspecific electrocardiographic abnormalities including complete right or left bundle branch blocks, A-V block, intraventricular conduction disturbance, "sick sinus syndrome," primary ST-T wave changes and ventricular arrhythmias are the main clinical features which are encountered.

(5) When the above four criteria are satisfied and when secondary myocardial disorders can be excluded, this strongly suggests that cardiomyopathy with electric disturbance is present (Table 1).

(6) To establish the diagnosis in such circumstances, it is useful to perform endomyocardial biopsy.[13] Findings of myocardial degeneration or fibrosis, when prominent, should be regarded as significant evidence of myocardial disease.[11,12] When hypertrophy of the myocytes is the only feature, it may be difficult to determine a basis of myocardial disease. Therefore, in only those cases which show, severer grades (more than 2-plus) of either degeneration of fibrosis or the myocardium should a positive diagnosis be made (Table 2).

SOME REFERENCE POINTS IN DIAGNOSIS

It is helpful to obtain a history of an influenza-like illness within about 10 days prior

TABLE 1.   Definition of the Electric Disturbance Type of Cardiomyopathy (ECM)

1. When patients with A-V block, CRBBB, CLBBB, IVCD, ventricular arrhythmia, atrial arrhythmia show
2. significant pathology of the RV, LV and/or RA endomyocardial biopsy and
3. a non-hypertrophic, non-dilated form is recognized, and
4. a non-significant coronary arteriogram is seen, diagnosis of ECM can be made.

IVCD: intraventricular conduction disturbance

TABLE 2.   Our Histopathologic Criteria for Defining Significant Pathology

A. Parameters	B. Criteria for Significant Pathology
1. Hypertrophy	1. At least one of A^{2-4} should exceed grade 2
2. Degeneration	2. Sum of A^{1-4} should exceed a score of 4
3. Interstitial fibrosis	
4. Disarrangement	

Grading

−	+	+ +	+ + +
0	1	2	3

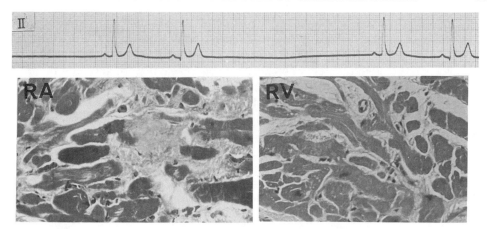

Fig. 1.   This 33-year-old male patient with sick sinus syndrome who suffered from diphtheria in childhood underwent a right atrial (RA) and right ventricular (RV) endomyocardial biopsy. The RA biopsy revealed more advanced interstitial fibrosis than the RV biopsy.

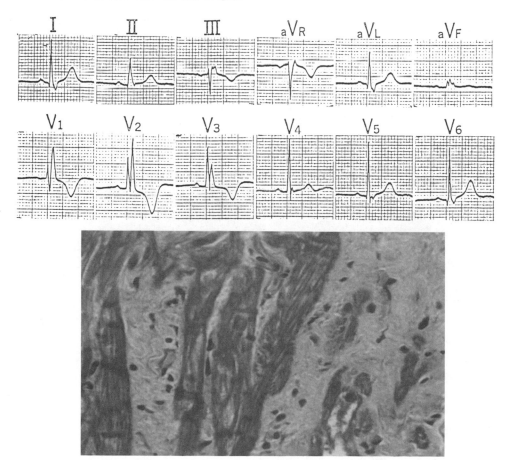

Fig. 2.   A case with a complete right bundle branch block (53-year-old male) which occurred intrafamilially. The right ventricular endomyocardial biopsy revealed marked interstitial fibrosis of the myocardium.

to the onset of cardiac symptoms.[15-19] In such a setting, viral myocarditis may be suspected. Familial occurrence of heart disorder is also a pointer.[4] Arrhythmia and conduction disturbance type of cardiomyopathy may be present intrafamilially.[4] Radionuclide studies using thallium or technetium may reveal abnormality in wall motion in cases of suspected cardiomyopathy. Thereafter a diagnosis can be finalized only by recourse to cardiac biopsy.[8-15,18-24] Arrhythmogenic right ventricular dysplasia[25,26] showing a defect in thalium scintigraphy may also be differentiated by endomyocardial biopsy.[23]

FREQUENCY OF OCCURRENCE AND SIGNIFICANCE

Analyzing our own case material, we have come to the conclusion that cases with

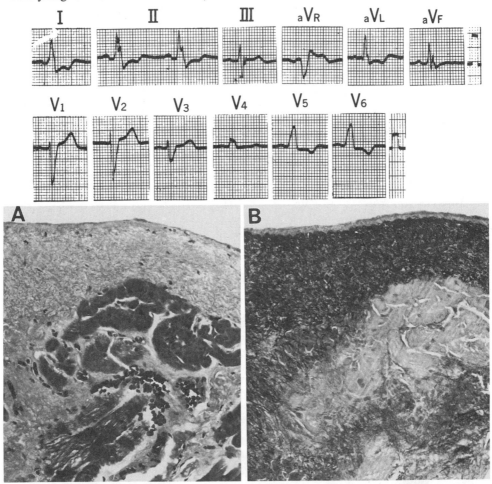

Fig. 3. This 16-year-old female developed faintings. Complete A-V block was recognized and a pacemaker was implanted. At the time of the A-V conduction, left bundle branch block was seen. A left ventricular endomyocardial biopsy revealed a marked endocardial thickening as well as subendocardial fibrosis (see H-E stain in B and elastic van-Giesson stain in B). This patient was later diagnosed as having familial cardiomyopathy of the non-hypertrophic, non-dilated electric disturbance form.

cardiomyopathy of the arrhythmia and conduction disturbance type are not infrequent.[6,7] Case examples are presented in Figs. 1–4, and the results of our case analysis are presented in Tables 2 and 3. In our series of endomyocardial biopsy in 573 cases, 264 were hypertrophic, 224 were dilated and 85 (14.8%) were classified into the ECM.

In our studies of cardiac involvement in sarcoidosis, we found many cases with atrioventricular conduction disturbance or bundle branch block.[27] Autopsy revealed sarcoid granulomata distributed throughout the ventricular wall and especially in the intraventricular septum. It was also confirmed at autopsy that cardiac sarcoidosis is not functionally classifiable into either the hypertrophic or dilated types of cardiomyopathy. While it is agreed that cardiac sarcoidosis is a specific heart muscle disease,[1,2] it is to be regarded as a pathologic model of myocardial disorder with arrhythmia or conduction disturbance as the major clinical manifestation.[27] It may, therefore, be inferred that a similar clinico-pathologic presentation may occur in other non-specific myocardial diseases.

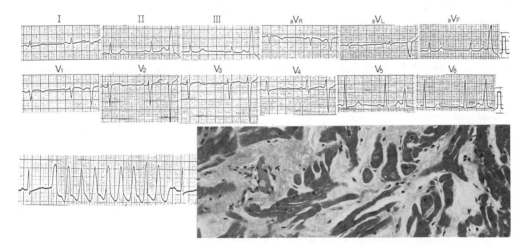

Fig. 4. A case of idiopathic ventricular tachycardia (VT) of LBBB-type underwent a right ventricular endomyocardial biopsy. A marked myocardial fibrosis and disarrangement of muscle bundles which are considered the cause of the VT are noteworthy.

TABLE 3. Incidence of Significant Pathology[6]

1. High degree of A-V block	13/50	26%
2. CRBBB	2/10	20%
3. CLBBB	2/8	25%
4. PVC	3/13	20%
5. LBBB type of VT	11/19	58%
6. SSS (RA biopsy)	13/27	48%
Total	44/127	35%

The incidence of significant pathology in various arrythmias or conduction disturbances. The high percentage of significant pathology may be due to the selection of patients for diagnosing heart muscle disease. Ages of the patients ranged from 11 to 68 with a mean ± S.D. of 32.2 ± 14.6.

In muscular dystrophy, the finding of increased amplitude of R waves in lead V_1 could be explained by regression of the myocardium in the posterolateral region of the ventricle.[28] Again heart muscle disease of muscular dystrophy type cannot be classified as the dilated type of heart muscle disease.

In our 14-year study of viral myocarditis, we have been able to recognize changes of acute myocarditis in biopsied specimens at a very early stage of the disease.[15-22] In those cases which have been followed for several years, right bundle branch block or left axis deviation persists even when the patient has clinically recovered and returned to full activity.[17] Patients who have recovered from myocarditis may also show persistent minor electrocardiographic changes or arrhythmias and various conduction disturbances.[19] A few of these cases may progress to dilated cardiomyopathy.[19]

When a biopsy is performed in cases of ventricular arrhythmia or bundle branch block as the main presenting features, postmyocarditic changes[20,22,23] are observed. A diagnosis of viral myocarditis is suggested on review of a history of an acute viral illness preceding the development of cardiac symptoms.

It is generally considered that sick sinus syndrome and advanced A-V block or fascicular block are diseases of the conduction system only and regarded as a gerontologic disorder as in Lev's disease.[29-32] Lenegre's disease is considered a disease of the conduction system in the young.[33] Both Lev's and Lenegre's disease can be differentiated from what we call ECM,[5] because we define ECM to be restricted in those cases where diffuse involvement of heart muscle disease is confirmed by endomyocardial biopsy.[6]

Acknowledgement

This study was supported by a grant from the Japan Research Promotion Society for Cardiovascular Diseases.

REFERENCES

1. Report of the WHO/ISFC task force on the definition and classification of cardiomyopathies. *Br. Heart J.* **44**: 672–673, 1980.
2. Olsen, E.G.J. Definitions of cardiomyopathies and specific heart muscle disease. In this volume, pp. i–vi.
3. Sekiguchi, M., Hiroe, M., Morimoto, S., and Kawagoe, Y. The contribution of endomyocardial biopsy to the diagnosis and assessment of cardiomyopathies. In: Hayase, S. and Murao, S., eds. International Congress Series No. 470. Proceedings of the VIII World Congress of Cardiology. Excerpta Medica., Amsterdam, pp. 583–590, 1979.
4. Sekiguchi, M., Hasegawa, A., and Ando, M. A proposal for analyzing the familial occurrence of cardiomyopathy in the clinical situation. In: Cardiomyopathy: Clinical, pathological and theoretical aspects. Sekiguchi, M. and Olsen, E.G.J. (eds.), Univ. of Tokyo Press, Tokyo, and Univ. Park Press, Baltimore, p. 445–453, 1980.
5. Sekiguchi, M., Hasumi, M , Hiroe, M., Kasanuki, H., Ohnishi, S., and Hirosawa, K. On the existence of non-hypertrophic, non-dilated cardiomyopathy as assessed by endomyocardial biopsy and a proposal for the term "electric disturbance type of cardiomyopathy". *Circulation* **72**: suppl. III-156. 1985 (abstr.)
6. Sekiguchi, M., Hiroe, M., Hasumi, M., Nishikawa, T., Ohnishi, S., Kasanuki, H., and Hirosawa, K. Endomyocardial biopsy approach to various arrhythmias and condition disturbances: In: Iwa T. (ed.) Proceedings of the Free Paper Session of the International Symposium on Cardiac Arrhythmias, Excerpta Medica, Amsterdam, pp. 76–79, 1987.
7. Hasegawa, A., Sekiguchi, M., Hasumi, M., Take, M., Hosoda, S., Nishikawa, T. and Hiroe, M. High incidence of significant pathology in endomyocardial biopsy and familial

occurrence in cases with arrhythmia and/or conduction disturbance. *Heart and Vessels* Suppl. 3: 24–26, 1990.

8. Sakakibara, S., and Konno, S. Endomyocardial biopsy. *Jap. Heart J.* 3: 537–543, 1962.

9. Konno, S., Sekiguchi, M., and Sakakibara, S. Catheter biopsy of the heart. *Radiol. Clin. North Am.* 9: 491–510, 1971.

10. Sekiguchi, M. and Konno, S. Diagnosis and classification of primary myocardial disease with the aid of endomyocardial biopsy. *Jpn. Circul. J.* 35: 737–754, 1971.

11. Sekiguchi, M., Hiroe, M., and Morimoto, S. On the standardization of histopathological diagnosis and semiquantitative assessment of the endo-myocardium obtained by endomyocardial biopsy. *Bull. Heart Inst., Japan*, 55–85, 1979–1980.

12. Sekiguchi, M., Hiroe, M., Ogasawara, S., and Nishikawa, T. Practical aspects of endomyocardial biopsy. *Ann. Acad. Med. Singapore* 10 Suppl.: 115–128, 1981.

13. O'Connell, J.B., Robinson, J.A., Subramanlian, R., and Scanlon, P.J. Endomyocardial biopsy: Technique and applications in heart disease of unknown cause. *Heart Transplantation* 3: 132–143, 1984.

14. Sekiguchi, M., Hiroe, M., Kasanuki, H., Ohnishi, S., and Hirosawa, K.: Experience of 100 atrial endomyocardial biopsy and the concept of atrial cardiomyopathy. *Circulation* 70: Suppl II-118, 1984 (abstract).

15. Sekiguchi, M., Hiroe, M., Take, M., and Hirosawa, K. Clinical and histopathological profile of sarcoidosis of the heart and acute myocarditis; II. Myocarditis. *Jpn. Circ. J.* 44: 264–273, 1980.

16. Take, M., Sekiguchi, M., Hiroe, M., and Hirosawa, K. Early clinical profiles of histopathologically proven cases with acute idiopathic myocarditis and a proposal for diagnostic criteria. *Jpn. Circul. J.* 45: 1415–1420, 1981.

17. Take, M., Sekiguchi, M., Hiroe, M., and Hirosawa, K. Long-term follow-up of electocardiographic findings in patients with acute myocarditis proven by endomyocardial biopsy. *Jpn. Circul. J.* 46: 1227–1234, 1982.

18. Sekiguchi, M., Hiroe, M., Yu, Z.-X., and Hasumi, M. A serial endomyocardial biopsy study on myocarditis. In: Pathogenesis of myocarditis and cardiomyopathy: Recent experimental and clinical studies. Kawai, C, and Abelmann, W.H. (eds.) Univ. of Tokyo Press, pp. 213–231, 1987.

19. Sekiguchi, M., Hiroe, M., Hiramitsu, S., and Izumi, T. Natural history of acute viral idiopathic myocarditis: A clinical and Endomyocardial biopsy follow-up. In: New Concepts in Viral Heart Disease: Virology, Immunology and Clinical Management. Schultheiss, H.-P. (ed) Springer, pp. 33–50, 1988.

20. Hasumi, M., Sekiguchi, M., Morimoto, S., Take, M., Hiroe, M., Ohnishi, S., Kasanuki, H., and Hirosawa, K. Catheter biopsy assessed cardiomyopathic and postmyocarditic changes in cases with atrioventricular or intraventricular conduction disturbance. In Cardiac Pacing, ed by Steinbach K et al., Steinkopf Verlag, Darmstadt, p. 101–108, 1983.

21. Hasumi, M., Sekiguchi, M., Morimoto, S., Take, M. and Hirosawa, K. Ventriculographic findings at the convalescent stage in eleven cases with acute myocarditis. *Jpn. Circ. J.* 47: 1310–1316, 1983.

22. Hasumi, M., Sekiguchi, M., Yu, Z.-X., Hirosawa, K., and Hiroe, M. Analysis of histopathologic findings in cases with dilated cardiomyopathy with special reference to formulating diagnostic criteria on the possibility of postmyocarditic change. *Jpn. Circ. J.* 50: 1280–1287, 1986.

23. Hasumi, M., Sekiguchi, M., Hiroe, M., *et al.* Endomyocardial biopsy approach to patients with ventricular tachycardia with special reference to arrhythmogenic right ventricular dysplasia. *Jpn. Circul. J.* 51: 242–249, 1987.

24. Hasumi, M., Sekiguchi, M., Morimoto, S., Ogasawara, S., Kasanuki, H., and Hirosawa, K. High incidence of detecting myocardial pathology with fatty tissue in cases with idiopathic ventricular tachycardia with and without right ventricular enlargement. A right ventricular

endomyocardial biopsy study. *Circulation* **72**: Suppl. III-46 1985 (abstr.)

25. Fontaine, G., Frank, R., Tonet, J.O., Guiraudon, G., Cabrul, C., Chomette, G., and Grosgogeat, Y. Arrhythmogenic right ventricular dysplasia: A clinical model for the study of chronic ventricular tachycardia. *Jpn. Circul. J.* **48**: 515–538, 1984.

26. Marcus, F.I., Fontaine, G., Guiraudon, G., Frank, R., Laurencear, J.L., Malergue, C., and Crosgogeat, Y. Right ventricular dysplasia: A report of 24 adult cases. *Circulation* **65**: 384–398, 1982.

27. Sekiguchi, M., Numao, Y., Imai, M., Furuie, T., and Mikami, R. Clinical and histopathological profile of sarcoidosis of the heart and acute idiopathic myocarditis. Concepts through employing endomyocardial biopsy I. Sarcoidosis. *Jpn. Circ. J.* **44**: 249–263, 1980.

28. Perloff, J.K., Roberts, W.C., deLeon, A.C., and O'Doherty, D. The distinctive electrocardiogram of Duchenne's progressive muscular dystrophy. *Am. J. Med.*, **42**: 179–188, 1967.

29. Gallagher, J.J. Mechanisms of arrhythmias and conduction abnormalities. In: The Heart Arteries and Veins. Hurst, J.W. (ed.). McGraw-Hill, 1984, pp. 489–519.

30. Ferrer, M. The sick sinus syndrome in atrial disease. *JAMA* **206**: 645–646, 1968.

31. Lev, M. The pathology of complete atrioventricular block. *Progr. Cardio. Dis.* **6**: 317–326, 1964.

32. Sugiura, M., Iizuka, H., Ohkawa, S., and Okada, R. Conduction system in 8 cases of AV conduction disturbances. *Jpn. Heart J.* **11**: 460–469, 1970.

33. Lenegre, J. Etiology and pathology of bilateral bundle braunch block in relation to complete heart block. *Progr. Cardiov. Dis.* **6**: 409–444, 1964.

The Cardiac Conduction System in Cardiomyopathy and Myocarditis

Thomas N. James

World Health Organization Cardiovascular Laboratory and the
Department of Medicine and Department of Pathology, University of Texas Medical Branch,
Galveston, Texas, U.S.A.

ABSTRACT

Arrhythmias and conduction disturbances are commonplace in both cardiomyopathy and myocarditis and are often blamed for sudden death. Accordingly, postmortem examination of the sinus node, AV node, and His bundle offers a special opportunity for meaningful correlation of clinical and pathologic observations. Three features of the morphology of the conduction system are useful in histologic evaluation. They are the special nutrient arteries of the conduction system, its remarkably rich innervation, and its anatomical proximity to normally abundant collagen. Just as the etiology of both cardiomyopathy and myocarditis varies greatly, so do the types of anatomical lesions to be found in the conduction system. However, the conduction system virtually always contains distinctive although varied lesions. There are other factors contributing to arrhythmogenesis in such patients, such as ventricular hypertrophy or focal myocardial lesions or extracardiac abnormalities of autonomic nerves or the brain, but the great frequency with which conduction system abnormalities exist in such cases suggests that they are of primary importance.

INTRODUCTION

Virtually every cardiac disease either causes or predisposes to electrical instability of the heart, some more than others. Cardiomyopathy and myocarditis are no exceptions; in fact, arrhythmias, conduction disturbances, syncope, and sudden death are characteristic of both diseases. Neither cardiomyopathy nor myocarditis is a single form of disease. On the contrary, each of them represents a wide assortment of processes, and each of them has been defined differently, depending upon the purpose of the definer.

To discuss abnormalities of the cardiac conduction system found in fatal cases of cardiomyopathy or myocarditis, this paper uses the following definitions. *Cardiomyopathy* includes those conditions in which the primary clinical problem resides in the myocardium. Valvular or arterial or pericardial abnormalities may coexist but they must be of lesser clinical importance. Specific diseases such as amyloidosis, scleroderma, and Friedreich's ataxia may cause cardiomyopathy, but myocardial abnormalities can also occur without apparent cause and should then be designated as idiopathic. Predictably, continued research will steadily reduce the numbers of idiopathic cases by discovering new explanations. For example, there is growing recognition that abnormalities of small coronary arteries may be the fundamental fault in an undetermined but possibly large percentage of cases of cardiomyopathy previously considered to be "idiopathic."[1-11]

Myocarditis encompasses all inflammatory diseases of the myocardium, whether caused by infection or not. Thus, the myocarditis of pheochromocytoma[12,13] and of Friedreich's ataxia[14] is manifested by inflammation secondary to multiple small foci of active degeneration or necrosis, and in both of these examples obstruction of multiple small coronary arteries is the probable mechanism. Other noninfectious forms of myocarditis include those found with collagen diseases or immunologic disorders such as lupus erythematosus,[15] polyarteritis nodosa,[16] and rheumatoid arthritis.[17] Infectious myocarditis may be diffuse (as seen with varicella or diphtheria) or focal and associated with granuloma formation (e.g., tuberculosis or Whipple's disease). Just as with cardiomyopathy, some cases of myocarditis remain unexplained despite careful investigation, and these also are best termed "idiopathic." In general, the presence of inflammation within the myocardium is necessary for the definition of myocarditis while it is unusual to find inflammation in cases of cardiomyopathy, although, as will be discussed below, there is nothing which would prevent genuine myocarditis from becoming superimposed upon cardiomyopathy.

INVOLVEMENT OF THE CARDIAC CONDUCTION SYSTEM

To the present author's knowledge there is no special affinity for the conduction system in myocarditis or cardiomyopathy, nor is there any known resistance or immunity to its involvement. Such involvement is largely a matter of chance,[18] whatever the underlying disease may be. The longer the disease exists, the greater the probability that the conduction system will be affected.

There are certain anatomical characteristics of the conduction system which help explain when and how it may become involved. First, rather consistent and specific nutrient arteries perfuse the sinus node[19] as well as the atrioventricular (AV) node and His bundle.[20] Thus, those protracted and progressive diseases known to cause narrowing of small coronary arteries may be expected sooner or later to involve arteries of the conduction system and consequently to destabilize the electrical activity of the heart (Figs. 1 and 2).

Second, both the sinus node and AV node are in close proximity to abundant normal collagen, with the entire framework of the sinus node being composed of an interwoven matrix of collagen,[19] while the AV node lies directly upon the mass of collagen forming the central fibrous body.[20] Whether the collagen in these 2 widely separated locations is of the same type is an unanswered and possibly important question. The His bundle for much of its course is completely surrounded by collagen, initially within the central fibrous body and then later at the base of the membranous interventricular septum. It is hardly surprising, therefore, that some diseases causing collagen abnormalities will have prominent effects upon the conduction system (Fig. 3). Within the AV junction the relationship between conduction tissue and fibroblasts is dynamic, accounting not only for normal postnatal morphogenesis of the AV node and His bundle,[21] but also for certain changes observed later in life.[22]

Third, the entire conduction system is richly innervated and all diseases with neurotropic features may include those special nerves of the heart which reside within or near the sinus node, AV node, or His bundle. Diseases of the cardiac neural structures (nerves, ganglia, and special neuroreceptors) are best collectively termed cardioneuropathies.[23] Cardioneuropathies are focal in nature, so that neural influence on the sinus node may become impaired while that to the AV node is preserved. This can lead to puzzling paradoxes. For example, with the reflex heart block occurring under such circumstances during any vagal reflex,[24] the functional abnormality (heart block) resides

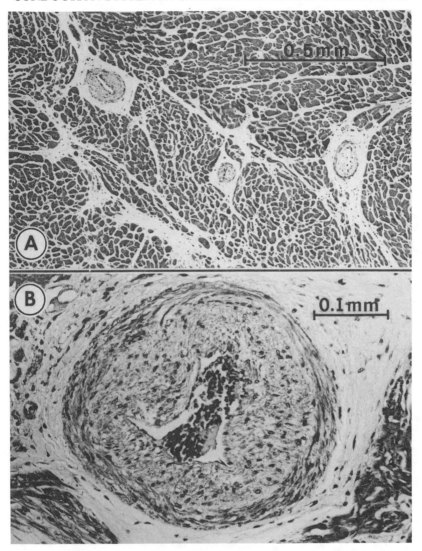

Fig. 1. Focal fibromuscular dysplasia is shown narrowing arteries in the interventricular septum (A) and in the AV node (B) from a fatal case of scleroderma heart disease. Goldner trichrome stain here and in all other photomicrographs unless otherwise indicated. All magnifications are indicated with reference bars. Reproduced from James[27] with permission of the publisher.

in a normal structure (AV node and His bundle) because of failure of the usually concomitant response by a diseased structure (sinus node and its local nerves) which has no primary responsibility for AV conduction.

CHARACTERISTICS AND PECULIARITIES OF CONDUCTION SYSTEM INVOLVEMENT BY CERTAIN DISEASES

A study of "idiopathic" cardiomyopathy in the form of asymmetrical hypertrophy of the heart demonstrated a variety of abnormalities in the conduction system.[25] Since

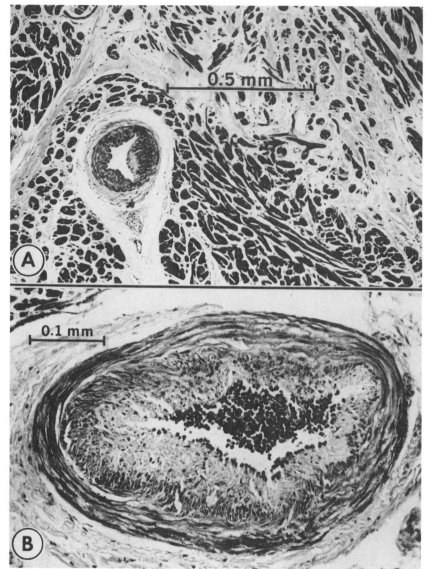

Fig. 2.   These 2 photomicrographs illustrate narrowed small coronary arteries
of 2 different fatal cases of asymmetrical hypertrophy of the heart. A is from
left ventricular myocardium and B is the AV node artery. Reproduced from
James and Marshall[25] with permission of the publisher.

the cases were chosen because they had all died suddenly and unexpectedly, one might
expect that there would be problems with the conduction system, but the variety of
their nature was surprising. Slightly less than half of the 22 hearts (10) exhibited narrowed small coronary arteries, including those supplying the conduction system. The
sinus node was sclerosed by excessive fibrosis in 12 of the 22, and the His bundle was
abnormally narrowed in 3. All 22 hearts exhibited fetal dispersion of the AV node and
His bundle,[26] and in 13 of these the dispersion was particularly conspicuous. Such a
wide assortment of abnormalities in the conduction system also suggests a variety of
possible mechanisms by which the heart may become electrically unstable.

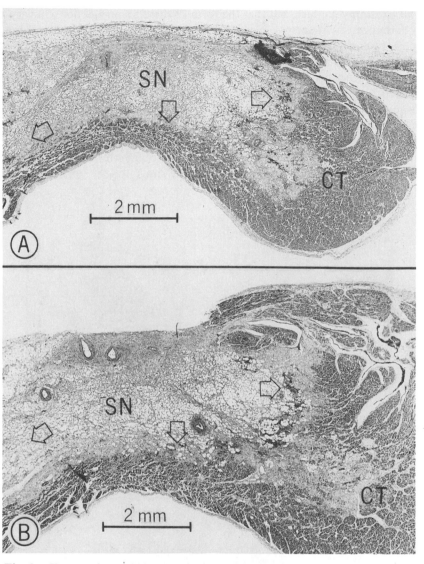

Fig. 3. Two sections of sinus node (A and B) have been photographed from sites about 2 mm apart in the heart of a fatal case of disseminated lupus erythematosus. Much of the substance of the sinus node (SN) has been destroyed by extensive cystic degeneration, with the margin (open arrows) of this process exhibiting recent hemorrhage and sweeping centrifugally into the nearby crista terminalis (CT) as well as toward the sinus intercavarum in the opposite direction.

Both asymmetric hypertrophy of the heart and the sudden death which so frequently accompanies it probably develop by a number of different pathogenetic mechanisms. Whether the heart in cardiomyopathy hypertrophies symmetrically or asymmetrically may only be a matter of chance, or at least there is no clear evidence of separate forms of pathogenesis. Given our present state of knowledge (or ignorance) of the matter, it is logical to anticipate that abnormalities of the conduction system may be characteristic of all cardiomyopathies, but that the form of these abnormalities will vary widely.

Scleroderma causes abnormal focal fibrosis throughout the myocardium, but this is often extraordinarily severe in the sinus node.[27] Scleroderma cardiomyopathy is also characterized by focal fibromuscular dysplasia of multiple small coronary arteries throughout the heart, including the nutrient arteries of the conduction system (Fig. 1). Abnormal collagen formation in the tunica media may be an etiologic factor in the focal fibromuscular dysplasia which narrows the small coronary arteries, which may in turn cause or exacerbate multifocal fibrosis in the myocardium.

Amyloidosis not only infiltrates myocytes directly, it also infiltrates the walls of both small and large coronary arteries and narrows or obliterates their lumens. Perhaps because it is in essence a periarterial structure, the sinus node is sometimes completely

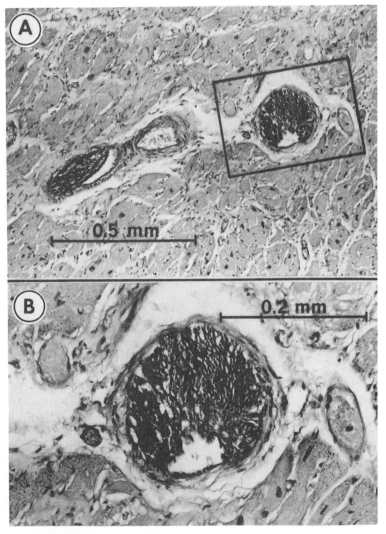

Fig. 4. Schiff-positive material is shown here narrowing the lumen of 2 small arteries of the right atrium near the sinus node of a patient dying of cardiomyopathy associated with Friedreich's ataxia. The artery boxed in A is seen at higher magnification in B. Periodic acid Schiff stain. Reproduced from James[2] with the permission of the publisher.

destroyed in cardiac amyloidosis.[28] Conversely, hemochromatosis rarely involves coronary arteries and seems conspicuously to spare the sinus node, although it prominently affects both the AV node and the His bundle, which helps explain the heart block so often recognized in cases of cardiac hemochromatosis.[29]

Cardiomyopathy is an important complication of several different heritable musculoskeletal or neuromuscular diseases such as Marfan's syndrome[30] and progressive muscular dystrophy.[31] The complex nature of these cardiomyopathies is well illustrated by Friedreich's ataxia (Figs. 4 and 5), where there are striking and possibly unique le-

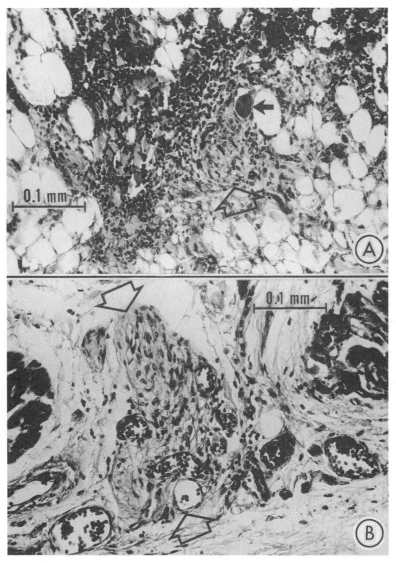

Fig. 5. Cardioneuropathy is illustrated here from 2 different sites near the sinus node of a second case of fatal cardiomyopathy associated with Friedreich's ataxia. Black arrow in A marks a degenerating neuron of a ganglion, while open arrows mark degeneration within nerves in both A and B. There is a mixture of local hemorrhage and infiltration of inflammatory cells. Reproduced from James et al.[32] with the permission of the publisher.

sions consisting of Schiff-positive deposits within the walls of small coronary arteries[32] accompanied by extensive cardioneuropathy, and these neurovascular lesions randomly involve any or all elements of the conduction system. Actually, an analogous explanation applies to the underlying morphologic abnormalities to be found in fatal cases of any disease associated with atrial fibrillation: there is no specific or unique abnormality characteristic of atrial fibrillation, but the cardiac conduction system is virtually never

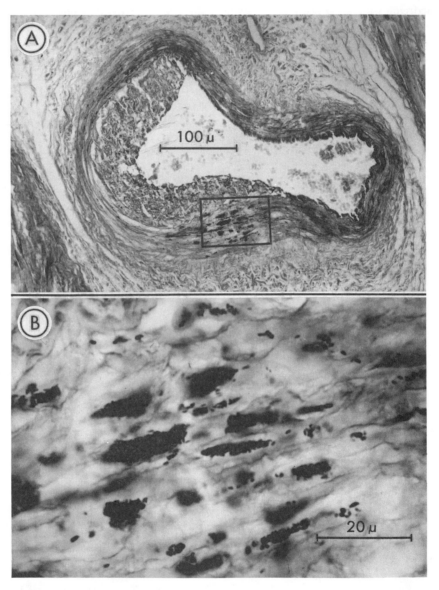

Fig. 6.   A small artery in the left ventricle of a patient with fatal cardiomyopathy due to Whipple's disease exhibits an arc of apparent atherosclerosis, but as seen in the boxed area of A with higher magnification in B, the tunica media is heavily infiltrated with Schiff-positive bacilli, some in dense clusters. Other bacilli are seen scattered throughout the tunica media. Periodic acid Schiff stain. Reproduced from James and Bulkley[37] with the permission of the publisher.

free of morphologic abnormalities plausibly contributing to the pathogenesis of atrial fibrillation.[33] It may be further noted that atrial fibrillation is a clinically serious complication of many cases of cardiomyopathy.[34]

Too often the exact etiology of myocarditis remains obscure. This is true not only for cases presumed to be viral in nature but also for some bacteria. Fortunately for the diagnostic clinician, extracardiac manifestations of the underlying disorder can provide valuable clues to its identification. Three notable examples are tuberculosis, diphtheria, and Whipple's disease, each of which can cause myocarditis and each of which may involve the conduction system. With diphtheria, which is frequently associated with heart block, not only is there active myocarditis involving sinus node and AV node, but cardioneuropathy is prominent, just as would be anticipated with a disease known for its neurotropic features.[35] Whipple's disease may be associated with Schiff-positive bacilli directly invading the conduction system and various nerves and ganglia, but the same type bacilli are also readily identified within the tunica media of small coronary arteries,[36,37] a surprising but intriguing observation of significance in a context broader than the rare recognized cases of Whipple's disease (Fig. 6).

GENERAL CONSIDERATION OF CONDUCTION SYSTEM ABNORMALITIES IN CARDIOMYOPATHY AND MYOCARDITIS

Among many hypotheses about the pathogenesis of idiopathic cardiomyopathy, 2 recurring ones are an abnormality of small coronary arteries[1-11] and some form of unusual neural influence upon the heart.[38-49] Of course, these 2 processes are not mutually exclusive, since the excessive sympathetic neural tone putatively causing myocardial hypertrophy is also a plausible explanation for focal fibromuscular dysplasia of small coronary arteries. Excessive sympathetic neural tone may be intermittent, but its recurring positive inotropic effect ending in hypertrophy of myocardium would be longer-lasting. Narrowed small coronary arteries could cause focal myocardial ischemic degeneration, each focus being small and individually unimportant but the eventual effect of many such foci would lead to compensatory myocardial hypertrophy of surviving myocytes for which the work load would inevitably be increased.

If an abnormal antibody is in some way responsible for either cardiomyopathy or myocarditis, it need not be primarily antimyocyte (for working myocardium) but could be antiarterial (either against endothelium or smooth muscle of tunica media or vascular collagen) or antineural, or combinations of these targets. Whether the etiologic hypothesis being considered is vascular or neural or antibody or a combination of these, the conduction still becomes vulnerable because of its normally rich innervation, its special arterial blood supply, and its composition of special myocytes.

With myocarditis, the etiologic considerations usually emphasize myocardial involvement, and perhaps correctly so. However, any disease with prominent neurotropic features could have its cardiac involvement primarily through focal inflammation or degeneration of the intracardiac nerves which are normally so widely distributed that the visualized lesions could be misinterpreted by the inexperienced as primarily myocardial in nature. The same concern may apply for coronary arteries, especially smaller ones, although lesions of the larger coronary arteries, at least, can be more readily identified correctly as primarily arterial in nature.

Having one disease seldom precludes the existence or development of another disease. A diagnosis of cardiomyopathy does not prevent the occurrence of myocarditis. Concerning the conduction system, there are several anatomical variants or distortions which by themselves may be relatively innocuous but could become functionally important in the subsequent presence of either cardiomyopathy or myocarditis. For example, a right-sided His bundle occurs normally in about 15% of human hearts,[50] but the remarkably narrow origin of the entire left bundle branch system in such cases (about 1 mm maximal dimensions) places all of the normal left ventricular activation at jeopardy if that narrow left bundle origin is by chance the site of a tiny focus of myocarditis; and cases of sudden unexpected death have exhibited exactly such lesions.[51]

Another important example of normal anatomical variation in the configuration of the AV node or His bundle is the persistence of fetal dispersion of fragments of conduction tissue throughout the central fibrous body.[21,22] Such dispersed fragments may be either few in number or very extensive, but in either case they sometimes form loops connecting one part of the AV node to another (Fig. 7), providing exactly the substrate for circus movement so dear to the hearts of both experimental and clinical electrophysiologists in their explanations of supraventricular tachycardias and related forms of electrical instability of the heart. Fragments detached from the AV node but remaining connected to the crest of the interventricular septum (Fig. 7) form an anatomically and physiologically ideal location for the genesis of parasystolic rhythms.[52] Myocarditis

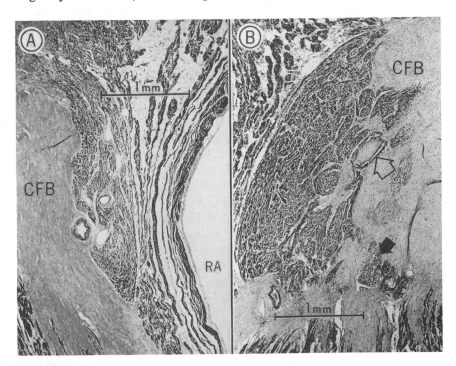

Fig. 7.   Persistent fetal dispersion of the AV node is shown in B from a case of sudden unexpected death. An open arrow indicates a loop of AV nodal tissue protruding into the central fibrous body (CFB); the cellular continuity of this loop was documented with serial sections. The black arrow indicates a fragment of AV nodal tissue detached from the AV node but in continuity with the crest of the interventricular septum below. For comparison a normal AV node is shown in A; note the absence of any dispersed fragments of AV node. Orientation of the two sections is reversed, with CFB to the left in A but to the right in B. RA marks the cavity of the right atrium in A. Reproduced from James and Marshall[26] with the permission of the publisher.

sometimes involves fragments of conduction tissue which are dispersed in the central fibrous body (Fig. 8). The essential point is that anatomical (and functionally important) variations or abnormalities of the conduction system may preexist or simply coincide with either cardiomyopathy or myocarditis.

Having claimed that the conduction system is often and perhaps always involved in fatal cases of cardiomyopathy or myocarditis, one must not ignore other arrhythmogenic features of these 2 conditions. Whether primarily hypertrophic or dilated, cardiomyopathy always provides a greater expanded geometric configuration of the heart, with a resultant increased dispersion of refractory periods and other features favoring the onset of arrhythmias. As a corollary, these same features make the treatment of arrhythmias more difficult. Hypertrophied hearts not only fibrillate more easily, but are more difficult to defibrillate.[53-57] Similarly, foci of fibrosis or of myocarditis make the heart electrically inhomogeneous even if the conduction system itself is normal. Some special forms of myocardial disease are notoriously associated with intractable arrhythmias, one example being sarcoid heart disease,[58] and in them arrhythmogenesis may be equally attributable to focal lesions in the ventricular myocardium as well as within the conduction system. Furthermore, for many systemic diseases causing either cardiomyopathy or myocarditis, the extracardiac involvement of either the autonomic nervous system or the brain could additionally have significant arrhythmogenic effects.

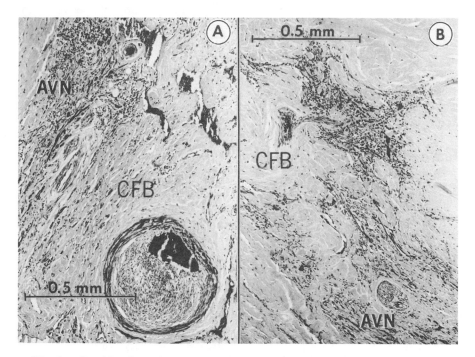

Fig. 8. Combination of multiple different abnormalities is shown here within the conduction system from a fatal case of myocarditis due to rheumatoid heart disease. Persistent fetal dispersion of the AV node (AVN) is present within the central fibrous body (CFB). Inflammatory infiltration of the AV node in A and throughout a large fragment dispersed within the CFB in B is accompanied by focal fibromuscular dysplastic narrowing of the AV node artery in A and of a smaller branch seen in B. Reproduced from James[17] with the permission of the publisher.

PRACTICAL SYNTHESIS CONCERNING INVOLVEMENT OF THE CONDUCTION SYSTEM IN CARDIOMYOPATHY AND MYOCARDITIS

For the clinician it is important to know that the conduction system is often and perhaps always involved in fatal cases of either cardiomyopathy or myocarditis, although the exact histological nature of the involvement varies. Additional factors contributing to electrical instability of the heart include myocardial hypertrophy or dilation, focal fibrosis or degeneration or inflammation of myocardium, and certain extracardiac problems originating in the autonomic nervous system or the brain. Most of these conditions not only favor the development of arrhythmias but also make them more difficult to treat. Since involvement of the conduction system in cardiomyopathy or myocarditis is probably a random circumstance, longer duration of the disease increases the chance of such involvement.

For the pathologist it should be mandatory to examine the conduction system in all fatal cases of cardiomyopathy or myocarditis, but especially when rhythm or conduction disturbances were documented or when death occurred suddenly and unexpectedly. Abnormalities of small arteries (especially those supplying the sinus node or the AV node and His bundle), of cardiac neural structures or of collagen may prominently involve the conduction system. Congenital or postnatal morphologic variations of the conduction system may preexist or simply coincide with either cardiomyopathy or myocarditis; these independent morphologic findings may become of special functional significance in the presence of either cardiomyopathy or myocarditis.

It is apparent that careful postmortem examination of the cardiac conduction system provides a special opportunity for meaningful correlation between clinical and pathological observations in cardiomyopathy and myocarditis. Unlike focal lesions distributed in the ventricular myocardium, those found in the conduction system more readily lend themselves to precise interpretation as to their functional significance. Such opportunities should never be dismissed.

ACKNOWLEDGMENT

This work was supported by the Pegasus Fund of the University of Texas Medical Branch in Galveston.

REFERENCES

1. James, T.N. An etiologic concept concerning the obscure myocardiopathies. *Prog. Cardiovasc. Dis.* **7**: 43–65, 1964.
2. James, T.N. Small arteries of the heart. The 36th George E. Brown Memorial Lecture. *Circulation* **56**: 2–14, 1977.
3. Andrade, Z.A. and Teixeira, A.R.L. Changes in the coronary vasculature in endomyocardial fibrosis and their possible significance. *Am. Heart J.* **86**: 152–158, 1973.
4. McReynolds, R.A. and Roberts, W.C. The intramural coronary arteries in hypertrophic cardiomyopathy. *Am. J. Cardiol.* **35**: 154, 1975.
5. Simons, M. and Downing, S.E. Coronary vasoconstriction and catecholamine cardiomyopathy. *Am. Heart J.* **109**: 297–304, 1985.
6. Factor, S.M. and Sonnenblick, E.H. Microvascular spasm as a cause of cardiomyopathies. *Cardiovasc. Rev. Rep.* **4**: 1177–1182, 1983.
7. Maron, B.J., Wolfson, J.K., Epstein, S.E., and Roberts, W.C. Intramural ("small vessel") coronary artery disease in hypertrophic cardiomyopathy. *J. Am. Coll. Cardiol.* **8**: 545–557, 1986.

8. Cohen, M.V. Coronary vascular reserve in the greyhound with left ventricular hypertrophy. *Cardiovasc. Res.* **20**: 182–194, 1986.

9. Cannon, R.O. III, Cunnion, R.E., Parrillo, J.E., Palmeri, S.T., Tucker, E.E., Schenke, W.H., and Epstein, S.E. Dynamic limitation of coronary vasodilator reserve in patients with dilated cardiomyopathy and chest pain. *J. Am. Coll. Cardiol.* **10**: 1190–1200, 1987.

10. Tanaka, M., Fujiwara, H., Onodera, T., Wu, D.-J., Matsuda, M., Hamashima, Y., and Kawai, C. Quantitative analysis of narrowings of intramyocardial small arteries in normal hearts, hypertensive hearts and hypertrophic cardiomyopathy. *Circulation* **75**: 1130–1139, 1987.

11. Zoneraich, S. Small-vessel disease, coronary artery vasodilator reserve, and diabetic cardiomyopathy. *Chest* **94**: 5–7, 1988.

12. Van Vleit, P.D., Burchell, H.B., and Titus, J.L. Focal myocarditis associated with pheochromocytoma. *N. Engl. J. Med.* **274**: 1102–1108, 1966.

13. James, T.N. De Subitaneis Mortibus. XIX. On the cause of sudden death in pheochromocytoma, with special reference to the pulmonary arteries, the cardiac conduction system and the aggregation of platelets. *Circulation* **54**: 348–356, 1976.

14. Russell, D.S. Myocarditis in Friedreich's ataxia. *J. Pathol. Bacteriol.* **58**: 739–748, 1946.

15. James, T.N., Rupe, C.E., and Monto, R.W. Pathology of the cardiac conduction system in systemic lupus erythematosus. *Ann. Intern. Med.* **63**: 402–410, 1965.

16. James, T.N. and Birk, R.E. Pathology of the cardiac conduction system in polyarteritis nodosa and its variants. *Arch. Intern. Med.* **177**: 561–567, 1966.

17. James, T.N. De Subitaneis Mortibus. XXIII. Rheumatoid arthritis and ankylosing spondylytis. *Circulation* **55**: 669–677, 1977.

18. James, T.N. Chance and sudden death. *J. Am. Coll. Cardiol.* **1**: 164–183, 1983.

19. James, T.N. The sinus node. Opening Plenary Address, American College of Cardiology. *Am. J. Cardiol.* **40**: 965–986, 1977.

20. James, T.N. Structure and function of the AV junction. The Mikamo Lecture for 1982. *Jpn. Circ. J.* **47**: 1–47, 1983.

21. James, T.N. Cardiac conduction system: Fetal and postnatal development. *Am. J. Cardiol.* **25**: 213–226, 1970.

22. James, T.N., Spencer, M.S., and Kloepfer, J.C. De Subitaneis Mortibus. XXI. Adult onset syncope, with comments on the nature of congenital heart block and the morphogenesis of the human atrioventricular septal junction. *Circulation* **54**: 1001–1009, 1976.

23. James, T.N. Primary and secondary cardioneuropathies and their functional significance. *J. Am. Coll. Cardiol.* **2**: 983–1002, 1983.

24. James, T.N., Urthaler, F., and Hageman, G.R. Reflex heart block. *Am. J. Cardiol.* **45**: 1182–1188, 1980.

25. James, T.N. and Marshall, T.K. De Subitaneis Mortibus. XII. Asymmetrical hypertrophy of the heart. *Circulation* **51**: 1149–1166, 1975.

26. James, T.N. and Marshall, T.K. De Subitaneis Mortibus. XVIII. Persistent fetal dispersion of AV node and His bundle within central fibrous body. *Circulation* **53**: 1026–1034, 1976.

27. James, T.N., De Subitaneis Mortibus. VIII. Coronary arteries and conduction system in scleroderma heart disease. *Circulation* **50**: 844–856, 1974.

28. James, T.N. Pathology of the cardiac conduction system in amyloidosis. *Ann. Intern. Med.* **65**: 28–36, 1966.

29. James, T.N. Pathology of the cardiac conduction system in hemachromatosis. *N. Engl. J. Med.* **271**: 92–94, 1964.

30. James, T.N., Frame, B., and Schatz, I.J. Pathology of the cardiac conduction system in Marfan's syndrome. *Arch. Intern. Med.* **144**: 339–343, 1964.

31. James, T.N. Observations on the cardiovascular involvement (including the cardiac conduction system) in progressive muscular dystrophy. *Am. Heart J.* **63**: 48–56, 1962.

32. James, T.N., Cobbs, B.W., Coghlan, H.C., McCoy, W.C., and Fisch, C. Coronary disease,

cardioneuropathy and conduction system abnormalities in the cardiomyopathy of Friedreich's ataxia. *Br. Heart J.* **57**: 446–457, 1987.

33. James, T.N. Diversity of histopathologic correlates of atrial fibrillation. In: Atrial Fibrillation. Kulbertus, H.E., Olsson, S.W., and Schlepper, M. (eds.), A.B. Hassle, Molndal, Sweden 1982, pp. 13–32.

34. Glancy, D.L., O'Brien, K.P., Gold, G.H., and Epstein, S.E. Atrial fibrillation in patients with idiopathic hypertrophic subaortic stenosis. *Br. Heart J.* **32**: 652–659, 1970.

35. James, T.N. and Reynolds, E.W., Jr. Pathology of the cardiac conduction system in a case of diphtheria associated with atrial arrhythmias and heart block. *Circulation* **28**: 263–267, 1963.

36. James, T.N. and Haubrich, W.S. De Subitaneis Mortibus. XIV. Bacterial arteritis in Whipple's disease. *Circulation* **52**: 722–731, 1975.

37. James, T.N. and Bulkley, B.H. Abnormalities of the coronary arteries in Whipple's disease. *Am. Heart J.* **105**: 481–491, 1983.

38. Laks, M.M., Morady, F., and Swan, H.J.C. Myocardial hypertrophy produced by chronic infusion of subhypertensive doses of norepinephrine in the dog. *Chest* **64**: 75–78, 1973.

39. Blaufuss, A.H., Laks, M.M., Garner, D., Ishimoto, B.M., and Criley, J.M. Production of ventricular hypertrophy stimulating "idiopathic hypertrophic subaortic stenosis" (IHSS) by subhypertensive infusion of norepinephrine (NE) in the conscious dog. *Clin. Res.* **23**: 77A, 1975.

40. Berg, R.A., Moss, J., Baum, B.J., and Crystal, R.G. Regulation of collagen production by the β-adrenergic system. *J. Clin. Invest.* **67**: 1457–1462, 1981.

41. Amorim, D.S. and Olsen, E.G.J. Assessment of heart neurons in dilated (congestive) cardiomyopathy. *Br. Heart J.* **47**: 11–18, 1982.

42. Tomanek, R.J., Bhatnager, R.K., Schmid, P., and Brody, M.J. Role of catecholamines in myocardial cell hypertrophy in hypertensive rats. *Am. J. Physiol.* **11**: H1015–H1021, 1982.

43. Kawai, C., Yui, Y., Hoshino, T., Sasayama, S., and Matsumori, A. Myocardial catecholamines in hypertrophic and dilated (congestive) cardiomyopathy: A biopsy study. *J. Am. Coll. Cardiol.* **2**: 834–840, 1983.

44. Downing, S.E. and Lee, J.C. Contribution of α-adrenoceptor activation to the pathogenesis of norepinephrine cardiomyopathy. *Circ. Res.* **52**: 471–478, 1983.

45. Cutilletta, A.F., Erinoff, L., Heller, A., Low, J., and Oparil, S. Development of left ventricular hypertrophy in young spontaneously hypertensive rats after peripheral sympathectomy. *Circ. Res.* **40**: 428–434, 1977.

46. Bernardi, D., Bernini, L., Cini, G., Ghione, S., and Bonechi, I. Asymmetric septal hypertrophy and sympathetic overactivity in normotensive hemodialyzed patients. *Am. Heart J.* **109**: 539–545, 1985.

47. Trimarco, B., Ricciardelli, B., De Luca, N., De Simone, A., Cuocolo, A., Galva, M.D., Picotti, G.B., and Condorelli, M. Participation of endogenous catecholamines in the regulation of left ventricular mass in progeny of hypertensive parents. *Circulation* **72**: 38–46, 1985.

48. Golf, S., Myhre, E., Abdelnoor, M., Anderson, D., and Hansson, V. Hypertrophic cardiomyopathy characterised by β-adrenoceptor density, relative amount of β-adrenoceptor subtypes and adenylate cyclase activity. *Cardiovasc. Res.* **19**: 693–699, 1985.

49. Ganguly, P.K., Dhalla, D.S., Innes, I.R., Beamish, R.E., and Dhalla, N.S. Altered norepinephrine turnover and metabolism in diabetic cardiomyopathy. *Circ. Res.* **59**: 684–693, 1986.

50. Massing, G.K. and James, T.N. Anatomical configuration of the His bundle and bundle branches in the human heart. *Circulation* **53**: 609–621, 1976.

51. James, T.N., Schlant, R.C., and Marshall, T.K. De Subitaneis Mortibus. XXIX. Randomly distributed focal myocardial lesions causing destruction in the His bundle or a narrow-origin left bundle branch. *Circulation* **57**: 816–823, 1978.

52. James, T.N. Normal and abnormal variations in anatomy of the atrioventricular node and His bundle and their relevance to the pathogenesis of reentrant tachycardias and para-

systolic rhythms. In: Cardiac Electrophysiology and Arrhythmias. Zipes, D.P. and Jalife, J. (eds.), Grune & Stratton, New York, 1985, pp. 301–310.

53. Anderson, K.P., Stinson, E.B., Derby, G.C., Oyer, P.E., and Mason, J.W. Vulnerability of patients with obstructive hypertrophic cardiomyopathy to ventricular arrhythmia induction in the operating room. *Am. J. Cardiol.* **51**: 811–816, 1983.

54. Messerli, F.H., Ventura, H.O., Elizardi, D.J., Dunn, F.G., and Frohlich, E.D. Hypertension and sudden death. Increased ventricular ectopic activity in left ventricular hypertrophy. *Am. J. Med.* **77**: 18–22, 1984.

55. Brandenburg, R.O. Cardiomyopathies and their role in sudden death. *J. Am. Coll. Cardiol.* **5**: 185B–189B, 1985.

56. Chapman, P.D., Sagar, K.B., Wetherbee, J.N., and Troup, P.J. Relationship of left ventricular mass to defibrillation threshold for the implantable defibrillator: A combined clinical and animal study. *Am. Heart J.* **114**: 274–278, 1987.

57. Kohya, T., Kimura, S., Myerburg, R.J., and Bassett, A.L. Susceptibility of hypertrophied rat hearts to ventricular fibrillation during acute ischemia. *J. Mol. Cell. Cardiol.* **20**: 159–168, 1988.

58. James, T.N. De Subitaneis Mortibus. XXV. Sarcoid heart disease. *Circulation* **56**: 320–326, 1977.

Pathology of Diseases of the Cardiac Conduction System

Ryozo Okada

Division of Cardiology, Department of Internal Medicine, Director of Research Laboratory for Cardiovascular Pathology, School of Medicine, Juntendo University, Tokyo, Japan

ABSTRACT

In this study, the conduction systems in patients with various arrhythmias were histologically examined using the serial sectioning method. The sinus node and sinoatrial junctions in the sick sinus syndrome show considerable fibrosis and adiposis. The His bundle and radicles of the bundle branches are infiltrated by adipose tissue and fibrosis, and have a close relationship to the sclerocalcific changes in the central fibrous body in Lev's disease. Both bundle branches are replaced by fibrosis in Lenegre's disease.

Paraconduction system bypass tracts, such as nodoventricular and fasciculoventricular fibers, occur in certain cases of postmyocarditic cardiomegaly.

The Purkinje cells are swollen and surrounded by fibrosis in the hereditary long QT syndrome. They are separated from the working myocytes by adipose tissue in arrhythmogenic right ventricular dysplasia.

Various pathologic lesions in the conduction system of those patients who die suddenly include hemorrhage, necrosis, adiposis, fibrosis, hypertrophy, and fibromuscular dysplasia of the supplying arteries; these could be influenced primarily and secondarily by abnormal nerve tonus and/or catecholamine stimulation.

INTRODUCTION

Clinicians are now able to make use of a variety of approaches to evaluate arrhythmias by using sophisticated electrophysiologic equipment to aid in the diagnosis and selection of the appropriate therapy. Yet, if clinicians lack a basic knowledge of the etiologies involved in the pathologic processes of the conduction system, they will not be able to prognosticate or select the appropriate therapy.

A pathologic study of the conduction system is essential in establishing the etiology of arrhythmias. Such research, however, requires many exhausting hours of labor to serially section the entire conduction system. The present author has examined histopathologically the conduction systems of more than 150 autopsied hearts, which during life showed numerous types of arrhythmias. All research was done using complete serial sectioning according to Lev's method,[1,2] as well as multiple-step sectioning of the internodal tracts and the Purkinje cell networks in the ventricles.

The present paper is based on that research, and focuses on several points of special interest. In every heart the main pathologic lesions were in the conduction system.

SINCK SINUS SYNDROME

The normal sinus node shows a gradual development of fibrosis and adiposis in and/or around the node. These are assumed to be part of the physiologic aging process.[3]

The sick sinus syndrome, which is partly related to changes in the sinus node and atrial myocardium due to aging, is pathologically divided into two types.[4] Type one, pure sinus node disease, has a high incidence among the elderly. It is characterized by sinus arrest and sustained bradycardia. The sinus node has shrunk and is severely fibrotic, with a significant loss of nodal cells. In the atrioventricular (AV) node, changes are characterized by severe fatty infiltration also accompanied by a considerable loss of nodal cells in a majority of cases. In such cases, the pathologic diagnosis is binodal disease and its etiology is still unknown. However, complications of ischemic heart disease, valvular disease, diabetes mellitus, and malignancies coexist in certain cases.

Type 2 is a sinoatrial (SA) junction disease, which has a high incidence among the middle-aged. It is usually associated with brady-tachyarrhythmia. In the sinus node, a fairly good number of nodal cells are preserved, with some fatty tissue infiltrated from the epicardial side. The main lesion is found at the SA junction. Severe fibrosis and adiposis have almost completely interrupted the anterior or posterior SA junction, as shown in Fig. 1, and have partially interrupted the other SA junctions. The internodal tracts have also lost a considerable number of their cells due to fatty infiltration and fibrosis in many locations. This unequal interruption between the anterior and posterior radiations of the sinus node could help to cause a circular circuit of excitation in the atrial myocardium, which then provokes episodes of tachycardia. Alternatively, a transient complete block at both sides of the sinus node could cause an SA block with bradycardia. The etiologies of this condition include inflammation, ischemia due to arteriosclerosis, and amyloid infiltration.

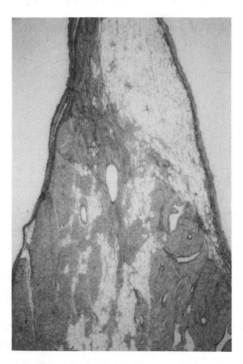

Fig. 1.   Sinus node from a patient with sick sinus syndrome. Note the fatty infiltration and fibrosis in the anterior SA junction. Weigert-van Gieson's stain, ×12.

ATRIOVENTRICULAR BLOCK AND BUNDLE BRANCH BLOCKS

AV block is known to have a variety of etiologies,[5] which include myocardial infarction, myocarditis, amyloidosis, and specific metabolic disorders. However, the etiology of the majority of the chronic AV blocks that usually occur in the elderly remains uncertain. Although sclerocalcific, primary degenerative, and idiopathic blocks have all been proposed for their nomenclature controversy as to exact pathologic process persists.[6,7]

Aging changes of the central fibrous body, which is located between the atrial and the ventricular myocardium and is penetrated by the His bundle, are strongly suspected to be responsible for AV block. With aging, collagen fibers show hyaline degeneration, focal accumulations of acid-mucopolysaccharides (aMPS), and irregular-shaped calcium deposition.[8] The His bundle and the proximal portions of the bundle branches appear to have been affected by aMPS infiltration from the surrounding central fibrous body. Also, both the degeneration and the disappearance of the conducting cells shown in Fig. 2 seem to have resulted from aMPS increase. Calcium deposition in and around the conduction system is also due to local aMPS pooling.

An increase in the calcium mass could press on and ultimately destroy the conducting cells as shown in Fig. 3. Thus, both sclerocalcific and primary degenerative changes may etiologically have a common base, and each affects the metabolic alteration of the

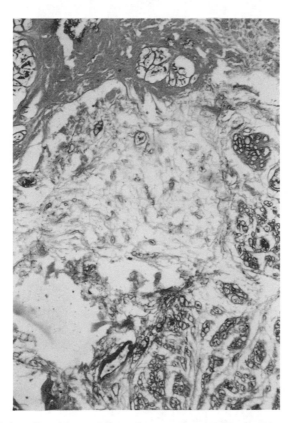

Fig. 2. His bundle with a primary degenerative AV block. Disappearing conducting cells are being replaced with fine connective tissue fibers. Bielschowsky-Maresch's stain, × 80.

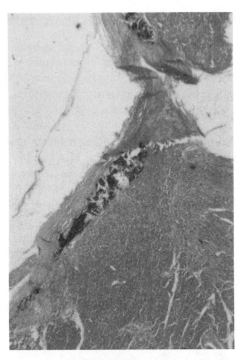

Fig. 3.   His bundle with a sclerocalcific block. A calcified mass in the central fibrous body occupies the bundle. Hematoxylin-eosin stain, × 13.

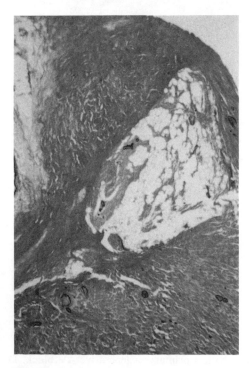

Fig. 4.   His bundle with adiposis. The lipomatous tissue replaces the conducting cells. Weigert-van Gieson's stain, × 40.

connective tissue in the elderly. Various conduction disturbances, such as a second- or a third-degree AV block or a bundle branch block, which includes an abnormal axis deviation, can be explained by the same mechanism. Myocyte loss from the penetrating

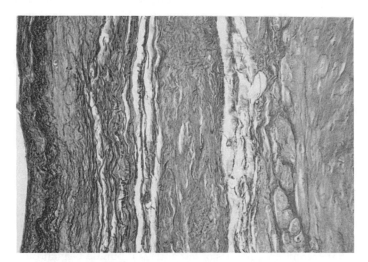

Fig. 5. Left bundle branch with fibrosis. Note the fibrous block of the bundle branch. Weigert-van Gieson's stain, × 80.

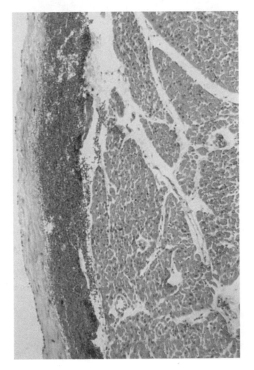

Fig. 6. Left bundle branch with hemorrhage. The subendocardial hemorrhage involves the anterior radiation of the left bundle branch. Hematoxylin-eosin stain, × 40.

portion of the His bundle to its branches, which include the radiations of both bundle branches, can cause any type of block. This disease group is known as Lev's disease.

Figure 4 shows severe infiltration of adipose tissue or a lipomatous lesion in the His bundle. The pathogenesis is still uncertain, but it may be an expression of chronic anoxia due to arteriolosclerosis or to excessive nervous stimulation, especially by catecholamines released from the nerve endings.

In Lenégre's disease, idiopathic bilateral bundle branch fibrosis is found (Fig. 5). The affected sites are several millimeters below the branching portions of the bundles instead of at the proximal portion, as in Lev's disease. Lenégre suggests that the etiology of this disease is due to microtrauma occurring in the subendocardial space, caused by friction as a result of too rapid a flow of blood in the ventricular outflow tract.[9]

Figure 6 shows a case of sudden-onset left-axis deviation.[10] The hemorrhage that has occurred in the subendocardial space on the left side of the ventricular septum extends throughout the territory of the proximal portion of the anterior radiation of the left bundle branch. If this patient had survived beyond the acute stage, the area of the hemorrhage would have become fibrotic and/or scar tissue would have formed. Assuming such a cause of events it can be speculated that a Lenègre type block, including both AV block and bundle branch block, could occur after hemorrhaging in the subendocardial space.

The author has encountered 2 types of left and right bundle branch block[11,12]: a proximal type derivative of Lev's disease, and a median type derivative of Lenegre's disease.

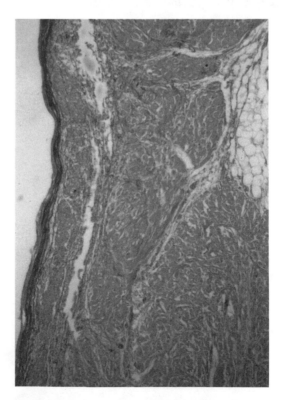

Fig. 7.   Bundle of Kent. Abnormal muscle band bridges between the right atrial and ventricular myocardium in a case of Ebstein's anomaly. Weigert-van Gieson's stain, × 32.

PREEXCITATION SYNDROMES

Preexcitation syndromes, including the W-P-W syndrome, L-G-L syndrome, and a bypass-conditioned tachycardial attack, bear a strict relationship to the existence of an abnormal myocyte connection between the atrial and ventricular myocytes. These preexcitation syndromes may also be due to an early connection of the AV conduction system to the atrial or ventricular myocardium.[13]

The bundle of Kent can be located anywhere near the atrioventricular valve rings. As shown in Fig. 7, this bundle usually contains 10 or more myocyte linings on both the atrial and ventricular sides, though the actual cell-to-cell connections over the fibrous rings can be distinguished only at a few points, i.e., 3 or 6 sites even in complete serial sections. The connecting cells resembling Purkinje cells, are hypertrophied especially on the ventricular side, and show a focal disarray around the fibrous ring.

Paraconduction system bypass tracts are composed of 3 types of fibers: James' fibers, nodoventricular or N-VS fibers,[14] and fasciculoventricular fibers or Mahaim's fibers. In certain cases of postmyocarditic cardiomegaly, multiple bypass tracts on the ventricular side have been detected along with preexcitation waves in EKG recordings. The AV conduction system of such cases, is usually hypertrophied, and cells of the bypass tracts are similar to those of the conduction system, as shown in Fig. 8.

In cases with no preexcitation waves, various types of blind bypass tracts were accidentally found. Some of them had an almost complete cellular connection between the atrial and ventricular myocytes. If such cases were to develop myocarditis, the abnormal stimulation could cause hypertrophy or even hyperplasia in the connecting cells. This would make preexcitation possible. Thus, an acquired preexcitation syndrome should be considered.

SUDDEN CARDIAC DEATH

Several special conditions such as the QT prolongation syndrome, arrhythmogenic

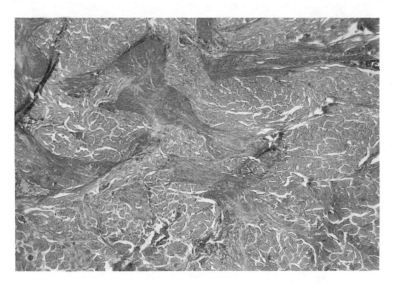

Fig. 8. Paraconduction system bypass. The AV node at the top is connected with the ventricular septum by zigzag running N-VS fibers. Weigert-van Gieson's stain, ×32.

right ventricular dysplasia, and Pokkuri disease have attracted interest in their relation to sudden death.

Figure 9 shows a case of the familial QT prolongation syndrome. The Purkinje cell networks on both the right and left ventricular sides are surrounded by extensive subendocardial fibrosis. The networks are interrupted irregularly and the Purkinje cells are swollen and degenerating.[15]

In cases of arrhythmogenic right ventricular dysplasia, free wall fatty infiltration in the right ventricle separates the subendocardial myocytes, including the Purkinje cells, from the middle and outer layers of the muscle.[16] A labyrinth of scattered myocytes can provoke ventricular arrhythmias through electrical reentry, in a manner similar to the QT prolongation syndrome. Strictly speaking, this type should be excluded from diseases of the conduction system. However, the presence of Purkinje cells in the subendocardial labyrinth, makes their participation in lethal arrhythmia highly suspect.

In cases of Pokkuri disease, some hearts show dual pathologic lesions in the conduction system. One is an advanced sinus node fibrosis associated with a U-turn or early multibranching of the sinus node artery which prevents direct blood supply to the node. Another is a fibrotic interruption of the right bundle branch and the anterior radiation of the left bundle branch, which is due to a sandwiched compression between a conal muscle bundle and the summit of the ventricular septum.[17]

In general, cases of sudden cardiac death with various etiologies often show a particular combination of pathologic lesions, such as fibromuscular dysplasia or minor anomalies of the sinus node and/or AV node arteries as shown in Fig. 10. Other pathologic lesions include: fibrosis of the sinus node; hypertrophy of the AV conduction system and of the occasional bypass tracts; fine, reticular fibrosis in the distal His bundle; and fibrosis, adiposis, or necrosis in and around the distal bundle branches and the Purkinje cells.[15]

A specific combination of pathologic lesions is also seen in patients who have been receiving L-Dopa therapy over a long period. This drug, acting as a catecholamine,

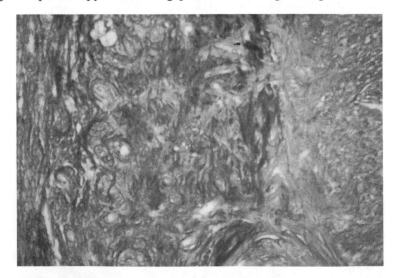

Fig. 9.   Purkinje cells of a case of hereditary long QT syndrome. The Purkinje cells surrounded by subendocardial fibrosis are swollen and degenerating. Azan stain, ×80.

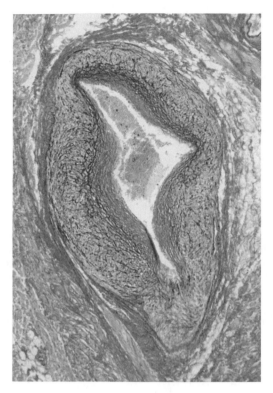

Fig. 10. AV node artery from a sudden death case. Note the fibromuscular dysplasia of the artery. Weigert-van Gieson's stain, × 32.

can cause sclerosis of the AV node artery, hypertrophy, and fibrosis in the AV conduction system, and focal myocardial lesions in the subendocardial area.

Diseases of the conduction system are greatly influenced by autonomic nerve activity, because of the presence of abundant nerve endings in the conduction system and their role in circulatory regulation.

The His bundle, an isolated, narrow muscle bundle, penetrates into the central fibrous body, which is a firm, connective tissue structure. Thus, pathologic changes in the connective tissue surrounding this bundle have a harmful effect on the conducting cells. Furthermore, the bundle branches can also be subjected to mechanical and/or hemodynamic stress as a result of the outflowing bloodstream from the ventricle, or stress from overstretching in cases involving dilatation or hypertrophy. The Purkinje cells and the Purkinje-working myocyte junctions may incur an altered sensitivity to catecholamines and to other active substances in the circulating blood. It is most likely that these factors work together in creating pathologic lesions in the conduction system, resulting in the tragedy of sudden death.

Although present knowledge of conduction system diseases is limited, it is hoped that the experience described above will encourage further research, leading to new therapies, enhancing the possibility of those prone to conduction system diseases to enjoy a normal, healthy life.

ACKNOWLEDGMENTS

This research was partly supported by a grant for group study of cardiomyopathies by the Ministry of Health and Welfare, Japan.

REFERENCES

1. Lev, M. and Watne, A.L. Method of routine histopathologic study of human sinoatrial node. *Arch. Pathol.* **57**: 168–177, 1954.
2. Lev, M., Widran, J., and Erickson, E.E. A method for the histological study of the atrio-ventricular node, bundle and branches. *Arch. Pathol.* **52**: 73–83, 1951.
3. Fujino, M., Okada, R., and Arakawa, K. The relationship of aging to histopathological changes in the conduction system of the normal human heart. *Jpn. Heart J.* **24**: 13–20, 1983.
4. Okada, R., Gotoh, K., Nakata, Y., and Kitamura, K. Pathology of the sick sinus syndrome. In: Cardiac Pacing. Proceedings of the Vth International Symposium, Tokyo, March 14–18, 1976, Watanabe, Y. (ed.), Excerpta Medica, Amsterdam, 1977, pp. 8–12.
5. Sugiura, M., Iizuka, H., Ohkawa, S., and Okada, R. Histological studies on the conduction system in 8 cases of A-V conduction disturbances. *Jpn. Heart J.* **11**: 460–469, 1970.
6. Davies, M.J. Pathology of Conducting Tissue of the Heart. Butterworth, London, 1971, pp. 63–119.
7. Lev, M. The conduction system. In: Pathology of the Heart and Blood Vessels, Gould, S.E. (ed.), 3rd ed., C.C. Thomas, Springfield, Ill., 1968, pp. 180–220.
8. Sugiura, M., Okada, R., Hiraoka, K., and Ohkawa, S. Histopathological studies on the conduction system in 14 cases of right bundle branch block associated with left axis deviation. *Jpn. Heart J.* **10**: 121–132, 1969.
9. Lenegre, J. Les blocs auriculo-ventricularis complets chronique. Etude des causes et des lesions a propos de 37 cas. *Mal. Cardiov.* **3**: 311–343, 1962.
10. Takagi, T. and Okada, R. An electrocardiographic pathologic correlative study on left axis deviation in hypertensive hearts. *Am. Heart J.* **100**: 838–846, 1980.
11. Sugiura, M., Okada, R., Ohkawa, S., and Shimada, H. Pathological studies on the conduction system in 8 cases of complete left bundle branch block. *Jpn. Heart J.* **11**: 5–16, 1970.
12. Fukuda, K., Nakata, Y., Okada, R., and Takagi, T. Histopathological study on the conduction system of complete right bundle branch block with special reference to configuration of QRS complex. *Jpn. Heart J.* **20**: 831–841, 1979.
13. Okada, R. Pathology of the pre-excitation syndrome. In: Etiology and Morphogenesis of Congenital Heart Disease, Van Praagh, R., and Takao, A. (eds.), Futura Publishing Co., New York, 1980, pp. 515–526.
14. Okada, R., Mizutani, T., and Mochizuki, S. A morphological study on the conduction system of an autopsy case with idiopathic myocardiopathy showing W-P-W type EKG change. *Shinzo* **6**: 630–640, 1974. (in Japanese)
15. Okada, R. and Kawai, S. Histopathology of the conduction system in sudden cardiac death. *Jpn. Circul. J.* **47**: 573–580, 1983.
16. Okada, R. Sudden cardiac death in the adolescents. *Rinsho to Kenkyu* **64**: 1701–1710, 1987. (in Japanese)
17. Okada, R. and Gotoh, K. Pathology of the conduction system in Pokkuri disease (sudden death of unknown etiology in young men). In: Cardiac Arrhythmias: Recent Progress in Investigation and Management. Iwa, T. and Fontaine, G. (eds.), Elsevier, Amsterdam 1988, pp. 177–188.

Histopathology in Arrhythmia and Conduction Disturbance Associated with Cardiomyopathies

Masaya Sugiura, ** and Shin'ichiro Ohkawa*

* Tokyo Metropolitan Institute of Gerontology, Tokyo, Japan
** Tokyo Metropolitan Hiroo General Hospital, Tokyo, Japan

ABSTRACT

The incidence and lesions of arrhythmias or conduction disturbances in 43 autopsied cases with cardiomyopathies (27 HCM, 9 HOCM, 7 DCM) were studied by histologic examination of the conduction system. Atrioventricular conduction disturbance was found in 14 and atrial fibrillation (AF) in 20 cases. The incidence of conduction disturbance was 30.6% (11/36) in HCM and 42.9% (3/7) in DCM, and that of AF was 41.7% (15/36) in HCM and 71.4% (5/7) in DCM. It was noteworthy that all 8 out of the 36 HCM cases which showed characteristic atrial dilatation at autopsy revealed AF or sick sinus syndrome clinically and myocardial fibrosis and degeneration which included the SA node at autopsy.

INTRODUCTION

It is well known that various kinds of arrhythmias or conduction disturbance occur in cardiomyopathies.[1-4] Sick sinus syndrome (SSS) is relatively rare, while the incidence of atrioventricular (AV) conduction disturbance is high. This paper presents the results of histologic analysis of the conduction system in AV conduction disturbance and atrial arrhythmia in patients with cardiomyopathies seen in Tokyo Metropolitan institute of Gerontology.

PATIENTS AND METHODS

This report describes a total of 43 patients (18 men and 25 women) with cardiomyopathies (Table 1). There were 27 cases of hypertrophic non-obstructive cardiomyopathy (HNOCM), 9 of hypertrophic obstructive cardiomyopathy (HOCM), and 7 of dilated cardiomyopathy (DCM) among a consecutive autopsy of 3,300 elderly patients. The 27 HNOCM cases included 8 of marked atrial dilatation, which was named atrial type HCM.[5] Atrial volume was especially dilated in these cases, beyond the upper limit of atrial volume in 133 cases of persistent atrial fibrillation.

There were 14 cases of AV conduction disturbances, including 2 cases of AV block, 1 of bilateral bundle branch block (BBBB), 8 of left bundle branch block (LBBB), and 3 of right bundle branch block (RBBB). There were also 20 cases of atrial fibrillation.

Serial sectioning was used for histologic study of the conduction system, as in our previous investigation.[6] The grades of lesions were classified as follows: complete destruction as 5, 75% lesion as 4, 50% lesion as 3, 25% lesion as 2, slight lesion as 1.

RESULTS

Incidence of Arrhythmias or Conduction Disturbances

TABLE 1. Arrhythmias and Conduction Disturbance in Cardiomyopathy

	No.	M	F	AV Conduction disturbance				Atrial arrhythmia	
				AVB	BBBB	LBBB	RBBB	af	SSS
HNOCM	19	8	11	1	1	5	2	7	
HNOCM (Atrial dilatation type)	8	7	1			1	1	7	1
HOCM	9	1	8						
DCM	7	2	5	1		2		5	
Total	43	18	25	2	1	8	3	19	1
						14		20	

HNOCM: hypertrophic nonobstructive cardiomyopathy, HOCM: hypertropic obstructive cardiomyopathy, AVB: atrioventricular block, BBBB: bilateral bundle branch block, LBBB: left bundle branch block, RBBB: right bundle branch block, af: atrial fibrillation, SSS: sick sinus syndrome.

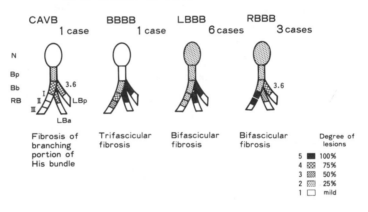

Fig. 1.   Lesions in AV conduction system in 11 cases of HCM. Abbreviations: those used in Table 1; N: AV node; Bp: penetrating portion of the AV bundle; Bb: branching portion of the AV bundle; RB: right bundle branch; LBp: posterior fascicle of left bundle branch; LBa: anterior fascicle of left bundle branch.

Conduction disturbances were noted in 30.6% of HCM cases (11/36), and in 42.9% of DCM cases (3/7). Incidence of atrial fibrillation was 41.7% (15/36) in HCM and 71.4% (5/7) in DCM, as shown in Table 1.

Arrhythmias or Conduction Disturbances in HCM

In the schematic presentation in Fig. 1, changes in the AV conduction system were shown in cases of HCM. A patient with complete AV block showed marked fibrosis at the branching portion of the AV bundle. A case of alternating bundle branch block showed severe damage to the first portion of the right bundle branch and complete interruption of the left bundle branch. In 6 cases of LBBB, interruption of the left

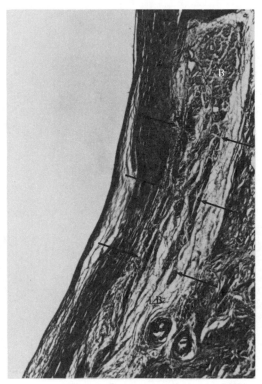

Fig. 2.   Branching portion of the AV bundle (B) in a case of complete AV block associated with HCM, which showed marked fibrosis (arrows) especially at the point of branching to the left bundle branch (LB). (Elastica van Gieson stain × 40)

bundle branch was complete. In 3 cases of RBBB, there was nearly complete interruption at the 1st or 2nd portion of the right bundle branch.

In a case of complete AV block, developing from a 2:1 block, His bundle electrogram showed an H-V block. Histologic sections in this case showed severe lesion (grade 4) at the branching portion of the AV bundle (Fig 2).

A 77-year-old woman, who had complete RBBB at the age of 72 and LBBB at the age of 74, developed torsade de pointes and advanced AV block necessitating implantation of a pacemaker, but she died suddenly. The posterior and anterior fascicles of the left bundle branch showed complete interruption at the branching portion. Severe fibrosis at the 1st portion of the right bundle branch was also revealed (Fig 3).

Histologic findings in 6 cases of LBBB showed fibrosis at the branching portion from the His bundle to the posterior and anterior fascicles of the left bundle branch. Fibrosis of the central fibrous body was evident, and persistence of the ghostlike remnants of the fascicles was additionally found. RBBB was found in 3 cases, showing interrupting lesions at the 1st or 2nd portion of the right bundle branch.

Arrhythmia in Atrial Dilatation Type of HCM

Histologic findings of atria in this particular type of HCM were fibrosis, degeneration, and endocardial fibroelastosis. Border zone between sinoatrial (SA) node and right atrium showed marked fibrosis, fatty infiltration in half of cases. In the SA node, there were fibrosis in 4 cases, reduced conduction cells in 3 cases.

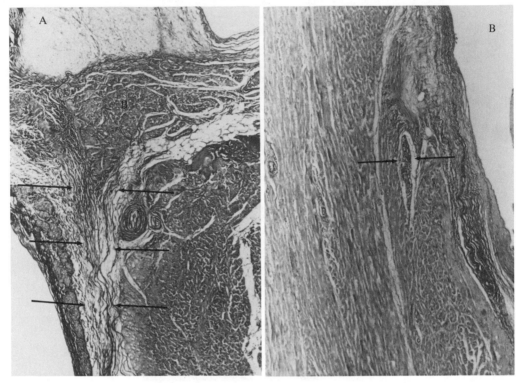

Fig. 3.   A case of BBBB associated with HCM. A: Fibrosis at the anterior fascicle of the left bundle branch (arrows). B: Fibrosis at the first portion of the right
bundle branch (arrows). (EvG × 40)

A case of a 71-year-old man was previously reported,[7] which was also considered
to be this type of HCM with atrial fibrillation and bradycardia. There was marked
fibrosis of the right atrium, including the SA node and the crista terminalis, and the
left atrial wall showed marked fibrosis and endocardial fibroelastosis.

A case of sick sinus syndrome in an 85-year-old man had sinus bradycardia and
junctional escape beats. His bundle electrogram showed prolongation of the P-A interval
to 70 msec, an A-H interval of 120 msec, and an H-V interval of 50 msec. The SA node
showed marked fibrosis that included the peripheral regions; the SA node artery showed
fibromuscular dysplasia with marked narrowing (Fig. 4).

Histologic findings in the usual type of HCM with atrial fibrillation revealed a con-
tiguity of the SA node with a normal right atrial myocardium, or the SA node surrounded by fatty tissues. In either case the right atrial muscle was devoid of marked
fibrosis, which could be the point of differentiation from the atrial type of HCM. The
atrial type of HCM shows markedly dilated atrial volume, with sick sinus syndrome
or atrial fibrillation, and is histologically characterized by fibrosis of the whole atria,
including the SA node.

Arrhythmias or Conduction Disturbances in Dilated Cardiomyopathy

The summary of pathologic findings in 7 cases of DCM was reported previously.[8]
Heart weight was 527g in average. Valvular ring was dilated, and atrial and ventricular
volumes were increased. Histological patterns were those of fibrosis in 3 cases, hyper-

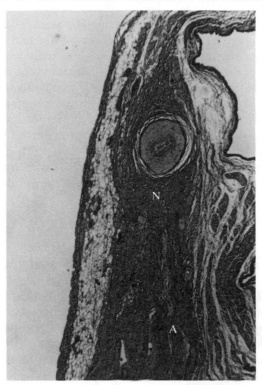

Fig. 4. A case of SSS associated with atrial type of HCM. Marked fibrosis of the whole atria (A), including SA node (N). SA node artery showed marked fibromuscular dysplasia. (EvG × 20)

LESIONS IN AV CONDUCTION SYSTEM IN 3 CASES OF DCM

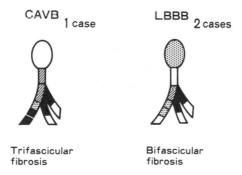

Fig. 5. Lesions in AV conduction system in 3 cases of DCM. Abbreviations: as in Fig. 1.

trophy in 2, degeneration in 1, and mixed type in 1.

Conduction disturbance was found in 3 out of 7 cases of DCM (Fig 5). A case of complete AV block showed fibrosis of both the left and the right bundle branch; that is, trifascicular fibrosis. Two cases of LBBB were both due to complete interruption of the left bundle branch.

A 60-year-old man had a long history of congestive heart failure and complete heart block, and showed a marked cardiomegaly weighing 590 g and globular shape at autopsy. The thickness of the ventricular septum was markedly reduced, to several mm. Histologic examination of the upper part of the interventricular septum showed marked fibrosis at the branching portion of the AV bundle to the left bundle branch. Survey of the right lower portion of the interventricular septum showed nearly complete loss of the right bundle branch. Lesions of the conduction system in this case were due to a secondary process from marked septal fibrosis, and not to primary changes in the conduction system itself.

Histologic findings of the conduction system in LBBB complicated with DCM showed that the lesions of the LBB were fibrotic in the middle of the His bundle or at the branching portion of the His bundle.

DISCUSSION

The incidence of complicating conduction disturbances was 30.6% (11/36) in HCM and 42.9% (3/7) in DCM. Incidence of atrial fibrillation was 41.7% (15/36) in HCM and 71.4% (5/7) in DCM, indicating higher incidence of both arrhythmias in DCM.[2,9]

The literature contains many reports concerning the conduction disturbances that complicate cardiomyopathy. But there have been few reports on the histological examination of the conduction system.[10-16] Fatal complications in cases with HCM were found in 2 cases of sudden death, and the presence of the accessory pathways was revealed by Krikler et al.[10] Bharati et al.[11] showed corresponding lesions in cases of LBBB. Maron et al.[12] found interruption of the His bundle in a case of congenital heart block; Hamamoto et al.[13] reported fibromuscular hyperplasia in the SA node artery in a patient with atypical hypertensive heart disease with asymmetric septal hypertrophy who died suddenly.

Concerning complication with DCM, Ohkawa et al.[14] reported a case of LBBB, showing fatty infiltration of the left bundle branch in histologic examination. Davies et al.[15] suggested the influence of diffuse myocardial lesions in 20 cases of AV block. Imamura et al.[16] reported fibrosis of the bilateral bundle branch in a case of complete AV block.

Lesions of the conduction system found in cases of HCM were not different from those in usual conduction disturbances, with fibrosis in various parts of the conduction system. Atrial dilatation in cases of atrial type HCM, accompanied by fibrosis of the whole atria including the SA node, resulted in the development of atrial fibrillation or sick sinus syndrome.

The conduction system in our cases of DCM was involved in severe myocardial fibrosis. In 2 cases of complete LBBB, fibrosis or cellular loss in the His bundle was considered as a causative factor.

REFERENCES

1. Savage, D.D., Seides, S.F., Clark, C.E. et al. Electrocardiographic findings in patients with obstructive and nonobstructive hypertrophic cardiomyopathy. Circulation 58: 402–408, 1978.
2. Mori, H. and Niki, T. Electrocardiograms, Vectorcardiograms. In: All of Idiopathic Cardiomyopathy. Kawai, C. (ed.), Nankodo, Tokyo, 1978, pp. 228–238.
3. Canedo, M.I., Frank, M.J., and Abdulla, A.M. Rhythm disturbances in hypertrophic

cardiomyopathy: Prevalence, relation to symptoms and management. *Am. J. Cardiol.* **45**: 848–855, 1980.

4. Toshima, Y. and Koga, Y. Hypertrophic cardiomyopathy (diagnosis and pathogenesis). In: Idiopathic Cardiomyopathy. Oda, T. (ed.), Nagai-shoten, 1981, pp. 121–155.

5. Ohkawa, S., Kimura, M., Kuboki, K. *et al.* Hypertrophic cardiomyopathy (HCM) in the elderly, especially atrial type of HCM. At the 31st Annual Meeting of Clinical Cardiography, in Sept. 1985.

6. Sugiura, M., Hiraoka, K., Ohkawa, S. *et al.* A clinicopathological study on 25 cases of complete left bundle branch block. *Jpn. Heart J.* **20**: 163–176, 1979.

7. Kuwajima, I., Sakai, M., Shiraki, M. *et al.* An autopsy case of idiopathic atrial dilatation with bradycardia and hyperkalemia. *Shinzo* **8**: 1236–1243, 1976. (in Japanese)

8. Ohkawa, S., Inoue, J., and Sugiura, M. A clinicopathologic study of dilated cardiomyopathy in the aged. *J. Cardiography* **16** (Suppl. IX): 35–47, 1986.

9. Seipel, L., Breihardt, G., and Kuhn, H. Involvement of the sinus node and the conduction system in myocarditis and cardiomyopathy. In: International Boehringer Mannheim Symposia, Myocarditis Cardiomyopathy, Selected problems of pathogenesis and clinic. Just, H. and Schuster, H.P. (eds.), Springer-Verlag, Berlin, 1983, pp. 233–243.

10. Krikler, D.M., Davies, M.J., Rowland, E. *et al.* Sudden death in hypertrophic cardiomyopathy: associated accessory atrioventricular pathways. *Br. Heart J.* **43**: 245–251, 1980.

11. Bharati, S., McAnulty, J.H., Lev, M. *et al.* Idiopathic hypertrophic subaortic stenosis with split His bundle potentials. Electrophysiologic and pathologic correlations. *Circulation* **62**: 1373–1380, 1980.

12. Maron, B.J., Connor, T.M., and Roberts, W.C. Hypertrophic cardiomyopathy and complete heart block in infancy. *Am. Heart J.* **101**: 857–860, 1981.

13. Hamamoto, H., Okada, R., Yamashita, S. *et al.* An autopsy case of atypical hypertensive heart disease associated with asymmetric septal hypertrophy and sudden death, with special reference to histopathological examination of the conduction system. *Shinzo* **16**: 1083–1089, 1984. (in Japanese)

14. Ohkawa, S., Sugiura, M., Iizuka, T. *et al.* Three cases of idiopathic cardiomegaly in the aged, with special reference to the morphological specificity and to the conduction system. *Jpn. Heart J.* **12**: 305–315, 1971.

15. Davies, M.J., Anderson, R.H., and Becker, A.E. The Conduction System of the Heart. Butterworths, London, 1983, pp. 244–248, p. 261.

16. Imamura, M., Fukuda, K., Koono, T. *et al.* A case of dilated cardiomyopathy with complete atrioventricular block from early period, and coronary artery disease was verified at autopsy. *Shinzo* **16**: 284–290, 1984. (in Japanese)

Left Ventricular False Tendons: Incidence and Clinical Implications

Michihiro Suwa, Yutaka Yoneda, Kiyotaka Kaku, Hikaru Nagao, Yuzo Hirota, and Keishiro Kawamura

Third Division, Department of Internal Medicine, Osaka Medical College, Osaka, Japan

ABSTRACT

Left ventricular false tendons are fibrous bands in the left ventricle that contain the Purkinje fibers. Since our first report indicated coexistence of false tendons and premature ventricular contractions (PVCs), we have continued to evaluate their relationship. This paper consists of 3 parts: the prevalence of false tendons in patients with PVCs and without organic heart disease is discussed in the first part; the prevalence of the coexistence of false tendons and PVCs evaluated prospectively in a large healthy population in the second; and thirdly the electrophysiologic aspect of PVCs with false tendons. Among 187 healthy subjects, false tendons were demonstrated echocardiographically in 133 (71%). False tendons were detected in 127 (71%) and PVCs in 48 (27%) in 179 healthy subjects, after the exclusion of 8 with mitral valve prolapse. Because this suggested that false tendons were not always associated with PVC, we evaluated the coexistence according to the thickness and the site of the attachment in the left ventricle. Consequently, it was found that PVCs were associated significantly with thick (≥ 2 mm in thickness) and longitudinal tendons. Furthermore, in 9 patients with this coexistence the origin of PVCs was examined electrophysiologically by pace mapping or mechanical stimulation using electrodes on the endocardial surface connected to false tendons because PVCs indicated left bundle branch block pattern in about 80% of the patients with false tendons. From this second study, it was suggested that PVCs of the left bundle branch block pattern did not necessarily originate from the right ventricle, but could be of left ventricular origin. Although it has not been conclusively demonstrated that left ventricular false tendons are arrhythmogenic, the prevalence of false tendons and PVCs in a large population, the special relation between PVCs and the type of false tendons, and the electrophysiologic aspect of PVCs with false tendons, suggest that false tendons may be strongly related to the genesis of PVCs in apparently healthy subjects.

INTRODUCTION

False tendons in the left ventricle (LV) are fibrous bands that traverse the chamber from the ventricular septum to the free wall, from the free wall to the free wall, or from the ventricular wall to the papillary muscles or between the papillary muscles.[1] For about 100 years, they have been recognized as anatomic variations at autopsy.[2] Also, it is well known that most false tendons contain the Purkinje fibers ever since the first description by Tawara in 1906,[3] and tendons in canine ventricles have been used in electrophysiologic studies of the Purkinje fibers.[4] Recently, some false tendons have been easily demonstrated *in vivo* by 2-dimensional echocardiography.[5-9] It has frequently been emphasized that caution must be exercised in the identification of the LV endocardium of the ventricular septum and in the differential diagnosis of mural thrombus, since the echo from the tendon may mimic these structures.[5] Thus, it has been considered that LV false tendons are normal structural variants of no clinical significance. It has been reported that 34% to 50% of healthy subjects without organic heart disease have premature ventricular contractions (PVCs), and some of them have frequent, consecutive, multiform PVCs or ventricular tachycardia.[10-13] In 1983, we had an opportunity to observe one young male who was referred to us for the examination of frequent PVCs and whose cardiac status was normal except for the presence of a false tendon. That case suggested to us that false tendons might be one cause of PVCs.[8]

This paper describes the relation between PVCs and false tendons.

METHODS

This survey consists of 3 parts. First, we examined the prevalence of the coexistence of PVCs and LV false tendons in patients with PVCs. Next, the prevalence of LV false tendons and PVCs was evaluated prospectively in a large healthy population. The third part consists of electrophysiologic studies in patients with PVCs and LV false tendons without organic heart disease.

The diagnosis of false tendons was made when a fibrous abnormal band was noted in the LV cavity with 2-dimensional echocardiography, and PVCs were documented with continuous 24-hr ambulatory ECG monitoring. The possibility of the presence of organic heart disease was eliminated by history, physical examination, chest X-ray, routine electrocardiogram, and exercise stress test in addition to echocardiographic examination in these 3 studies. Cardiac catheterization including coronary cineangiogram was also performed in the third study.

RESULTS

Prevalence of False Tendons in Patients with PVCs

For the survey of the prevalence of LV false tendons in patients with PVCs, we examined 113 patients who consulted the outpatient clinic for the evaluation of PVCs. The prevalence of false tendons and the features of PVCs among these 113 patients are shown in Table 1. False tendons were detected in 85 (75%). In patients with false tendons, the focus of PVCs was single in 69% and bifocal in the rest. All patients with PVCs and without false tendons had a single focus, except for one patient. Coupled PVCs were seen in both groups, but sustained ventricular tachycardia was recorded only in patients with false tendons. In these 113 patients, all PVCs were suppressed by the exercise stress test; PVCs with false tendons were suppressed at a significantly (p < 0.05) lower heart rate than those without false tendons.

Prevalence of PVCs and False Tendons in Healthy Subjects

In the second study, the prevalence of LV false tendons and PVCs were prospectively evaluated in 187 healthy volunteers who underwent a complete cardiovascular examination: 118 men and 69 women aged 21 to 50 years (mean 36 ± 9). These healthy volunteers were the employees of an electric company, who participated in this study with informed concent.

Eight subjects were excluded because of the presence of silent mitral valve prolapse. False tendons were detected in 133 (71%) and PVCs were recorded in 48 subjects (24%). The study subjects were divided into 4 groups according to the presence or absence of

TABLE 1. Comparison of Premature Ventricular Contractions (PVCs) between Subject with and without False Tendons

	False tendon (+)	False tendon (−)
Total patients	113	
Number of patients	85 (75%)	28 (25%)
Age (mean)	40 ± 15 years	43 ± 13 years
Frequency of PVC	mean: 7095 beats/24 hr (10–44,589 beats)	mean: 10,659 beats/24 hr (10–40,632 beats)
Focus of PVC	single focus: 59 (69%) bifocus: 26 (31%)	single focus: 27 (96%) bifocus: 1 (4%)
Type of PVC	single: 42 couplets: 22 ($n=74$) salvos: 7 sustained ventricular tachycardia: 3	single: 14 couplets: 5 ($n=21$) salvos: 2
Suppressed heart rate of PVC on exercise stress test	118 ± 29/min*	143 ± 20/min

*: $p<0.05$, + : present, − : absent.

TABLE 2. Prevalence of False Tendons and PVCs in 179 Healthy Subjects

	False tendon (+)	False tendon (−)
PVC	40/127 (32%)*	8/52 (15%)

*: $p<0.05$. Reprinted with permission from Suwa et al.[17]

TABLE 3. Frequency and Form of PVCs in Subjects with and without False Tendons

	False tendon (+)	False tendon (−)
Frequency		
<1/hr	31	8
1 to 9/hr	5	0
10 to 29/hr	2	0
≧30/hr	2	0
Mean	96 beats/24 hr	3 beats/24 hr
Form		
Uniform	29	7
Multiform	6	1
Couplets	4	0
Ventricular tachycardia	1	0

Reprinted with permission from Suwa et al.[17]

false tendons and PVCs. PVCs and false tendons coexisted in 40 of the 179 subjects as shown in Table 2, and the presence of PVCs was significantly related to the presence of false tendons ($p<0.05$).

Among 48 subjects with PVCs, the frequency and the form of PVCs were compared

154   SUWA *ET AL.*

between those with and without false tendons. PVCs were less frequent in 8 subjects
without false tendons. In contrast, there was a wide variation in frequency in 40 subjects with false tendons and the mean frequency was 96 beats/24 hr. Among these 40
subjects with PVCs and false tendons, 29 had uniform, 6 had multiform, and 4 had
coupled PVCs, and one had nonsustained ventricular tachycardia (maximum 18 beats).
In contrast, 7 of 8 subjects with PVCs and without false tendons had uniform PVCs
(Table 3).

Among these 179 healthy volunteers, false tendons were detected in 127, 40 of whom

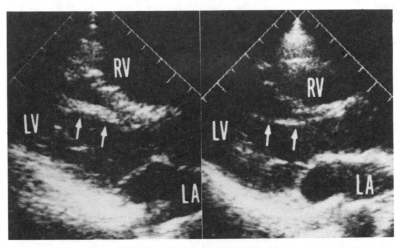

Fig. 1.   Two-dimensional echocardiograms of thick (≧2 mm) (left) and thin
(< 2mm) (right) false tendons (FT). LA, left atrium; LV, left ventricle; RV,
right ventricle. Reprinted with permission from Suwa *et al.*[17]

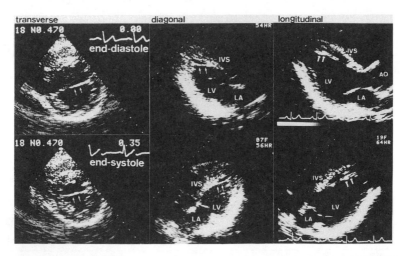

Fig. 2.   Two-dimensional echocardiograms of various types of false tendons.
False tendons are classified into 3 types according to their points of adherence
to the endocardium of the LV: 1) transverse type (left), a tendon is attached to
the interventricular septum (IVS) and the lateral wall transversely; 2) diagonal
type (middle), from the midportion of the IVS to the apical wall diagonally; and
3) longitudinal type (right), from the base of the ventricular septum to the apex
of the free wall longitudinally. Reprinted with permission from Suwa *et al.*[17]

TABLE 4.   Prevalence of PVCs in Relation to 6 Types of False Tendons in Patients with False Tendons

	Longitudinal type	Diagonal type	Transverse type
Thick type	76	14	4
PVC (+)	35 (46%)*	4 (29%)	1 (25%)
Thin type	21	6	6
PVC (+)	0	0	0

*: p < 0.005. Reprinted with permission from Suwa et al.[17]

had PVCs. This suggested that false tendons were not always associated with this arrhythmia. Therefore, we evaluated the coexistence according to the thickness and the site of the attachment of false tendons. False tendons were classified into 6 types according to the thickness and the sites of the attachment to the LV wall. We termed those 2 mm or greater in thickness "thick" and those less than 2 mm "thin" false tendons (Fig. 1). The 3 patterns of the attachment were: 1) transverse type; 2) diagonal type; and 3) longitudinal type (Fig. 2). Of the 127 subjects with false tendons, 94 had thick and 33 had thin tendons. PVCs were detected in 40 (43%) of the 94 subjects with thick tendons, but in none of the 33 with thin tendons. Accordingly, the presence of PVCs was significantly associated with thick tendons by chi-square analysis (p < 0.005). Longitudinal tendons were seen in 97 subjects, and transverse or diagonal tendons in 30 subjects. PVCs were noted in 35 subjects (36%) with longitudinal type, and in only 5 subjects (17%) with diagonal or transverse type. Thus, the occurrence of PVCs was significantly associated with the longitudinal type by chi-square analysis (p < 0.05). There were 76 subjects with both longitudinal and thick false tendons, and PVCs were observed in 35 (46%) of them. The coexistence of false tendons and PVCs was significantly higher than in the other 5 groups. Thus, the occurrence of PVCs was significantly related to longitudinal and thick tendons by chi-square analysis (p < 0.005) (Table 4).

Electrophysiologic Aspect of PVCs with False Tendons

In patients with PVCs and false tendons in the first study, about 80% of PVCs showed a left bundle branch block pattern on surface electrocardiograms, which was usually considered as originating from the right ventricle (Fig. 3). In patients without false tendons, PVCs also showed a left bundle branch block pattern in about 90% of them.

When all left bundle branch block pattern PVCs originate from the right ventricle, it is difficult to explain false tendons as a possible etiologic factor for them. Therefore, we performed an electrophysiologic study in 9 patients who had frequent PVCs or sustained ventricular tachycardia in association with false tendons. Endocardial stimulation, mechanical and/or electrical, was performed using a Josephson's mapping electrode with 2-dimensional echocardiography. The stimulations were carried out at 2 endocardial sites corresponding to the septal and free wall ends of the tendon. Spontaneous PVCs or ventricular tachycardia indicated left bundle branch block pattern in 6, right bundle branch block pattern in 2, and an intermediate pattern in one according to standard 12-leads electrocardiograms. The stimulations at the free wall end of the tendon provoked right bundle branch block pattern PVCs in all cases (9/9: 100%), but left bundle branch block pattern PVCs were also provoked on different occasions (2/9: 22%). Stimulation at the septal end was performed in 8 patients, and right bundle branch block pattern PVCs were provoked in 6 patients (6/8: 75%), left bundle branch block pattern PVCs

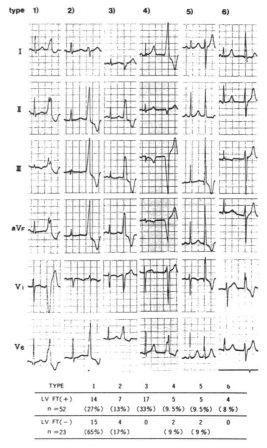

TYPE	1	2	3	4	5	6
LV FT(+) n =52	14 (27%)	7 (13%)	17 (33%)	5 (9.5%)	5 (9.5%)	4 (8%)
LV FT(−) n =23	15 (65%)	4 (17%)	0	2 (9%)	2 (9%)	0

Fig. 3. Electrocardiographic patterns of premature ventricular contractions (PVCs) with or without LV false tendons. In the 75 patients with PVCs and without underlying heart disease, PVCs were classified into 6 patterns according to bundle branch block pattern and QRS electrical axis of surface electrocardiograms (indicated by standard leads I, II, and III and precordial leads V_1 and V_6). Without relation to the presence (+) or the absence (−) of false tendons, more than 80% of PVCs showed a left bundle branch block pattern, but there was no presence of types 3 and 6 of PVCs in patients without false tendons.

TABLE 5. Relationship between QRS Pattern of PVCs Provoked by Stimulation and Stimulation Site of False Tendons

QRS pattern of PVC provoked by stimulation	Stimulation site of false tendons	
	Septal side ($n=8$)	Free wall side ($n=9$)
RBBB	6	9
LBBB	3	2
Intermediate	2	0

LBBB: left bundle branch block, RBBB: right bundle branch block.

in 3 (3/8: 38%), and intermediate pattern PVCs in 2 (2/8: 25%) (Table 5). From these results, it was suggested that left bundle branch block pattern PVCs did not necessarily originate from the right ventricle, but could be of left ventricular origin.

DISCUSSION

The Anatomical Aspects of False Tendons

The presence of LV false tendons has been recognized for a long time, since their first description as "moderator bands" by Turner.[2] The prevalence of LV false tendons has been reported to be about 50% in various autopsy studies. In a series of 483 autopsy specimens of human hearts from subjects evenly distributed by sex and age, Luetmer et al.[1] reported that the prevalence was 55%; the incidence was 48% in 636 children's hearts with various congenital cardiac malformation and 52% in the hearts of 50 adults who underwent surgery for acquired heart disease in the report by Gerlis et al.[14] LV false tendons were also present in 95% of 159 hearts from animals of 6 species.[14] From the fact that false tendons were present in about one-half of the human hearts examined and at all ages, it has been considered that this is a normal anatomic structure.

Echocardiographic Aspects of False Tendons

With the progress in the equipment for and skill in echocardiographic examination, we have been able to detect various intracardiac structures more easily. Nishimura et al.[5] and Okamoto and his colleagues[6] first revealed the echocardiographic features of LV false tendons in 1981. The echocardiographic importance of LV false tendons has been emphasized for the differential diagnosis from abnormal echoes in LV outflow tract or in the identification of the LV endocardium of the interventricular septum because the motion of the tendons is similar to that of the interventricular septum.[5,6]

The reported prevalence of LV false tendons demonstrated by 2-dimensional echocardiography varies from 0.4% to 71%,[5-9,15-17] and the prevalences were lower in echocardiographic studies than were found at autopsy. The variation in the reported prevalence is probably related to: 1) whether false tendons are noted incidentally during routine diagnostic examination or are intentionally searched for; and 2) differences in the skill or experience of the examiner in detecting false tendons. In 2 reports of false tendons from our department, the prevalence was 6.4% in the initial study[8] and 71% in the second study.[17] The tendons were examined intentionally in multiple echocardiographic cross-sections, such as a laterally angled long-axis view and a rotated 4-chamber view, in addition to routine observations in the latter. For detection, the examiner must understand that false tendons are frequently positioned eccentrically in the LV cavity. Figure 4 shows a routine parasternal long-axis section where false tendons are not seen (upper panel), but a thick false tendon is demonstrated on a laterally angled long-axis view in the same patient (lower panel). Also, the variable detection rate may be related to the quality of the transducer, but we think that this contribution is not so high.

Relationship between PVCs and False Tendons

The data suggest that the occurrence of PVCs is significantly related to the presence of false tendons in healthy subjects, and that there is a causal relation between them.

Left bundle branch block pattern PVCs are generally considered to originate from the right ventricle. In the first study, over 80% of the patients had PVCs of left bundle

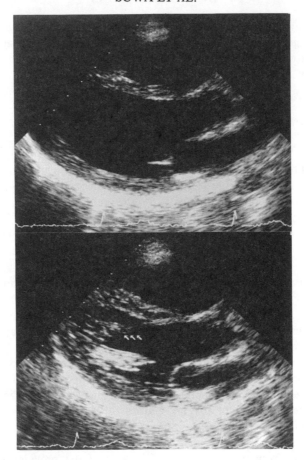

Fig. 4. Two-dimensional echocardiograms of routine parasternal (top) and laterally angled (bottom) long-axis views in a patient with a longitudinal tendon. A thick and longitudinal false tendon was detected on laterally angled long-axis view, but it could not be seen on routine parasternal long-axis view.

branch block pattern without relation to the presence or absence of false tendons. Although the electrophysiologic studies were performed in only 9 subjects, it was suggested that left bundle branch block pattern PVCs did not necessarily originate from the right ventricle, but could be of left ventricular origin. This may suggest that epicardial breakthrough is related to the occurrence or the conduction of PVCs associated with the tendons, especially those of left bundle branch block pattern.

Two hypotheses can be considered as possible mechanisms of PVCs related to false tendons. It is well known that the stretching of the Purkinje fibers increases the slope of phase 4 depolalization of transmembrane action potentials, and results in the development of PVCs in the LV.[18] Therefore, the stretching of false tendons may produce PVCs by increasing the slope of the resting potential of the Purkinje fibers. The other possibility is direct mechanical stimulation of the LV wall at the site of attachment. As thick false tendons may contain more Purkinje fibers and longitudinal false tendons are generally associated with greater stretching of the tendon and the adjacent tissue, this stretching theory is strongly suggestive of a mechanism for the production of PVCs. As electrocardiographic features, in the patients with false tendons 31 % revealed bifocal PVCs, suggesting 2 foci corresponding to 2 adhesion sites of the tendon. Also, PVCs were easily suppressed by exercise stress test in the patients with the tendon, as the tension of the tendon might be reduced by the reduction of LV size due to the increase of heart rate on exercise test. We consider that this evidence may also support the stretching mechanism hypothesis.

CONCLUSIONS

Although we cannot conclude definitely that LV false tendons are arrhythmogenic from these investigations, these indirect evidences strongly suggest that false tendons play an important role in the genesis of ventricular arrhythmias in apparently healthy subjects.

REFERENCES

1. Luetmer, P., Edwards, W.D., Seward, J.B., and Tajik, J.A. Incidence and distribution of left ventricular false tendons: An autopsy study of 483 normal human hearts. *J. Am. Coll. Cardiol.* **8**: 179–183, 1986.
2. Turner, W. A human heart with moderator band in left ventricle. *J. Anat. Physiol.* **27**: 19–20, 1893.
3. Tawara, S. Die Entwickelung der Leher von den Purkinjeschen Faden. In: Das Reizleitungsystem des Saugtierherzens. Gustav Fischer Verlags, Jena. 1906, pp. 158–189.
4. Katholi, R.E., Woods, W.T., Kawamura, K., Urthaler, F., and James, T.N. Dual dependence in both Ca^{2+} and Mg^{2+} for electrical stability in cells of canine false tendons. *J. Mol. Cell. Cardiol.* **11**: 434–445, 1979.
5. Nishimura, T., Kondo, M., Umadome, H., and Shimono, Y. Echocardiographic features of false tendons in the left ventricle. *Am. J. Cardiol.* **48**: 177–183, 1981.
6. Okamoto, M., Nagata, S., Park, Y.D., Masuda, Y., Beppu, S., Yutani, C., Sakakibara, H., and Nimura, Y. Visualization of the false tendon in the left ventricle with echocardiography and its clinical significance. *J. Cardiogr.* **11**: 265–270, 1981.
7. Perry, L.W., Ruckman, R.N., Shapiro, S.R., Kuehl, K.S., Galioto, F.M., and Scott, L.P. Left ventricular false tendons in children: Prevalence as detected by 2-dimensional echocardiography and clinical significance. *Am. J. Cardiol.* **52**: 1264–1266, 1983.
8. Suwa, M., Hirota, Y., Nagao, H., Kino, M., and Kawamura, K. Incidence of the coexistence of left ventricular false tendons and premature ventricular contractions in apparently healthy subjects. *Circulation* **70**: 793–798, 1984.
9. Keren, A., Billingham, M.E., and Popp, R.L. Echocardiographic recognition and implication of ventricular hypertrophic trabeculations and aberrant bands. *Circulation* **70**: 836–842, 1984.
10. Bethge, K.P., Bethge, D., Meiners, B.G., and Lichtlen, P.R. Incidence and prognostic significance of ventricular arrhythmias in individuals without detectable heart disease. *Eur. Heart J.* **4**: 338–346, 1983.
11. Dickinson, D.F. and Scott, O. Ambulatory electrocardiographic monitoring in 100 healthy teenage boys. *Br. Heart J.* **51**: 179–183, 1984.
12. Romhilt, D.W., Chaffin, C., Chol, S.C., and Irby, E.C. Arrhythmias on ambulatory electrocardiographic monitoring in women without apparent heart disease. *Am. J. Cardiol.* **54**: 582–586, 1984.
13. Brodsky, M., Wu, D., Denes, P., Kanakis, C., and Rosen, K.M. Arrhythmias documented by 24 hour continuous electrocardiographic monitoring in 50 male medical students without apparent heart disease. *Am. J. Cardiol.* **39**: 390–395, 1977.
14. Gerlis, L.M., Wright, H.M., Wilson, N., Erzengin, F., and Dickinson, D.F. Left ventricular bands. A normal anatomical feature. *Br. Heart J.* **52**: 641–647, 1984.

15. Brenner, J.I., Baker, K., Ringel, R.E., and Berman, M.A. Echocardiographic evidence of left ventricular bands in infants and children. *J. Am. Coll. Cardiol.* **3**: 1515–1520, 1984.

16. Malouf, J., Gharzuddine, W., and Kutayli, F. A reappraisal of the prevalence of clinical importance of left ventricular false tendons in children and adults. *Br. Heart J.* **55**: 587–591, 1986.

17. Suwa, M., Hirota, Y., Kaku, K., Yoneda, Y., Nakayama, A., and Kawamura, K. Prevalence of the coexistence of left ventricular false tendons and premature ventricular complexes in apparently healthy subjects: A prospective study in the general population. *J. Am. Coll. Cardiol.* **12**: 910–914, 1988.

18. Hoffman, B.F. and Cranefield, P.F. The Purkinje fibers. In: Electrophysiology of the Heart, McGraw-Hill, New York, 1960, pp.175–210.

Influence of Underlying Heart Disease upon Utility of Electrophysiologic Study

Jay W. Mason, Kelley P. Anderson, Roger A. Freedman, and David A. Rawling

Cardiology Division, University of Utah Medical Center, Salt Lake City, Utah, U.S.A.

INTRODUCTION

Ventricular tachyarrhythmias may result from coronary artery disease or from various myocardial diseases. The incidence of coronary artery disease is low in Japan. Ten years ago and probably at the present time its incidence was 8 times less frequent than in the U.S.A. and several other Western countries.[1] The purpose of this paper is to develop the hypothesis that geographic variations in the ratio of coronary to other cardiac disease incidences influence the applicability of electrophysiologic study for selection of therapy for ventricular tachyarrhythmias.

VULNERABILITY OF VENTRICULAR TACHYARRHYTHMIAS IN RELATION TO UNDERLYING HEART DISEASE

During the past 10 years electrophysiologic study has been used widely to select therapy. Patients with previously documented sustained ventricular tachyarrhythmias, including monomorphic ventricular tachycardia and ventricular fibrillation, undergo electrophysiologic study, while they are not receiving antiarrhythmic drugs, to evaluate their vulnerability to induction of ventricular tachyarrhythmias. Typically, arrhythmia induction is attempted with a right ventricular electrode catheter through which up to 2 extrastimuli are delivered. Results after positioning the catheter in additional right ventricular sites and in the left ventricle, use of more than 2 ventricular extrastimuli, and infusion of isoproterenol or other agents to enhance arrhythmia inducibility are interpreted with care because of the risk of nonspecific responses. After ventricular arrhythmias are reproducibly induced (at least 2 or 3 times), antiarrhythmic therapies are assessed. If, under the influence of an antiarrhythmic agent, usually administered orally and brought to a therapeutic concentration over a few days, the tachyarrhythmia is no longer induced, the therapy is predicted to be effective. On the other hand, if arrhythmias are still inducible, then inefficacy is predicted and other drugs are evaluated until the arrhythmia can no longer be induced. Good evidence exists that use of this protocol provides accurate prediction of antiarrhythmic drug efficacy both for patients with recurrent tachycardia and for those with aborted sudden death. In a group of 239 subjects with recurrent ventricular tachyarrhythmias, Swerdlow and colleagues[2] demonstrated a markedly lower incidence of sudden death and cardiac death in patients who had a drug efficacy prediction compared to those who did not. In that study an efficacy prediction by electrophysiologic study was an independent predictor of arrhythmia-free survival. It is noteworthy that most subjects in the study had coronary artery disease as the underlying cause of ventricular tachyarrhythmias.

CORONARY ARTERY DISEASE VS CARDIOMYOPATHY AS A CAUSE OF VENTRICULAR TACHYARRHYTHMIAS

The underlying etiologies of ventricular tachyarrhythmias appear to be markedly different in patients in the U.S.A. compared to Japan. In the previously noted study of Swerdlow and colleagues from the U.S.A.,[2] 68% of patients with ventricular tachyarrhythmias had coronary artery disease and 65% had a previous myocardial infarction. Only 22% had idiopathic cardiomyopathy or other heart muscle diseases. On the other hand, Suyama and colleagues[3] found an incidence of coronary artery disease in patients with ventricular tachyarrhythmias of only 39%. Fifty-one percent had heart muscle disease or various causes. The demographic findings reported by Swerdlow and colleagues have been reiterated in numerous other studies in Western countries. There are no sizable published studies from Japan of which we are aware other than that of Suyama. Thus, it does appear that the low incidence of coronary artery disease in Japan has had an impact upon the etiology of ventricular tachyarrhythmias. Does this low prevalence of coronary disease affect the utility of electrophysiologic study?

Swerdlow and colleagues[4] and Spielman and coworkers[5] found that indices of coronary artery disease were strong predictors of outcome in a group of patients predominated by coronary disease as the etiology for ventricular tachyarrhythmias. In both of those studies as well as in others the presence and greater degrees of severity of coronary disease were strong predictors of subsequent failure of antiarrhythmic therapy. Freedman and colleagues[6] studied prognostic indicators in 150 patients resuscitated from sudden cardiac death. They also found several univariate predictors of outcome which were related to coronary disease. In a multivariate analysis the second strongest predictor was previous myocardial infarction, and, again, it was a negative predictor of outcome. Thus, there is considerable evidence that subjects who have ventricular tachyarrhythmias do more poorly if coronary disease is the underlying etiology than if other diseases are etiologic. One interpretation of these data is that electrophysiologic study might be less frequently required in patients with ventricular tachyarrhythmias in Japan because more of those patients have a better prognosis due to the low incidence of coronary disease and higher incidence of myocardial disease. This better prognosis could reduce the need for aggressive assessment by electrophysiologic study.

INDUCIBILITY OF VENTRICULAR TACHYCARDIA

The low incidence of coronary disease among patients with ventricular tachyarrhythmias has other implications. Schoenfeld and colleagues[7] have demonstrated that inducibility of ventricular tachyarrhythmias is highly reproducible over long periods of time in patients with coronary disease, but not in those with cardiomyopathy. Thus, tachyarrhythmia inducibility appears to be less specific, because it is not as reproducible, in patients with etiologies of ventricular tachycardia other than coronary artery disease.

Inducibility rates of ventricular tachycardia are also different in populations with or without coronary artery disease. In a study of 311 patients with ventricular tachyarrhythmias Mason and colleagues[8] found that ventricular tachyarrhythmias were inducible in 93% of patients who had spontaneous episodes of sustained ventricular tachycardia and in 85% of patients resuscitated from sudden death episodes. Freedman,[9] Swerdlow,[10] and Schoenfeld[11] and their colleagues have all demonstrated that previous myocardial infarction is a strong predictor of ventricular tachyarrhythmia inducibility. On the other hand, Naccarelli and coworkers[12] found ventricular tachycardia to be inducible in only 69% and Poll and colleagues[13] in only 52% of patients with cardiomyopathy who had previously had spontaneous episodes of ventricular tachyarrhythmia. The considerably lower incidence of tachyarrhythmia inducibility in subjects without coronary disease would be expected to further reduce the utility of electrophysiologic study in the Japanese patient population.

There are specific myocardial diseases in which ventricular tachyarrhythmia induction has virtually no value. For example, Anderson and colleagues[14] demonstrated that ventricular tachyarrhythmias were inducible in nearly all patients with hypertrophic cardiomyopathy, even though they did not have spontaneous tachyarrhythmia. It is certainly possible that nonspecificity of arrhythmia induction occurs in other myocardial diseases such as the apical hypertrophy syndrome which is seen primarily in Japan.

For a number of reasons the utility of electrophysiologic study in patients with recurrent ventricular tachycardia or aborted sudden death could be less in Japan than in the West. This speculation is heavily based upon the reduced incidence of coronary disease in Japan with an accompanying lower incidence of coronary disease among subjects with spontaneous ventricular tachyarrhythmias. These conclusions should be applicable to other countries with a low incidence of coronary disease. Needless to say, these conclusions will not be valid if coronary disease as the underlying etiology of ventricular tachyarrhythmias in Japan approaches approximately 70%, as in the U.S.A. and other Western countries.

It is important to note that these comments regarding the utility of electrophysiologic study are conjectural. Proof does not exist that electrophysiologic study is less frequently applicable in Japan. It is also important to note that there is no reason to suspect that the validity of electrophysiologic study would be any lesser or greater than in the U.S.A. in subjects with similar characteristics. An examination of the influence of the underlying etiology of ventricular tachyarrhythmias upon applicability and the predictive value of electrophysiologic study performed prospectively and in multiple countries would be of considerable interest.

REFERENCES

1. Levy, R.I. and Feinleib, M. Risk factors for coronary artery disease and their management. In: Heart Disease, A Textbook of Cardiovascular Medicine. Braunwald, E. (ed.), W.B. Saunders Company, Philadelphia, 1984, p. 1208.
2. Swerdlow, C.D., Winkle, R.A., and Mason, J.W. Determinants of survival in patients with ventricular tachyarrhythmias. *N. Engl. J. Med.* **308**: 1436–1442, 1983.
3. Suyama, A., Anan, T., Araki, H., Takeshita, A., and Nakamura, M. Prevalence of ventricular tachycardia in patients with different underlying heart diseases: A study by Holter ECG monitoring. *Am. Heart J.* **112**: 144, 1986.
4. Swerdlow, C.D., Gong, G., Echt, D.S., Winkle, R.A., Griffin, J.C., Ross, D.L., and Mason, J.W. Clinical factors predicting successful electrophysiologic-pharmacologic study in patients with ventricular tachycardia. *J. Am. Coll. Cardiol.* **1**: 409–416, 1983.
5. Spielman, S.R., Schwartz, J.S., McCarthy, D.M., Horowitz, L.M., Greenspan, A.M., Sadowski, L.M., Josephson, M.E., and Waxman, H.L. Predictors of the success or failure of medical therapy in patients with chronic recurrent sustained ventricular tachycardia: A discriminant analysis. *J. Am. Coll. Cardiol.* **1**: 401–408, 1983.
6. Freedman, R.A., Swerdlow, C.D., Soderholm-Difatte, V., and Mason, J.W. Prognostic significance of arrhythmia inducibility or noninducibility at initial electrophysiologic study in survivors of cardiac arrest. *Am. J. Cardiol.* **61**: 578–582, 1988.

7. Schoenfeld, M.H., McGovern, B., Garan, H., and Ruskin, J.N. Long-term reproducibility of responses to programmed cardiac stimulation in spontaneous ventricular tachyarrhythmias. *Am. J. Cardiol.* **54**: 564–568, 1984.

8. Mason, J.W., Swerdlow, C.D., Winkle, R.A., Ross, D.L., Echt, D.S., Anderson, K.P., Mitchell, L.B., and Clusin, W.T. Ventricular tachyarrhythmia induction for drug selection: Experience with 311 patients. In: Clinical Pharmacology of Antiarrhythmic Therapy, Lucchesi, B.R., Dingell, J.V., and Schwarz, R.P., Jr., (eds.), Raven Press, New York, 1984, pp. 229–239.

9. Freedman, R.A., Swerdlow, C.D., Soderholm-Difatte, V., and Mason, J.W. Clinical predictors of arrhythmia inducibility in survivors of cardiac arrest: Importance of gender and prior myocardial infarction. *J. Am. Coll. Cardiol.* **12**: 973–978, 1988.

10. Swerdlow, C.D., Bardy, G.H., McAnulty, J., *et al.* Determinants of induced sustained arrhythmias in survivors of out-of-hospital ventricular fibrillation. *Circulation* **76**: 1053–1060, 1987.

11. Schoenfeld, M.H., McGovern, B., Garan, H., Kelly, E., Grant, G., and Ruskin, J. Determinants of the outcome of electrophysiologic study in patients with ventricular tachyarrhythmias. *J. Am. Coll. Cardiol.* **6**: 298–306, 1985.

12. Naccarelli, G.V., Prystowsky, E.N., Jackman, W.M., Heger, J.J., Rahilly, G.T., and Zipes, D.P. Role of electrophysiologic testing in managing patients who have ventricular tachycardia unrelated to coronary artery disease. *Am. J. Cardiol.* **50**: 165–171, 1982.

13. Poll, D.S., Marchlinski, F.E., Buxton, A.E., and Josephson, M.E. Usefulness of programmed stimulation in idiopathic dilated cardiomyopathy. *Am. J. Cardiol.* **58**: 992–997, 1986.

14. Anderson, K.P., Stinson, E.B., Derby, G.C., Oyer, P.E., and Mason, J.W. Vulnerability of patients with obstructive hypertrophic cardiomyopathy to ventricular arrhythmia induction in the operating room. Analysis of 17 patients. *Am. J. Cardiol.* **51**: 811–816, 1983.

Endomyocardial Biopsy Findings in Cases with Idiopathic Ventricular Tachycardia

Motonari Hasumi,* Morie Sekiguchi,* Michiaki Hiroe,** and Koshichiro Hirosawa*

*The Heart Institute of Japan, Tokyo Women's Medical College, Tokyo, Japan
**Department of Radiology, Tokyo Women's Medical College, Tokyo, Japan

ABSTRACT

Various attempts have been made to clarify the pathogenetic mechanism of idiopathic ventricular tachycardia (VT). Performing right ventricular endomyocardial biopsy in 34 cases with VT of left bundle branch block morphology in the electrocardiogram, we were able to find a high incidence (74%) of myocardial pathology characterized by an increase in fatty tissue and advanced myocardial fibrosis. We were able to classify the VT cases into 3 groups, i.e., group A: right ventricular enlargement ($n=8$), group B: left ventricular dysfunction and/or left ventricular enlargement ($n=7$), and group C: without bi-ventricular enlargement ($n=19$). Since we found the pathology in 11/19 cases (58%) of group C, the existence of a non-hypertrophic, non-dilated, electric disturbance type of cardiomyopathy is proposed.

INTRODUCTION

Various attempts have been made to clarify the pathogenetic mechanism of idiopathic ventricular tachycardia.[1-5,8,11,15-22,25,26] Some of the cases show a fatal outcome.[1-5] Clinical analyses employing ambulatory electrocardiograms and/or electrophysiological studies, various experiments using animals, and studies at the cellular level are now in progress.[15,18-20]

One of the clinical methods to investigate the pathogenetic mechanism of this disease is to perform endomyocardial biopsy.[6-14,16,17] Performing right ventricular endomyocardial biopsy in patients with ventricular tachycardia of left bundle branch block morphology in the electrocardiogram (LBBB-VT) is considered a reasonable approach to clarify the morphological aspects of the myocardial changes in cases with idiopathic ventricular tachycardia.

We analyzed the cases which we have studied in the past 15 years, and a high incidence of myocardial pathology characterized by an increase in fatty tissue and advanced myocardial fibrosis was found.[11,26]

PATIENTS AND METHODS

In the present study,[26] we analyzed pathological findings of the right ventricular endomyocardium by right endomyocardial biopsy in order to clarify the morphological background of the left bundle branch block type of ventricular tachycardia.[16,17] Josephson[18,20] and others[19,21] have reported that most of the idiopathic LBBB-VT cases originate in the right ventricular myocardium. Yet other investigators have reported that the LBBB-VT is not always of right ventricular origin.[25] Another report

TABLE 1.   Semiquantitative Assessment of Biopsy Findings

A. Parameters
    (1) Interstitial fibrosis
    (2) Disarrangement
    (3) Degeneration
    (4) Hypertrophy
    (5) Fatty tissue infiltration
    (6) Other
B. The criteria for significant pathology
    (1) At least one of A_{1-3} should exceed grade 2.
    (2) The sum of A_{1-4} should exceed a score of 4.

Grading			
−	+	‖	⧣
0	1	2	3

Modified from Hasumi et al.[9]

states that LBBB-VT is not usually due to organic heart disease.[4] However, Pietras et al.[4] reported that there is a spectrum of diseases among cases with VT. In our cases, the VT was proved by coronary arteriography not to be due to ischemic heart disease and could not be classified as either hypertrophic or dilated cardiomyopathy. There are

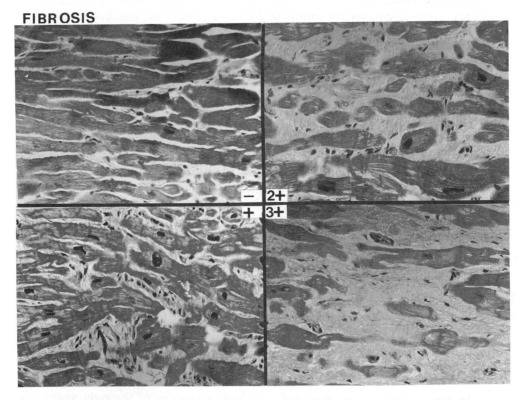

FIBROSIS

Fig. 1.   Model micrographs of the interstitial fibrosis grading (−) to (3+). (×200)
    All pictures with grades (−) to (3+) were specimens biopsied from patients with DCM. In each picture of (−), (+), (2+) and (3+), the percentage of interstitial fibrosis was 9%, 20%, 35% and 62%, respectively. In grading, we made reference to these models. (From Hasumi et al.,[11] reproduced with permission.)

FATTY TISSUE

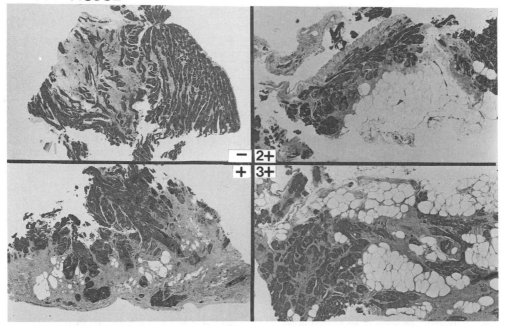

Fig. 2.   Model micrographs of the fatty tissue infiltration grading (−) to (3+),
which also show some examples of the findings for a semiquantitative
assessment. (×60)

The percentage of fatty tissue infiltration was 1% in (−), 6% in (+), 22% in
(2+) and 34% in (3+). All specimens except the picture (−) were biopsied
from patients with ARVD; (−) from a case of DCM. (From Hasumi *et
al*.,[11] reproduced with permission.)

many cases where wall contractions and/or slight ventricular volume abnormalities are
recognized. In our study, cases with LBBB-VT were classified into the following three
groups.[26]

1) Arrhythmogenic right ventricular dysplasia;[11] 8 cases, group A.

2) Decreased left ventricular function and/or enlarged left ventricle; 7 cases, group B.

3) Cases without apparent enlargement of either ventricle; 19 cases, group C.

All patients underwent right and left cardiac catheterization, ventriculography and
coronary arteriography. Our own criteria for a semiquantitative analysis were applied
(Table 1; Figs. 1 and 2).

RESULTS AND DISCUSSION

Our analysis revealed that 74% of the total of 34 cases with LBBB-VT showed distinct
pathologic myocardial changes (Figs. 3, 4, and 5). In groups A and B, significant pathology (Table 1) was found in 100% and 86% of the cases, respectively. It can be suggested
that such a change may be due to mechanical influence of ventricular dilatation. However, it is noteworthy that even in group C, 58% of the cases showed a similar pathology,
and this seemed to be an important background factor in the analysis of idiopathic
ventricular tachycardia without ventricular dilatation. There are at least two reports

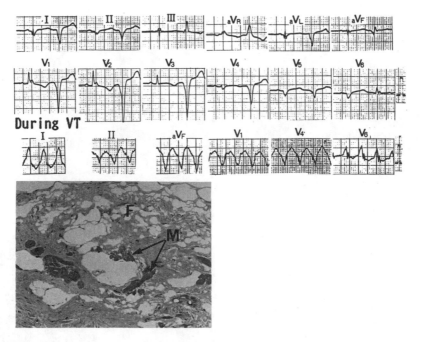

Fig. 3.   A case of arrhythmogenic right ventricular dysplasia (ARVD) (53-year-old female in group B). Note electrocardiographic changes and a biopsy finding. Cardiac myocytes are scarcely seen, and marked interstitial fibrosis mixed with fatty tissue showing a vacuolated appearance is observed.

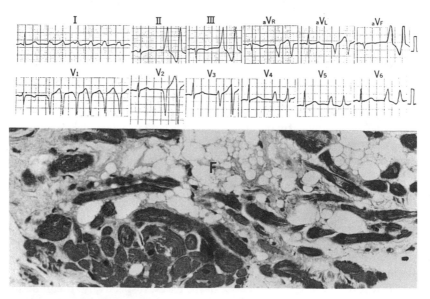

Fig. 4.   A case of idiopathic LBBB-VT without dilatation of both ventricles showing a significant pathology with a marked fatty tissue in the myocardium (42-year-old female in group C).

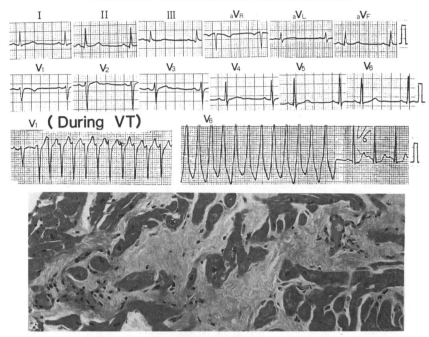

Fig. 5. A case of idiopathic LBBB-VT without dilatation of both ventricles showing an advanced interstitial fibrosis in the myocardium (50-year-old male in group C).

which clarify the evidence of myocardial changes in cases with VT.[16,17] However, further analysis using a control specimen or semiquantitative assessment was not carried out in these studies. Our analysis has detailed the pathomorphological assessment, using the method of assessing significant pathology and classifying the changes in regard to postmyocarditic change using various control specimens from patients with normal and dilated ventricular cavities (Fig. 6).[11-14] The changes we have seen in patients with LBBB-VT were the same as in cases with DCM when the findings were assessed by the degree of significant pathology.[12] The incidence of detection of significant pathology was less in patients with RBBB-VT, signifying that the changes seen in the right ventricle in patients with LBBB-VT are related to the development of the LBBB-VT. However, we have not accumulated data on the left ventricular biopsy findings in cases with RBBB-VT, and this should be investigated in the future.

The details of the group A patients were reported by us and revealed that 7 out of 8 patients showed typical findings, including advanced interstitial fibrosis as well as a great increase in fatty tissue in right ventricular biopsy.[11] One of the 8 patients had only marked endocardial thickening, sub-endocardial fibrosis and no apparent myocardial tissue. This may be due to the limitations of the biopsy where we are unable to obtain a specimen from the deeper layer. Furthermore, this typical ARVD type-histology was not observed in any of the control group patients and was seen in one group B patient and in two group C patients. The high incidence of fatty tissue infiltration may signify that this pathology is a contributory factor for the genesis of VT. The real mechanism of the high occurrence of fatty tissue remains obscure.

Another important finding was the postmyocarditic change that we have defined.[12,13] Employing serial endomyocardial biopsy, we were able to define the histopathologic

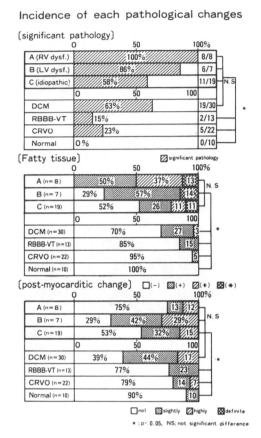

Fig. 6.   The incidence of each pathologic change in cases with or without
VT.[11, 26] The upper part of the figure shows significant pathology, the middle
part shows fatty tissue, and the lower part shows the incidence of factors suggestive of postmyocarditic change. The incidence of significant pathology was 100%
in group A (A), 86% in group B (B), and 58% in group C (C). The incidence of
significant pathology in groups A, B, and C was apparently higher than in VT
with RBBB morphology (RBBB-VT), chronic right ventricular overloading
(CRVO), and normal controls. The incidence of fatty tissue was 100% in group
A, 71% in group B, and 48% in group C, which was also significantly higher than
in CRVO and normal controls. The incidence of findings "highly suggestive"
of postmyocarditic change in patients with LBBB-VT was as high as the incidence in the dilated cardiomyopathy (DCM) group. Biopsy findings from
subjects who showed no evidence of apparent heart disease were used as "normal" controls. In this study, consecutive DCM cases without VT were chosen
as controls.

criteria of postmyocarditic change, and, accordingly, the criteria for assessing the sug-
gestiveness of myocarditis were formulated. The criterion "highly suggestive" is noteworthy as it signifies the preceding existence of myocarditis.[12,27] It was seen in one
group A patient, 2 group B patients and 3 group C patients. The incidence of "highly
suggestive" amounted to 18% of the cases in this study. Also worthy of note is that
fatty tissue infiltration was often seen in cases with previous myocarditis where the

biopsy was proven at the acute stage; the low incidence of significant pathology in the non-VT control myocardium may also signify that in LBBB-VT cases, the pathology that we have seen is of a characteristic nature and will very likely contribute to the development of VT due to re-entry, abnormal automaticity, and triggered activity. The pathologic findings that we have seen in group C may be those of latent arrhythmogenic ventricular dysplasia without ventricular dilatation.

In 27% of the cases, the biopsy findings were almost normal, possibly because the pathology was not evenly distributed in the myocardium or was mild. This may be a limitation of the endomyocardial biopsy approach.

ACKNOWLEDGEMENT

This work was supported in part by a Research Grant from the Intractable Diseases Division, Public Health Bureau, Ministry of Health and Welfare, Japan.

REFERENCES

1. Hair, T.E., Eagan, J.T., and Orgain, E.S. Paroxysmal ventricular tachycardia in the absence of demonstrable heart disease. *Am. J. Cardiol.* **9**: 209–214, 1962.
2. Lesch, M., Lewis, E., Humphries, J.O.N., *et al.* Paroxysmal ventricular tachycardia in the absence of organic heart disease. *Ann. Int. Med.* **66**: 950–960, 1967.
3. Vetter, V.L., Josephson, M.E., and Horowitz, L.N. Idiopathic recurrent sustained ventricular tachycardia in children and adolescents. *Am. J. Cardiol.* **47**: 315–322, 1981.
4. Pietras, R.J., Mautner, R., Denes, P., *et al.* Chronic recurrent right and left ventricular tachycardia. Comparison of clinical, hemodynamic and angiographic findings. *Am. J. Cardiol.* **40**: 32–37, 1977.
5. Reiter, M.J., Smith, W.M., and Gallagher, J.J. Clinical spectrum of ventricular tachycardia with left bundle branch block morphology. *Am. J. Cardiol.* **51**: 113–121, 1983.
6. Konno, S., and Sakakibara, S. Intracardiac heart biopsy. *Dis. Chest.* **44**: 345–350, 1963.
7. Sekiguchi, M., and Konno, S. Diagnosis and classification of primary myocardial disease with the aid of endomyocardial biopsy. *Jpn. Circul. J.* **35**: 737–754, 1971.
8. Sekiguchi, M., Hasumi, M., and Hiroe, M., *et al.* On the existence of non-hypertrophic, non-dilated cardiomyopathy as assessed by endomyocardial biopsy and a proposal for the term "Electric disturbance type of cardiomyopathy." *Circulation* **72**: Suppl. III-156, 1985. (abstr.)
9. Hasumi, M., Sekiguchi, M., and Morimoto, S., *et al.* Catheter biopsy assessed cardiomyopathic and postmyocarditic changes in cases with atrioventricular or intraventricular conduction disturbance. In: Cardiac Pacing. (Steinbach, K. *et al.* (eds.), Steinkopf Verlag, Darmstadt, 1983, pp. 101–108.
10. Sekiguchi, M., Hiroe, M., Ogasawara, S., *et al.* Practical aspects of endomyocardial biopsy. *Ann. Acad. Med. Singapore* **10**: Suppl. 115–128, 1981.
11. Hasumi, M., Sekiguchi, M., Hiroe, M., *et al.* Endomyocardial biopsy approach to patients with ventricular tachycardia with special reference to arrhythmogenic right ventricular dysplasia. *Jpn. Circul. J.* **51**: 242–249, 1987.
12. Hasumi, M., Sekiguchi, M., Yu, Z.-X., *et al.* Analysis of histopathologic findings in cases with dilated cardiomyopathy with special reference to formulating diagnostic criteria on the possibility of postmyocarditic change. *Jpn. Circul. J.* **50**: 1280–1287, 1986.
13. Yu, Z.-X., Sekiguchi, M., Hiroe, M., *et al.* Histopathological findings of acute and convalescent myocarditis obtained by serial endomyocardial biopsy. *Jpn. Circul. J.* **48**: 1368–1374, 1984.
14. Hasumi, M., Sekiguchi, M., Morimoto, S., *et al.* Ventriculographic findings at the convalescent stage in eleven cases with acute myocarditis. *Jpn. Circul. J.* **47**: 1310–1316, 1983.

15. Josephson, M.E., and Wellens, H.J.J. Tachycardias. Lea and Febiger, Philadelphia, 1984, pp. 61–89.

16. Strain, J.E., Grose, R.M., Factor, S.M., *et al.* Results of endomyocardial biopsy in patients with spontaneous ventricular tachycardia but without apparent structural heart disease. *Circulation* **68**: 1171–1181, 1983.

17. Morgera, T., Salvi, R.M., Alberti, E., *et al.* Morphological findings in apparently idiopathic ventricular tachycardia. An echocardiographic haemodynamic and histologic study. *Eur. Heart J.* **6**: 323–334, 1985.

18. Josephson, M.E., Horowitz, L.N., Waxman, H.L., *et al.* Sustained ventricular tachycardia: Role of the 12-lead electrocardiogram in localizing site of origin. *Circulation* **64**: 257–272, 1981.

19. Lewis, S., Kanakis, C., Rosen, K.M., *et al.* Significance of site of premature ventricular contraction. *Am. Heart J.* **97**: 159–164, 1979.

20. Josephson, M.E., Horowitz, L.N., Spielman, S.R., *et al.* Comparison of endocardial catheter mapping with intraoperative mapping of ventricular tachycardia. *Circulation* **61**: 395–404, 1980.

21. Marcus, F.I., Fontaine, G., Guiraudon, G., *et al.* Right ventricular dysplasia: A report of 24 adult cases. *Circulation* **65**: 384–398, 1982.

22. Fontaine, G., Frank, R., Tonet, J.L., *et al.* Arrhythmogenic right ventricular dysplasia: A clinical model for the study of chronic ventricular tachycardia. *Jpn. Circul. J.* **48**: 515–538, 1984.

23. Take, M., Sekiguchi, M., Hiroe, M., *et al.* Long-term follow up of electrocardiographic findings in patients with acute myocarditis proven by endomyocardial biopsy. *Jpn. Circul. J.* **46**: 1227–1234, 1982.

24. Sekiguchi, M., Hiroe, M., Take, M., *et al.* Clinical and histopathological profile of sarcoidosis of the heart and acute idiopathic myocarditis. Concepts through a study employing endomyocardial biopsy. II. Myocarditis. *Jpn. Circul. J.* **44**: 264–273, 1980.

25. Kennedy, H.L., Pescarmona, J.E., Bouchard, R.J., *et al.* Objective evidence of occult myocardial dysfunction in patients with frequent ventricular ectopy without clinically apparent heart disease. *Am. Heart J.* **104**: 57–65, 1982.

26. Hasumi, M., Sekiguchi, M., Morimoto, S., Ogasawara, S., Kasanuki, H., Hirosawa, K. High incidence of detecting myocardial pathology with fatty tissue in cases with idiopathic ventricular tachycardia with and without right ventricular enlargement. A right ventricular endomyocardial biopsy study. *Circulation* **72**: Suppl. III-46, 1985. (abstr.)

27. Sekiguchi, M., Hiroe, M., Yu, Z.-X. and Hasumi, M. A serial endomyocardial biopsy study on myocarditis. In: Pathogenesis of Myocarditis and Cardiomyopathy: Recent experimental and clinical studies. Kawai, C., and Abelmann, W.H. (eds.) Univ. of Tokyo Press, Tokyo, 1987, pp. 213–231.

Acquired and Transmitted Dysplasia

G. Fontaine, F. Fontaliran, P. Mesnildrey, J.P. Fauchier, J.C. Daubert, B. Olsson, G. Chomette, and Y. Grosgogeat

Service de Rythmologie et de Stimulation Cardiaque, Hôpital Jean Rostand, Ivry

Arrhythmogenic right ventricular dysplasia (ARVD) has been identified from clinical data as well as surgical biopsies obtained in 3 patients who underwent surgical operation for the treatment of resistant ventricular tachycardia originating in the right ventricle. Three other suggestive clinical cases were also included in the same original description.[1]

A more thorough study of 24 consecutive cases observed in the same institution was the basis of a composite consistent pattern despite the fact that no pathognomonic signs could be established.[2] Identification of this syndrome proved important, however, since some cases of sudden death have been reported.[3-5]

Typically, the diagnosis should be suspected in a young male patient suffering from ventricular tachycardia with a left ventricular delay, in the absence of signs of coronary artery disease or obvious signs of dilated cardiomyopathy. Data from gross pathology as well as histologic studies obtained from surgical biopsies have shown that in most cases, only the right ventricle is involved by a pathologic process replacing the subepicardial as well as working myocardial fibers by fibro-adipose tissue.[6] Infiltrations by lymphocytes reported by Marcus *et al.*[2] suggested inflammatory reactions for which different etiologies can be responsible.[7]

This disease, which is exclusively limited to the right ventricle, also suggests a very rare cardiac congenital anomaly, called Uhl's anomaly. Therefore 2 cases pertaining to this entity were originally included in the ARVD syndrome.[2,8]

The dysgenetic basis of dysplasia was suggested when we learned that the brother of one of our patients also had episodes of ventricular tachycardia.[2] Since the original description, other familial cases of dysplasia have been reported in the literature.[9-12] The heredofamilial feature of dysplasia is also well established in Uhl's anomaly.[13,14] In the 52 consecutive cases of probable dysplasia recorded at Jean Rostand Hospital, abnormal ventricular rhythms have been found in the brothers of 4 patients.

The systematic identification of the disease in members of the same family has been also undertaken using summation-averaging ECG techniques, in order to show delayed potentials originating in a possible latent arrhythmogenic substrate. An increase in the sensitivity of the technique was achieved in terms of identifying patients with overt cardiac arrhythmias.[1,2,10] Despite the fact that specific criteria for detection of delayed potentials have not been clearly identified in arrhythmogenic right ventricular dysplasia, we gained the impression that 4 other families could fulfill the criteria for inclusion in the syndrome.

These elements tend to confirm the initial impression which suggests that ARVD is a cardiac anomaly due to a derangement in heart development restricted to the right ventricle. This anomaly has few or no hemodynamic consequences. However, it could set up an arrhythmogenic substrate which could remain quiescent during long periods of time, and could finally manifest itself clinically in episodes of ventricular arrhythmias and, in exceptional cases, sudden death.

However, we observed delayed potentials at the surface of the left ventricle during the recording of epicardial maps, suggesting that at least in some cases the dysplastic process is not restricted to the right ventricle.[1] Involvement of the left ventricle could explain why some patients in whom the diagnosis of dysplasia was suggested, was in fact initially the result of sequelae of myocarditis or a particular form of dilated cardiomyopathy.[15,16] Biopsies obtained at the time of surgery in 3 of 6 patients in whom the clinical pattern of ARVD was recently studied in Tours, France, and identified by angiography and nuclear scintigraphy, showed lymphoplasmocyte granulomas suggesting sequelae of myocarditis.[17] At the end of 1987 we were the faculty opponents of a medical thesis presented at the University of Göteborg in Sweden.[18] Beforehand, we obtained authorization to review the histology of the 10 cases, which represented the

TABLE 1. Patient Characteristics

No.	Sex	Age	Diagnosis	Histological diagnosis
1	M	38	ARVD	SOM
2	M	40	ARVD	ARVD
3	M	23	ARVD	ARVD+SOM
4	F	49	ARVD	loc UHL
5	M	49	ARVD	IDCM
6	F	45	IVT-ARVD	SOM
7	F	36	ARVD	ARVD
8	M	22	ARVD	SOM
9	F	19	ARVD	SOM
10	M	29	ARVD	ARVD+SARC
11	M	42	ARVD	LIP C
12	F	51	UHL	UHL
13	M	22	ARVD	SOM
14	M	50	IDCM-ARVD	SOM IDCM
15	M	42	ARVD	SOM
16	M	33	ARVD	SOM
17	M	44	ALVD	SOM
18	M	53	ARVD	SOM SA
19	F	9	CHF	LIP C
20	M	63	ARVD	IDCM
21	M	28	ARVD	SOM IDCM
22	M	29	ARVD	SOM
23	M	33	ARVD	SOM
24	F	36	UHL	UHL
25	M	19	ARVD	SOM
26	M	24	ARVD	IDCM
27	M	58	ARVD	SOM

ARVD: arrhythmogenic right ventricular dysplasia, ALVD: arrhythmogenic left ventricular dysplasia, SOM: sequelae of myocarditis, loc UHL: localized Uhl's anomaly, IVT: idiopathic ventricular tachycardia; SARC: sarcoidosis; IDCM: idiopathic dilated cardiomyopathy, LIP C: lipomatosis cordis, CHF: congestive heart failure, SA: subacute.

material used in this thesis. In this series, 4 patients had autopsies, and in the 6 remaining patients myocardial biopsies were taken at the time of surgery. We reviewed the data concerning 5 of these 10 patients, and in 3 lymphoplasmocyte infiltrates were found.

The retrospective analysis of the histologic data obtained in cases at La Salpêtrière and Jean Rostand Hospitals, in addition to 5 cases from Tours and one from Rennes, finally comprised 27 cases, of which the main histologic features are shown in Table 1. Only 2 suggested the original ARVD pattern. One suggested dysplasia, whilst some histologic data favored sarcoidosis (no. 10); one case suggested dysplasia associated with sequelae of myocarditis (no. 3) (Fig. 1), and 2 cases had previously been reported as definite Uhl's anomaly.[19] Thirteen cases suggested sequelae of myocarditis, one in its subacute form (no. 18) (Fig. 2). In 3 cases a possible diagnosis of dilated cardiomyopathy was considered. Two cases suggested sequelae of myocarditis associated with cardiomyopathy (nos. 14, 21). Two cases suggested lipomatosis cordis (nos. 11, 19), and one case a localized Uhl's anomaly (no. 4). Therefore, we were led to the conclusion that among patients with ARVD several subgroups can be identified, of which

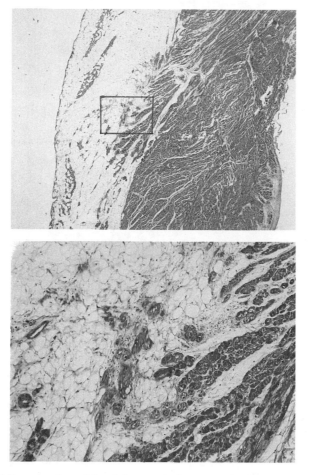

Fig. 1. Oblique section of the right ventricular apex of patient no. 3. The upper part of this figure shows at low power ($G=20$) a typical pattern of dysplasia on the right ventricular free wall. However, at high power ($G=100$) infiltrates of mononuclear cells suggest sequelae of endocarditis.

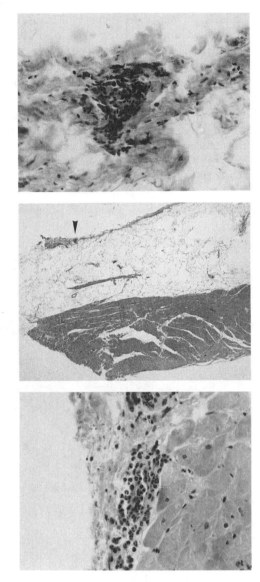

Fig. 2. Surgical sample of the right ventricle in a patient (patient no. 18) considered to have arrhythmogenic right ventricular dysplasia, with some unclear clinical symptoms including chest pain, poor general condition, and possible myocardial infarction. Review of histologic samples taken at surgery indicates in the middle picture at low power ($G = 20$) normal endocardium and fatty tissue on the subepicardial layers where a strand of surviving fibers is clearly seen. On the epicardium (arrow) a localized infiltrate better observed at high amplification (upper picture, $G = 400$) in a zone of fibrosis suggests sequelae of myocarditis. In the same preparation in another area (lower picture, $G = 400$), leukocytes and inflammatory cells are clearly seen inside fibrous tissue and suggest a subacute form of myocarditis.

one, and probably the most frequent, suggests that the original basis of the disease was the result of an infectious process.

Recent advances mainly in analyzing endocardial biopsies have opened new avenues in understanding the primary myocardial disease by the identification of myocarditis and the changes resulting therefrom.[15,20] In acute myocarditis (and probably also in its chronic forms) the myocardial involvement varies from case to case and can be either diffuse or localized.[21] When the disease is confined to the right ventricle, the clinical symptoms can be minor and the cardiac arrhythmia can be the first presenting symptom of the disease without impairment of left myocardial function.[22] In the diffuse form, the left ventricle can be involved, with subsequent impairment of myocardial contraction in addition to cardiac arrhythmias. However, in the diffuse as well as in the localized forms, myocardial involvement is the result of an acquired heart disease.[22]

Therefore two completely different pathogenetic mechanisms can be proposed: (1) the "transmitted dysplasia" form when a determinant heredofamilial factor can be identified, and (2) "acquired dysplasia" when the disease is the result of a previous inflammatory or infectious process. These have been considered 2 independent entities by Iwa and Okada[16] based on histologic samples obtained at surgery in patients operated on for ventricular tachycardia of a right ventricular origin not related to coronary artery disease. In fact, in their study, which comprised 25 patients, 3 patients demonstrated a typical form of dysplasia. In 2 others, the diagnosis was suspected. One suggested the association of myocarditis with dysplasia, and 13 cases suggested sequelae of myocarditis. In this subgroup, 5 cases exhibited fatty transformation of the right ventricular myocardium. Thiene et al.[5] have recently reported gross pathologic as well as histologic data obtained from young subjects dying suddenly in the Venetian area. These authors have described 2 main histologic patterns: adipose and fibro-adipose. This form of cardiomyopathy involving the right ventricle seems close to the concept of ARVD. However, some cases also showed mononuclear infiltrates and contraction bands suggesting previous myocarditis.[5]

Sekiguchi et al. have reported on their experience at the Women's Medical College of Tokyo in a series of 9 patients studied by endocardial biopsies with quantitative assessment.[23] ARVD was easily distinguished from the other forms of primary myocardial disease, in particular, dilated cardiomyopathy and right ventricular overload. The main features of dysplasia found by these authors were interstitial fibrosis, fatty infiltration, hypertrophy, and degeneration of myocytes. Other changes suggested sequelae of myocarditis found in 37% of the patients. This proportion which is lower than that in the series of Iwa and Okada[16] as well as in our own series, may be explained by the smaller amount of myocardial tissue studied due to the limitations of endocardial biopsy. Inflammation as the cause of cardiac arrhythmia could also explain some forms suggesting dysplasia localized to the left ventricle.[24] In the same way, when there is an impairment of left ventricular function, either at rest or during exercise, sequelae of myocarditis can be suspected.[25]

It is therefore suggested that when several members of a family including symptomatic as well as nonsymptomatic cases a heredofamilial disease seems likely. It is nevertheless theoretically possible that a viral origin could have affected several members of the same family. As a result, the differential diagnosis between acquired and transmitted dysplasia can be difficult. These 2 pathogenetic mechanisms could lead to a clinical pattern which has not been sufficiently separated by the current diagnostic approaches.[2]

The combination of myocarditis and ARVD due to a derangement in heart development was first discussed by Bharati et al.[7] and by Iwa et al.[16] In one of our patients (Fig. 3), this combination was also found. Histologic signs of sarcoidosis were observed with giant cells including asteroid bodies, although the lack of histologic examination

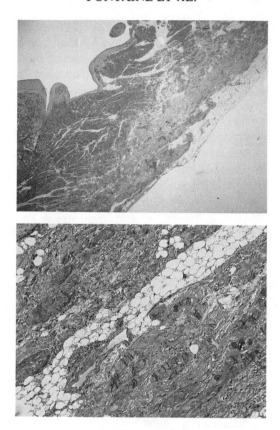

Fig. 3.   Surgical sample of the right ventricle in a patient (patient no. 5) referred for probable arrhythmogenic right ventricular dysplasia. The upper part
of the picture at low amplification ($G=10$) shows thickening of the endocardium, fibrous infiltration of the subendocardial layers, and fatty tissue infiltration. At high power ($G=400$) fatty infiltration and fibrous tissue with contraction
bands are seen. Also note the large number of cells inside the fibrous tissue,
suggesting idiopathic dilated cardiomyopathy as a result of sequelae of myocarditis.

of other organs makes this diagnosis somewhat uncertain.[26] The combination of these
two diseases could be more easily explained if the myocardial changes in abnormal
transmitted dysplasia were due to infectious or inflammatory courses.

The diffuse or localized pattern of the succeeding myocarditis could produce different
histologic patterns as compared with transmitted dysplasia.[27] However, the histologic
criteria established in the differential diagnosis have not yet been defined.[7]

Some forms of dysplasia could therefore be the result of myocarditis or minor
forms of cardiomyopathy. This concept has led to the suggestion that the two diseases
could be related. If it is accepted that myocarditis could lead to some form of
dysplasia, it is also well established that myocarditis could also lead in time to the
development of histologic patterns of dilated cardiomyopathy[20,28,29] in which the initial
signs of infection have disappeared.[15] Endocardial biopsy is at the present time the
most effective means to distinguish these 2 forms, but this approach was not used in
our study.[30]

This mechanism could be suggested in cases with dilated cardiomyopathy in which the heart shows only minor dilatation and in which the first presenting symptom is ventricular tachycardia with a left ventricular delay.[31] In such cases, left ventricular function is only moderately impaired and therefore a stress test could be valuable. It is therefore possible to suggest that dilated cardiomyopathy histologically proven could be considered as cases with ARVD.[25,32] The histology of one of our patients (no. 21) showed areas of fibrosis located in the myocardium of both ventricles, in which only few inflammatory cells could be found. This can be interpreted as being a sequelae of myocarditis leading to cardiomyopathy.[6,27]

Therefore, if dysplasia can either be transmitted or be acquired, let us discuss cases of transmitted cardiomyopathies. Familial forms of cardiomyopathies have been well documented in humans,[31,33,34] as well as in animals.[35,36] But in such cases, fibrosis is not a major feature, in contrast to the changes we have seen in cases of previous myocarditis. The absence of fibrosis could therefore constitute the distinguished feature of transmitted dysplasia.

The consequences of these findings could be important for the management of patients as well as for their families. New insights provided by endocardial biopsy and electro-cardiogram analyses using summation averaging techniques as well as magnetic nuclear resonance will prove to be great help.[20,23,37]

ACKNOWLEDGMENTS

This study was supported in part by a grant from Centre de Recherche sur les Maladies Cardiovasculaires de l'Association Claude Bernard, La Fondation de Cardiologie, and L'Institut National de la Santé et de la Recherche Médicale (INSERM Contract No. 865005).

REFERENCES

1. Fontaine, G., Guiraudon, G., Frank, R., Vedel, J., Grosgogeat, Y., Cabrol. C., and Facquet, J. Stimulation studies and epicardial mapping in ventricular tachycardia: Study of mechanisms and selection for surgery. In: Reentrant Arrhythmias, Kulbertus, H.E. (ed.), MTP Pub., Lancaster, 1977, pp. 334–350.

2. Marcus, F.I., Fontaine, G., Guiraudon, G., Frank, R., Laurenceau, J.L., Malergue, M.C., and Grosgogeat, Y. Right ventricular dysplasia: A report of 24 cases. *Circulation* **65**: 384–399, 1982.

3. Olsson, S.B., Edvardsson, N., Emanuelsson, H., and Enestrom, S. A case of arrhythmogenic right ventricular dysplasia with ventricular fibrillation. *Clin. Cardiol.* **5**: 591–596, 1982.

4. Virmani, R., Robinowitz, M., Clark, M.A., and McAllister, H.A. Sudden death and partial absence of the right ventricular myocardium. *Arch. Pathol. Lab. Med.* **106**: 163–167, 1982.

5. Thiene, G., Nava, A., Corrado, D., Rossi, L., and Pennelli, N. Right ventricular cardiomyopathy and sudden death in young people. *N. Engl. J. Med.* **318**: 129–133, 1988.

6. Fontaine, G., Fontaliran, F., Martin de la Salle, E., Pavie, A., Cabrol, C., Chomette, G., and Grosgogeat Y. Right ventricular dysplasias. In: Ventricular Tachycardias: From Mechanism to Therapy. Aliot, E. and Lazzara, R. (eds.), Martinus Nijhoff, Dordrecht, 1987, pp. 113–133.

7. Bharati, S., Feld, A.W., Bauernfeind, R.A., Kattus, A.A., and Lev, M. Hypoplasia of the right ventricular myocardium with ventricular tachycardia. *Arch. Pathol. Lab. Med.* **107**: 249–253, 1983.

8. Uhl, H.S. A previously undescribed congenital malformation of the heart: Almost total

absence of the myocardium of the right ventricle. *Bull. John Hopkins Hosp.* **91**, 197–205, 1952.

9. Nava, A., Scognamiglio, R., Thiene, G., Canciani, B., Daliento, L., Buja, G., Stritoni, P., Fasoli, G., and Dallavolta, S. A polymorphic form of familial arrhythmogenic right ventricular dysplasia. *Am. J. Cardiol.* **59**: 1405–1409, 1987.

10. Blomstrom-Lundqvist, C., Enestrom, S., Edvardsson, N., and Olsson, S.B. Arrhythmogenic right ventricular dysplasia presenting with ventricular tachycardia in a father and a son. *Clin. Cardiol.* **10**: 277–283, 1987.

11. Ruder, M.A., Winston, S.A., Davis, J.C., Abbott, J.A., Eldar, M., and Scheinman, M.M. Arrhythmogenic right ventricular dysplasia in a family. *Am. J. Cardiol.* **56**: 799–800, 1985.

12. Rakovec, P., Rossi, L., Fontaine, G., Sasel, B., Markez, J., and Voncina, D. Familial arrhythmogenic right ventricular disease. *Am. J. Cardiol.* **58**: 377–378, 1986.

13. Diggelmann, U. and Baur, H.R. Familial Uhl's anomaly in the adult. *Am. J. Cardiol.* **53**: 1402–1403, 1984.

14. Hoback, J., Adicoff, A., From A.H.L., Smith, M., Shafer, R., and Chesler, E. A report of Uhl's disease in identical adult twins: Evaluation of right ventricular dysfunction with echocardiography and nuclear angiography. *Chest* **79**: 3, 1981.

15. Quigley, P.J., Richardson, P.J., Meany, B.T., Olsen, E.G.J., Monaghan, M.J., Jackson, G., and Jewitt, D.E. Long-term follow-up of acute myocarditis: Correlation of ventricular function and outcome. *Eur. Heart J.* **8**: Suppl. J, 39–42, 1987.

16. Iwa, T., Misaki, T., Mukai, K., Kamata, E., and Ishida, K. Surgical management of nonischemic ventricular tachycardia. In: Cardiac Arrhythmias. Recent Progress in Investigation and Management. Iwa, T. and Fontaine, G. (eds.), Elsevier Science Pub., The Hague, 1988, pp. 271–292.

17. Fontaine, G., Frank, R., Tonet, J.L., Gallais, Y., Touzet, I., Todorova, M., Baraka, M., and Grosgogeat, Y. Treatment of resistant ventricular tachycardia by endocavitary fulguration associated with antiarrhythmic therapy as compared to antiarrhythmic therapy alone. Experience of 117 consecutive patients with a mean follow-up of 20 months. In: Cardiac Arrhythmias. Recent Progress in Investigation and Management. Iwa, T. and Fontaine, G. (eds.), Elsevier Science Pub., The Hague, 1988. (in press)

18. Blomstrom-Lundqvist, C. The syndrome of arrythmogenic right ventricular dysplasia, diagnostic and prognostic implications. *Medical Thesis*, 1987, Göteborg.

19. Vedel, J., Frank, R., Fontaine, G., Drobinski, G., Guiraudon, G., Brocheriou, C., and Grosgogeat, Y. Tachycardies ventriculaires recidivantes et ventricule droit papyrace de l'adulte (A propos de deux observations anatomo-cliniques). *Arch. Med. Coeur.* **71**: 973–981, 1978.

20. Richardson, P.J. Endomyocardial biopsy: Technique and evaluation of a new disposable forceps and catheter sheath system. In: Viral Heart Disease. Bolte, H.D. (ed.), Springer-Verlag, Berlin, 1984, pp. 173–176.

21. Goodwin, J.F. Myocarditis and peri-myocarditis. Historical survey, epidemiology and clinical features. *Eur. Heart J.* **8**: Suppl. J, 7–9, 1987.

22. Billingham, M.E. Is acute cardiac rejection a model of myocarditis in humans? *Eur. Heart J.* **8**: Suppl. J, 19–23, 1987.

23. Hasumi, M., Sekiguchi, M., Hiroe, M., Kasanuki, H., and Hirosawa, K. Endomyocardial biopsy approach to patients with ventricular tachycardia with special reference to arrhythmogenic right ventricular dysplasia. *Jpn. Circ. J.* **51**: 242–249, 1987.

24. Fontaine, G., Guiraudon, G., Frank, R., Tereau, Y., Pavie. A., Cabrol, C., Chomette, G., and Grosgogeat, Y. Surgical management of ventricular tachycardia not related to myocardial ischemia. In: Tachycardias, Mechanisms, Diagnosis and Treatment. Josephson, M.E. and Wellens, H.J.J. (eds.), Lea & Febiger, Philadelphia, 1984, pp. 451–473.

25. Manyari, D.E., Gulamhusein, S.S., Boughner, D.R., Kostuk, W.J., Purves, P., Guiraudon, G., and Klein, G.J. Arrhythmogenic right ventricular dysplasia: A generalized cardiomyopathy. *Circulation* **66**: Suppl. II, 1372, 1982.

26. Roberts, W.C., McAllister, H.A., and Ferrans, V.J. Sarcoidosis of the heart. A clinicopathologic study of 35 necropsy patients (group I) and review of 78 previously described necropsy patients (group II). *Am. J. Med.* **63**: 86–108, 1977.

27. Fontaine, G., Fontaliran, F., Linares-Cruz, E., and Chomette, G. The arrhythmogenic right ventricle. In: Cardiac Arrhythmias. Recent Progress in Investigation and Management. Iwa, T. and Fontaine, G. (eds.), Elsevier Science Pub., The Hague, 1988, pp. 189–202.

28. Dec, G.W., Palacios, I.F., and Fallon, J.T. Active myocarditis in the spectrum of acute dilated cardiomyopathy. *N. Engl. J. Med.* **312**: 885–890, 1985.

29. Meany, B.T., Quigley, P.J., Olsen, E.G.J., Richardson, P.J., and Jewitt, D.E. Recent experience of endomyocardial biopsy in the diagnosis of myocarditis. *Eur. Heart J.* **8**: Suppl. J, 17–18, 1987.

30. Hasumi, M., Sekiguchi, M., Yu, Z.X., Hirosawa, K., and Hiroe, M. Analysis of histopathologic findings in cases with dilated cardiomyopathy with special reference to formulating diagnostic criteria on the possibility of postmyocarditic change. *Jpn. Circ. J.* **50**: 1280–1287, 1986.

31. Ibsen, H.H.W., Baandrup, U., and Simonsen, E.E. Familial right ventricular dilated cardiomyopathy. *Br. Heart J.* **54**: 156–159, 1985.

32. Sugrue, D.D., Edwards, W.D., and Olney, B.A. Histologic abnormalities of the left ventricle in a patient with arrhythmogenic right ventricular dysplasia. *Heart Vessels* **1**: 179–181, 1985.

33. Ross, R.S., Bulkley, B.H., and Hutchins, G.M. Idiopathic familial myocardiopathy in three generations: A clinical and pathologic study. *Am. Heart J.* **96**: 170–179, 1978.

34. Harveit, F., Maehle, B.O., and Pihl T. A family with congestive cardiomyopathy. *Cardiology* **68**: 193–200, 1981.

35. Homburger, F., Baker, J.R., Nixon, C.W., and Whitney, R. Primary generalized polymyopathy and cardiac necrosis in an inbred line of Syrian hamsters. *Med. Exp.* **6**: 339–345, 1962.

36. Bajusz, E. Hereditary cardiomyopathy: A new disease model. *Am. Heart J.* **77**: 686–696, 1969.

37. Nishikawa, T., Sekiguchi, M., Kunimine, Y., Momma, K., Ando, M., and Takao, A. An infant with dilated cardiomyopathy confirmed as myocarditis by endomyocardial biopsy. *Heart Vessels* **3**: 108–110, 1987.

Extent of Tissue Involved in Arrhythmogenic Right Ventricular Dysplasia Using Electrophysiologic and Angiographic Studies

Hiroshi Kasanuki, Satoshi Ohnishi, and Saichi Hosoda

The Heart Institute of Japan, Tokyo Women's Medical College, Tokyo, Japan

ABSTRACT

Ten cases with ARVD were studied (9 male, 1 female, average age 47). All cases had RV enlargement, wall motion abnormality and dysfunction. LV enlargement, wall motion abnormality and dysfunction were found in four of ten cases. Endocardial mapping delayed potentials in all cases. Localization of delayed potential was as follows: RV inflow tract in all, RV outflow in eight, RV apex in two cases, and LV apex in two cases. In conclusion, the extent of cardiac tissue involved in ARVD can include a part of LV, as well as various sites within RV.

INTRODUCTION

In 1977, Fontaine *et al.* described a recurrent ventricular tachycardia (VT) which was characterized by a left bundle branch block (LBBB) pattern, right ventricular (RV) cardiomyopathy of unknown causes, and RV dilatation with hypokinesis, in which the RV musculature is replaced by fatty and fibrous tissue.[1,2] Although this disease, termed arrhythmogenic right ventricular dysplasia (ARVD), has since attracted considerable attention,[3-12] its pathogenesis, treatment and prognosis have yet to be clarified.

The purpose of this study is to investigate the extent of cardiac tissue involved in ARVD using angiographic and electrophysiologic studies.

SUBJECTS AND METHODS

Subjects: 10 patients had ARVD with associated recurrent sustained VT. Nine cases were male, and one case was female. Their average age was 47.3 years, ranging from 23 to 78 years.

Methods: All had intracardiac mapping of both ventricles, VT induction tests, cardiac catheterizations, angiography, and signal averaged ECGs.

Our electrical stimulation protocol consisted of delivering single and double extra stimuli during paced rhythm (basic cycle length, 600, 500, 400 msec), rapid pacing and burst pacing from the right atrium and the right ventricle (apex, outflow, and inflow).

The stimulation and the pharmacologic protocol of our laboratory have been reported in detail in other reports.[13]

Endocardiac mappings of delayed potentials were made by the potentials recorded from both ventricles, using cinefilm under bidirectional fluoroscopy. Signal averaged ECGs were recorded by a high resolution electrocardiograph (produced by Marquette Company) through the band pass filter from 100 to 300 Hz.

The mean follow-up period was 7.2 years (range, 1–15 years).

RESULTS

1. Clinical Findings (Table 1)

The initial symptom was palpitation attack in all cases. The onset of VT ranged between ages 19–63, average age 22.6. During VT, 5 cases complained of syncope, and one had faintness. None had congestive heart failure and all were class 1 of the NYHA cardiac function classification. The cardiac-thoracic ratio ranged from 44 to 63%, average ratio 54.5%. Seven cases had ratios over 50%.

2. ECG Findings (Table 2)

During normal sinus rhythm ECGs, 3 cases showed left axis deviation (LAD), 2 cases had right axis deviation, 2 cases showed incomplete right bundle branch block (RBBB) and one case showed low voltage. In nine cases, negative T waves in precordial leads (V,–V4) were found. Post excitation wave (PEW) was observed in all cases. All cases showed an LBBB pattern on ECG during VT. As far as the QRS axis is concerned, nine cases showed LAD, five cases showed normal axis deviation, and 4 cases should

TABLE 1.   Clinical Findings

Case	Sex	Age	Age of VT onset	CTR	NYHA	Symptom
1	M	46 y	36 y	44%	class I	faintness
2	M	45	39	47	I	syncope
3	M	56	47	48	I	palpitation
4	M	32	27	51	I	palpitation
5	M	48	35	62	I	palpitation
6	F	55	30	63	I	palpitation
7	M	23	19	53	I	syncope
8	M	78	63	63	I	syncope
9	M	41	24	58	I	syncope
10	M	49	40	56	I	syncope

TABLE 2.   ECG Findings during Sinus Rhythm and Ventricular Tachycardia

Case	During sinus rhythm			During VT
	PEW	QRS wave	Neg T	QRS configulation
1	−	normal		LBBB+LAD, LBBB+NAD
2	+	normal	V_{1-4}	LBBB+LAD*
3	+	LAD	V_{1-4}	LBBB+LAD, LBBB+NAD
4	+	low voltage	V_{1-4}	LBBB+LAD*, LBBBB+NAD, LBBB+RAD
5	+	normal	V_{1-5}	LBBB+RAD
6	+	rBBB+LAD	V_{1-4}	LBBB+LAD, LBBB+RAD
7	−	RAD	V_{1-4}	LBBB+LAD
8	+	rBBB+LAD	V_{1-5}	LBBB+LAD, LBBB+NAD
9	+	RAD	V_{1-4}	LBBB+LAD*, LBBBB+NAD, RBBB+NAD
10	−	normal	V_{1-4}	LBBB+LAD

PEW=post excitation wave, LAD=left axis deviation, RAD=right axis deviation, NAD= normal axis deviation, rBBB=incomplete right bundle branch block, RBBB=complete right bundle branch block, LBBB=complete left bundle branch block. Asterisk indicates two kinds of ventricular tachycardia.

right axis deviation. One case exhibited a RBBB pattern. In 7 of 10 cases, more than two kinds of VT were found.

In single averaged ECGs, late potentials were recorded in all cases. Maximum amplitude ranged from 1.1 to 1.9 uV, (average, 1.7 uV), the duration ranging from 6.9 to 250 msec (average, 111.9 msec).

TABLE 3.   Cardiac Catheterization and Angiographic Findings

Case	RV				LV			
	EF(%)	EDVI	Wall motion	EDP	EF(%)	EDVI	Wall motion	EDP
1	22	113	hypokinetic outflow: dyskinetic	5	62	76	normal	12
2	34	136	hypokinetic	5	56	82	normal	10
3	20	170	hypokinetic outflow: dyskinetic	7	55	52	normal	12
4	24	210	hypokinetic	13	62	87	normal	12
5	25	255	hypokinetic	11	55		normal	5
6	16	154	hypokinetic	12	31	129	apex: none	12
7	23	191	hypokinetic	8	54	98	normal	13
8	20	261	hypokinetic	5	48	103	hypokinetic	8
9	22	209	hypokinetic	6	35	113	apex: hypo	9
10	21	188	hypokinetic	7	48	82	apex: hypo	10

EF = ejection fraction, EDVI = end-diastolic volume index, EDP = end-diastolic pressure.

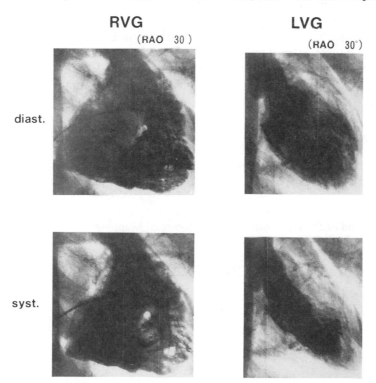

RVG
(RAO 30)

LVG
(RAO 30°)

diast.

syst.

Fig. 1.   Case 9, in which LVEF abnormalities (35%), LV enlargement (EDVI, 113 ml/m²), and LV wall motion abnormalities (hypokinesis of apex) were found. RVEF was 22%, and RVEDVI was 209 ml/m².

3. *Cardiac Catheterization and Angiography* (*Table 3*)

RV ejection fraction (EF) decreased in all cases, average value being 22.7% (range, 16–34%). RV end-diastolic volume index (EDVI) increased in all cases, average value being 188.7 ml/m² (range, 113–225 ml/m²). RV end diastolic pressure ranged from 5 to 13 mmHg, average 7.9-mmHg. All patients exhibited a RV wall motion abnormality as follows: all had hypokinesis, and 2 had dyskinesis of RV outflow tract.

LV wall motion abnormalities were found in 4 of 10 cases. LV enlargement was found in 3 cases. LVEF ranged from 31 to 62%, average 50.6%. LVEDVI ranged from 52 to 113 ml/m², average 91.3 ml/m². Two had tricuspid regurgitation, and one had mitral regurgitation. Coronary angiogram revealed no abnormalities in any of the cases. Figure 1 shows a case in which LVEF abnormalities, LV enlargement and LV wall motion abnormalities were found.

4. *Endocardiac Mapping* (*Table 4*)

Endocardiac mapping showed delayed potentials in all cases. Localization of delayed potential was as follows: RV inflow tract in all, RV outflow tract in 8, RV apex in 2 cases, and LV apex in 2 cases. Delayed potentials in more than two sites were observed in all cases except one. For example, localization of delayed potential was RV outflow/inflow in 6 and RV outflow/inflow/apex in 2. VT of LBBB pattern originating in the RV was found in all 10 patients. Figure 2 shows a case in which delayed potentials were found in RV outflow/inflow/apex.

5. *Induction and Termination of VT*

Sustained monomorphic VT could be induced by cardiac pacing in 9 cases and by administering Aprindine in one case. VT was inducible by single extrastimuli in the RV in 2 cases, double extrastimuli in 6 cases, and burst pacing in 2 cases. A morphology of induced VT was similar to that of spontaneous VT in every case. VT was terminated by RV burst pacing in 3 cases, by RV single extrastimuli in one case, and by DC shock in one case.

DISCUSSION

The pathogenesis, progress, therapy and prognosis of ARVD remain widely disputed.[1-12] The relation between ARVD and Uhl's anomaly, parchment heart syndrome

TABLE 4. Location of Delayed Potential on Endocardial Mapping.

Case	RV Inflow	Inflow-apex	Apex	Apex-outflow	Outflow	LV
1	+	−	−	−	+	−
2	+	−	−	−	+	−
3	+	+	+	−	+	−
4	+	−	−	−	+	−
5	+	+	+	+	+	−
6	+	−	−	−	−	+
7	+	−	−	−	−	−
8	+	+	−	+	+	−
9	+	+	−	+	+	+
10	+	−	−	−	+	−

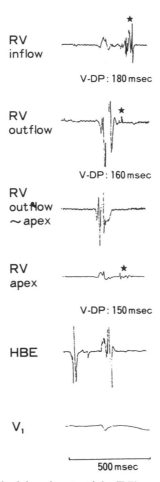

Fig. 2.   Case 3, in which delayed potentials (DP) were found in RV inflow/outflow/apex. Asterisk shows delayed potential.

and RV dilated cardiomyopathy (RVDCM) is not always clear.[13-17] Of 24 cases ARVD, Marcus *et al.* reported 2 cases without VT.[4] Fitchett *et al.* proposed the concept of RV dilated cardiomyopathy (RVDCM) defined as myocardial disease of unknown cause with RV enlargement and RVEF abnormalities.[17] These authors suggested that RVDCM and LVDCM represented two extremes of one continuous spectrum. We defined ARVD as the myocardial disease of unknown cause composed primarily of recurrent sustained VT originating from RV without heart failure. There are few reports which evaluate the extent of tissue involved in ARVD using angiographic and electrophysiologic findings.

1. Clinical Findings

Of 24 cases reported by Marcus *et al*, 16 cases were male and 6 were female, the average age being 39 years (range, 17–65),[4] and of 14 cases reported by Fitchett *et al* none were male and 5 were female, the average age being 28 years (range, 9–62).[17] In this study, males outnumbered females 9 to one, the average age of VT onset being about the same, ranging from 16 to as old as 63 years. It is apparent that further sex and age analysis is necessary to clarify the etiology of ARVD, and especially genetic factors. In Fitchett's study, only 6 of 14 cases had VT, but 11 cases had heart failure.[17] Thus the pathogenesis of their cases were considered to be different from that of our cases.

2. ECG Findings

Marcus *et al.* reported for ECGs at rest T wave inversion in precordial leads in 19 of 22 cases, similar to in 90% in our studies.[4] Although, the QRS morphology showed incomplete RBBB, LAD, right axis deviation, and low voltage in our study, many cases with RBBB or low voltage and fewer cases with LAD or right axis deviation have been reported. On ECG during VT, all cases exhibited a LBBB pattern with various axes, and 7 cases had more than 2 types of VT. Marcus *et al.* also reported identical results.[4] Therefore the origin of VT is considered to be at various sites of the RV, especially at the RV inflow tracts. Post excitation wave (also called Epsilon potential) on standard 12 leads ECG and late potential on signal-averaged ECG are considered to request the presence of conduction delay areas in the ventricle. According to Marcus *et al.*, post excitation waves were observed in 7 of 22 cases, and late potentials were recorded in 13 of 16.[4] In our study, they were observed in 90% and 100%, respectively. As these findings, especially late potentials, are considered to be important for the diagnosis of ARVD and the analysis of its pathogenesis, further investigation is necessary.

3. Cardiac Catheterization and Angiographic Findings

Although RV enlargement, hypokinesis and EF abnormalities were recognized in all cases, their degree varied in individual cases. One had marked hypokinesis of entire RV, changing hemodynamically to mimic function of the right atrium. Two other patients had dyskinesis of RV outflow tract. Marcus *et al.* also reported one case with systolic bulging of RV infundibulum. As for involvement of LV tissue, Marcus *et al.* reported one case with hypokinesis of LV diaphragmatic wall in one case of right ventricular dysplasia,[4] and Fitchett *et al.* reported two cases with slight LV enlargement in 2 cases of RVDCM.[17] Manyari *et al.* observed latent LV dysfunction using radionuclide angiography in all cases of ARVD.[11] Although all cases had normal LV end-diastolic diameter at rest, during exercise, two cases showed a decrease of LVEF and an enlargement of the end-diastolic diameter. All cases exhibited segmental contraction abnormalities (interventricular septum, 5 cases; infero-apical region, 4 cases). Therefore, these authors proposed the concept of a generalized cardiomyopathy. In our study of ARVD, LV enlargement and LV wall motion abnormalities (one case with hypokinesis of the entire LV, one case with hypokinesis, two cases dyskinesis of LV apex) were also found in four cases. Therefore, the extent of tissue involved in ARVD is considered to be different in the LV and the RV. In other words, ARVD might constitute one continuous spectrum with LV dilated cardiomyopathy, characterized by congestive heart disease. However, one case showed normal LV function and wall motion in spite of marked RV enlargement and dysfunction on follow-up over a period of 15 years, indicating the pathogenesis localization only in the RV. Therefore, the possibility exists that ARVD is not due to only one etiology, one pathogenesis is not suggested.

4. Endocardial Mapping and VT Induction

Delayed potentials on endocardial and epicardial mapping are considered to show directly the presence of a slow conduction area. In cases in which the time from V wave to the delayed potential of the less than 100 msec, which frequently occurs during the QRS waves. As a consquence neither post excitation wave nor late potential can be recorded. Therefore delayed potential on endocardial mapping is the best indicator which shows electrophysiologic lesions of localized conduction delay. Marcus *et al.* recognized delayed potentials on epicardial mapping in all 22 cases, but found delayed potentials on endocardial mapping in only four cases (18%).[4] On the other hand, in our study, all cases had delayed potentials on endocardial mapping. Its detection ratio depends on the methods employed. The reason for our high detection ratio is probably due to our endocardial mapping in more than 20 sites under bidirectional fluoroscopy. Previous pathologic studies[18,19] and observations made during operation[1,2,4,10] had found that the most frequent areas affected by dysplasia are in the anterior infundibulum, the RV apex, and the inferior wall of the RV, often referred to as the "triangle of dysplasia." Our findings on endocardial mapping confirmed this pattern of distribution, especially at RV inflow tract. Furthermore, in our study, although all cases had wall motion anomalies of entire RV, localizations of delayed potential were found. It is clinically important that wall motion anomalies and the presence of delayed potential are not always consistent. This is because slow conduction at the area of delayed potential may cause reentry, resulting in VT. In our study, delay potentials spread widely in all but two cases. Although the presence of delayed potential does not mean reentrant circuit, there is a possibility it will cause reentrant VT. There are few reports of delayed potential of the LV in cases with ARVD. In our study, two cases with LV wall motion anomalies should delayed potentials in LV apex. One case exhibited non-sustained VT of RBBB pattern originating in the delayed potential region of the LV apex. Therefore, in cases with ARVD, electrophysiologic lesion as well as angiographic abnormality is considered to extend to the LV, indicating the occurrence of sustained VT originating in the LV.

Reentry and triggered activity due to late after potentials are considered as causes for VT which can be induced by programmed stimulation.[19] According to Marcus *et al.*, VT could be induced by extrastimulation in 18 of 22 cases.[4] In our study, clinical sustained VT was inducible by electrical stimulation in nine cases except for one case, in which Aprindine markedly prolonged the time from V wave to delayed potential, resulting in sustained VT. In all cases, entrainment phenomenon was found, indicating the reentrant mechanism. Furthermore, delayed potentials were recorded at the earliest excitation sites of VT, suggesting that the delayed potential related to the reentry circuit.

REFERENCES

1. Fontaine, G.H. *et al.* Stimulation studies and epicardial mapping in ventricular tachycardia: Study of mechanisms and selection for surgery. In: Reentrant Arrhythmias, Kulbertus, H. (ed.), MTP Press, Lancaster, 1977, p. 334.
2. Frank, R. *et al.* Electrocardiologie de quatre cas de dysplasie ventriculaire droite arrhythmogene. *Arch. Mal. Coeur.* **71**: 963, 1978.
3. Dungan, W.T. *et al.* Arrhythmogenic right ventricular dysplasia: A cause of ventricular tachycardia in children with apparently normal hearts. *Am. Heart J.* **102**: 745, 1981.
4. Marcus, F.I. *et al.* Right ventricular dysplasia: A report of 24 adult cases. *Circulation* **65**: 384, 1982.
5. Rossi, P. *et al.* Arrhythmogenic right ventricular dysplasia: Clinical features, diagnostic techniques, and current management. *Am. Heart J.* **103**: 415, 1982.
6. Higuchi, S. *et al.* 16-year follow up of arrhythmogenic right ventricular dysplasia. *Am. Heart J.* **108**: 1363, 1984.

7. Robertson, J.H. *et al.* Comparison of two-dimensional echo cardiographic and angiographic findings in arrhythmogenic right ventricular dysplasia. *Am. J. Cardiol.* **55**: 1506, 1985.

8. Olsson, S.B. *et al.* A case of arrhythmogenic right ventricular dysplasia with ventricular fibrillation. *Clin. Cardiol.* **5**: 591, 1982.

9. Sevick, R.J. *et al.* Long-term management of arrhythmogenic right ventricular dysplasia. *Can. Med. Assoc. J.* **128**: 418, 1983.

10. Guiraudon, G.M. *et al.* Total disconnection of the right ventricular free wall: Surgical treatment of right ventricular tachycardia associated with right ventricular dysplasia. *Circulation* **67**: 463, 1983.

11. Manyari, D.E. *et al.* Arrhythmogenic right ventricular dysplasia: A generalized cardiomyopathy, *Circulation* **68**: 251, 1983.

12. Webb, J.G. *et al.* Left ventricular abnormalities in arrhythmogenic right ventricular dysplasia. *Am. J. Cardiol.* **58**: 568, 1986.

13. Kasanuki, H. *et al.* Availability of electrophysiological approach to the selection and assessment of antiarrhythmic drugs for recurrent ventricular tachycardia. *Jpn. Circ. J.* **47**: 105, 1983.

14. Gaffney, F.A. *et al.* Noninvasive recognition of the parchment right ventricule (Uhl's anomaly arrhythmogenic right ventricular dysplasia) syndrome. *Clin. Cardiol.* **6**: 235, 1983.

15. Uhl, H.S.M. A previously undescribed congenital malformation of the heart: Almost total absence of the myocardium of the right ventricle. *Bulletin of the Johns Hopkins Hospital* **91**: 197, 1952.

16. Waller, B.F. *et al.* Congenital hypoplasia of portions of both right and left ventricular myocardial walls. *Am. J. Cardiol.* **46**: 885, 1980.

17. Fitchett, P.H. *et al.* Right ventricular dilated cardiomyopathy. *Br. Heart J.* **51**: 25, 1984.

18. Cherrier F. *et al.* Les dysplasies ventriculaires droites: A propos de 7 observations. *Arch. Mal. Coeur.* **72**: 766, 1979.

19. Gould, L. *et al.* Partial absence of the right ventricular musculature. A congenital lesion. *Am. J. Med.* **42**: 636, 1967.

Surgical Experience of Ventricular Tachycardia Unrelated to Ischemic Heart Disease

Takashi Iwa,* Takuro Misaki,* Makoto Tsubota,* Kazuki Ishida,* and Ryozo Okada**

* Department of Surgery (I), Kanazawa University School of Medicine, Kanazawa, Japan
** Department of Internal Medicine, Research Laboratory for Cardiovascular Pathology, Juntendo University School of Medicine, Tokyo, Japan

ABSTRACT

Resection and cryocoagulation of the origin of ventricular tachycardia (VT) in the right ventricle and incision and cryocoagulation of the left ventricular nonischemic VT are our procedures of choice based on pre- and intraoperative electrophysiologic studies. Surgical results in 38 patients with nonischemic VT refractory to drug therapy were satisfactory. Five patients had delayed potentials during VT, which formed a macroreentry circuit. Histopathologic studies of surgical specimens revealed the specific cause of VT in every case. So-called idiopathic VT is unlikely to exist. Chronic myocarditis is the most common cause of nonischemic VT. Arrhythmogenic right ventricular dysplasia showed no inflammatory cell infiltrate in the myocardium by serial histopathologic study.

INTRODUCTION

With increasing knowledge and experience of electrocardiophysiology, surgical management of ventricular tachycardia (VT) has now become a practical proposition. Most efforts, however, have been directed to ischemic VT[1-3] and reports of surgical management of VT unrelated to ischemic heart disease have been extremely rare.[4-7] We have been treating patients with nonischemic VT from the start of our surgical intervention since ischemic VT is much less common in Japan compared with Western countries. Surgical experience of nonischemic VT has revealed several new findings such as myocarditis as the cause of so-called idiopathic VT, and macroreentry proved by epicardial mapping. These as well as surgical results are the subjects of this paper.

PATIENTS AND METHODS

We operated on a 15-year-old girl with VT of left ventricular origin on April 15, 1975, one of the first such operations reported. However, the VT was not cured due to insufficient electrophysiologic studies obtained during the surgery.

We resumed direct surgery for VT on February 6, 1978, and by the end of August 1988 had performed such a procedure on 38 patients with nonischemic VT, with sufficient pre- and intraoperative electrophysiologic studies. Twenty-four patients had VT of right ventricular origin and 14 of the left side. Thirty patients were males and 8 females, aged between 9 and 66 years old (average 32.1 years). Seven patients were 15 years old or below that age. The time from onset of VT was between 4 months to 23 years (average 6 years and 2 months).

All patients were referred to us as having idiopathic VT except 6 with arrhythmogenic right ventricular dysplasia(ARVD)with typical clinical findings[8] and one with postoperative status of tetralogy of Fallot. They were all referred to us by cardiologists throughout Japan, and had been treated with various antiarrhythmic drugs except Amiodarone which is not yet commercially available in Japan. The VT was judged refractory to drug therapy. Four patients were sent to us as emergencies by helicopter or airplane with attending doctors, intravenous infusion of antiarrhythmic drugs, and DC countershocks in hand, and even under general anesthesia in one patient.

1. Preoperative Diagnostic Studies

Twelve-lead electrocardiograms and electrocardiophysiology studies were performed in all patients. Vector cardiography, body surface mapping, the nuclear medical cardiography method, catheterization, and cardio- and coronary angiography were undertaken in almost every case.

Programmed pacing resulted in sustained VT in 25 of the 38 cases. Eight had VT of multiple origins. Only uniform premature ventricular contractions (PVC) were produced during the study in 12 patients despite the presence of sustained VT documented by ECG before admission. In those patients the QRS direction of the PVC in the 12-lead ECG was the same as those in previous VT, which indicates that the origin of both was the same site.[9] In one patient, PVCs but no sustained VT were detected before or after admission to our hospital. She had 40,000 PVCs per day as confirmed by Holter monitoring study.

2. Epicardial Mapping

We employ the largest polychannel recorder available in Japan, a 16-channel recorder, and implant bipolar platinum electrodes in 5 × 3 rows with one lead as reference in silicone rubber to make large, medium, and small mats. The large mat is 12 × 6 cm, covers 70% of one ventricle and is able to cover completely the whole ventricle in one move. It is possible to determine the earliest excitation site by reading the time delay of the potential on a personal computer and following mapping in about 30 sec.[9] We often encounter one or 2 PVCs during surgery without sustained VT. The earliest excitation site can be determined with the above polypolar mat from PVC, based on the finding that such a PVC is similar to VT in terms of detailed QRS polarity. This means that the origin of PVC is the same as that of VT.

3. Delayed Potentials

Delayed potentials were found during normal sinus rhythm in 12-lead ECGs in 4 of 6 ARVD patients. During VT, delayed potentials or potentials in diastolic phase were recorded in 5 patients, which formed macroreentry. Three patients had ARVD, one myocarditis, and one postoperative status of tetralogy of Fallot. The first ARVD patient has been reported previously.[10] During tachycardia, delayed potentials were recorded over the right ventricular anterior wall. It was evident that delayed potentials formed diastolic bridging through the cardiac cycle in the opposite direction of essential epicardial activation. We plotted essential epicardial activation and delayed potentials separately, although both potentials were taken at the same time. This was not done with the other 4 patients. The electrophysiologic data suggested a macroreentrant loop, which was the movement of the excitation wave of electrical activity starting near the right ventricular apex and returning slowly to the same point through the delayed potentials as the reentry circuit.[10]

Since we started using a 15-channel bipolar silicone mat for epicardial mapping in

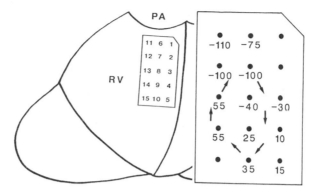

Fig. 1. A medium-sized silicone mat (5 × 3 cm) was placed on the outflow tract of the right ventricle longitudinally. Serial numbers indicate sites of bipolar electrodes and correspond to the numbers in the left column in Fig. 2. Numbers in the enlarged figure shown on the right indicate time intervals measured after the onset of the QRS complex and are expressed in msec. RV, right ventricle; PA, pulmonary artery.

1983, we have mapped 4 patients. They all showed delayed potentials during VT, forming diastolic bridging. Findings attributed to postoperative tetralogy of Fallot were revealed using the method described below.

A medium-sized 15-bipolar silicone mat, 5 × 3 cm in size, 16-channel polygraphy MIC 9800 S (Fukuda Denshi), 159–500 Hz, paper speed 200 mm/min, with direct ink jet writing, were utilized. After opening the chest by longitudinal sternum incision, the reference lead was placed on the midanterior wall of the right ventricle. The medium-sized silicone mat was placed on the outflow tract of the right ventricle longitudinally (Fig. 1) and VT was induced by programmed electrical stimulation of the right ventricle.

Epicardial mapping (Fig. 2) revealed fragmented activity on leads 13, 12, and 11 and late potentials on 7, 6, and 3 in the diastolic phase. They then connected to 4, 5, 9, 10, and 14 in that order in the systolic phase forming a reentry circuit. Low polarities at 8, 11, 12, and 13 were probably due to scar formation around an incision in the right ventricle after previous surgery for tetralogy of Fallot.

A 2 × 2.5 cm area of the whole thickness of the right ventricle at 3 as the center was resected. Then cryocoagulation of the surrounding area, where the delayed potentials and fragmented activity occurred, was done at 60°C for 2 min and the defect was closed with a Gore-Tex® patch of the same size. VT did not recur spontaneously or upon electrical stimulation after the surgery.

4. Surgical Method

The principle of our surgical method for VT is to excise the whole thickness of the myocardium of the right ventricle at the site of origin and cryocoagulate sites of delayed potential if present, or by a simple incision at the earliest excitation site of the left ventricle and cryocoagulation of early excitation sites. For VT of right ventricular origin, resection of the whole thickness of the myocardium at the earliest excitation site, 2 × 2.5 cm on average, is performed. The surrounding area of the excised portion is cryocoagulated to abolish delayed potentials, which are usually scattered in a wide area, particularly in ARVD.

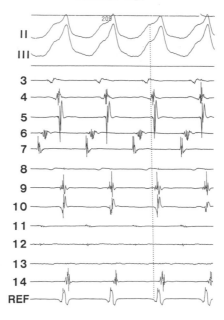

Fig. 2. Electrocardiographic leads II and III are shown with electrograms recorded at the mid-right ventricular anterior wall as the reference (REF). The dotted line indicates the onset of the QRS complex. All time interval measurements are expressed in msec after the onset of the QRS complex and listed in Fig. 1. Potentials at 13, 12, 11, 7, 6, and 3 are seen in that order in the diastolic phase. Then the potential connects to 4, 5, 9, 10, and 14 in that order in the systolic phase. They form a reentry circuit as shown by arrows in Fig. 1.

In nonischemic VT of left ventricular origin, an incision of approximately 3 cm in length is made at the site of earliest excitation. Cryocoagulation is applied from the endocardial side after performing endocardial mapping with a pencil type of catheter electrode. Cardiac muscle is usually not resected to avoid reduction of the size of the left ventricle, which is normal in nonischemic VT patients. This is a major difference from ischemic VT. Only a thin slice of the incised face of the myocardium is taken as the surgical specimen. A specially made cryoprobe is applied on the left septal VT through a 3-cm incision in the left ventricle.

Excision plus cryocoagulation is used mainly in right ventricular VT, and incision plus cryocoagulation for left ventricular VT (Table 1).

TABLE 1. Operative Procedure for Nonischemic VT

Procedure	RV	LV	Total
Excision + Cryocoagulation	19	3	22
Excision	3	0	3
Incision + Cryocoagulation	2	10	12
Removal of tumor	0	1	1
Total	24	14	38

RV : right ventricle, LV : left ventricle.

RESULTS

The results of surgery in our patients were more favorable than expected. Thirty-six of 38 patients were cured (Table 2). In 27 patients, frequent preoperative VT, even with heavy antiarrhythmic drug therapy, disappeared completely without the use of anti-arrhythmic agents. VT disappeared on medication in 2. Three had no VT but PVCs. In the other 4 patients, VT attacks decreased considerably, but PVCs still occurred. Two patients died. In one with ARVD, myocardial resection in 3 portions and cryocoagula-tion brought about a cure initially, but the first attack of VT 5 months postoperatively resulted in death. The other patient had undergone emergency surgery. Nonischemic left ventricular aneurysm was resected as an emergency measure without sufficient pre-operative electrocardiophysiologic study. VT was not cured, and the patient died one week after the surgery. Of the 38 patients, 36 were cured, and 2 cases died from congestive heart failure 2 years and 2 years and 4 months later, respectively. The results are more favorable than expected in view of the seriousness of the disease and unestablished operative procedures.

HISTOPATHOLOGY

Since we excised part of the myocardium from the earliest excitation area, interesting pathologic findings were obtained. Surgical biopsy specimens were taken from 34 of 38 patients, and pathologic study was completed in 28. A stay suture was stitched to indicate the earliest excitation site of either ventricle. On average, a 2×2.5 cm area of the thickness of whole the right ventricular myocardium including the stay suture, or a much smaller area of the left ventricle, was resected as a specimen for pathologic study. Serial sections of all specimens were undertaken.

The study revealed 6 patients had ARVD, 2 suspected ARVD without typical clinical findings, 17 chronic myocarditis, 2 abnormal muscle band, and one a cardiac fibroma (Table 3). Figure 3 shows the relationship between the histopathologic findings in each patient and the site of the lesions.

1. Myocarditis

In most patients with myocarditis, in addition to fibrosis or fatty degeneration, diffuse inflammatory cell infiltration mainly consisting of lymphocytes was detected in the

TABLE 2. Results of Surgery for Nonischemic VT

Cured	36	Without medication	29	
		With medication	2	
		VT ($-$), PVC ($+$)	3	#
		VT ($\downarrow$), PVC ($+$)	4	$*$
Died	2	Sudden death	1	(5 Mo)
		VT + LOS	1	(1 W)
Total	38		38	

\# 1 died, cardiac failure (2 years and 4 months).
$*$ 1 died, cardiac failure (2 years).
PVC: premature ventricular contraction, LOS: low cardiac output syndrome, Yr: year, Mo: month, W: week.

TABLE 3. Pathology of Nonischemic VT

Pathology	Site of origin	
	RV	LV
ARVD	6	0
ARVD suspected	2	0
Myocarditis	6	11
Abnormal muscle band	2	0
Tumor	0	1
Subtotal	16	12
Under pathologic study	6	0
Without specimen	2	2
Total	24	14

RV: right ventricle, LV: left ventricle.

VT origins and operative procedures

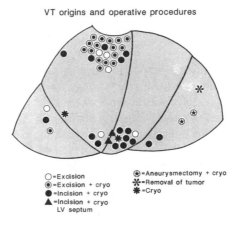

○ =Excision
◉ =Excision + cryo
● =Incision + cryo
▲ =Incision + cryo
       LV septum

⊛ =Aneurysmectomy + cryo
✳ =Removal of tumor
✱ =Cryo

Fig. 3.   VT origins and surgical procedures.

whole region of resected myocardial tissue. The myocarditis group can be divided into 2 subtypes based on pathologic features. One has mainly fatty infiltration and the other mainly fibrosis.

(1) Six of 17 patients had extensive fatty infiltration with myocarditis (Fig. 4). Every specimen showed moderately severe fatty infiltration in the right ventricle, particularly in the outflow tract. In addition a marked infiltration of inflammatory cells, fatty tissue infiltration, and disarray of muscle bundles was noted (Fig. 5).

(2) Eleven of 17 patients showed mainly fibrosis with myocarditis (Fig. 6), all in the left ventricle. Degeneration and disarrangement of myocytes was also found—as well as scattered fibrosis and inflammatory cell infiltration, consisting predominantly of lymphocytes (Fig. 7).

2. ARVD

Six patients had ARVD, with marked infiltration of fatty tissue in the right ventricular wall, which was very thin. On light microscopic examination almost transmural fat replacement was found. Some of the residual myocardial cells were coarsely arranged

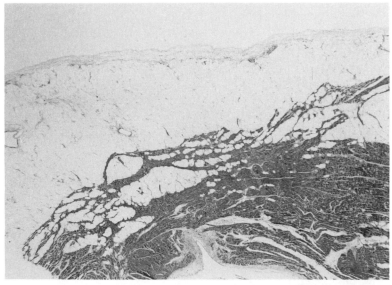

Fig. 4.   Patient no. 6, 34 years old, male, myocarditis I. Surgical biopsy speci-men was taken from the right ventricular outflow tract. There was marked fatty infiltration on the epicardial side and fibrous thickening of both the epi- and endocardium. Diffuse lymphocyte infiltration in the interstitium was noted. Hematoxylin-eosin stain, × 20.

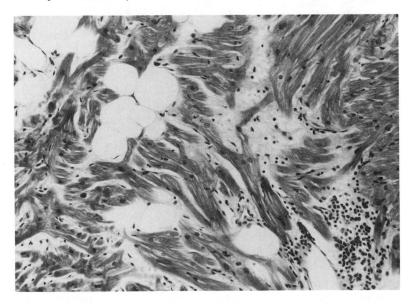

Fig. 5.   Higher magnification of specimen from patient no. 6 revealed disar-rangement of myocardial fiber, fatty infiltration, and diffuse infiltration of in-flammatory cells, mostly lymphocytes. Hematoxylin-eosin stain, × 200.

indicating a characteristic wafer-like layer between the thickened endo- and epicardium. An increase of medial thickness of the peripheral coronary arteries was often seen. No inflammatory cell infiltration was observed in any of the serial sections (Fig. 8).

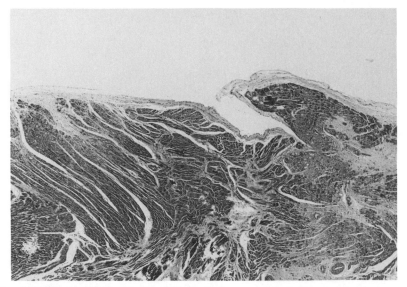

Fig. 6. Patient no. 18, 10 years old, male, myocarditis II. Specimen taken from the left ventricular apex. There was disarrangement of myocardial fibers and scattered fibrosis. Hematoxylin-eosin stain, × 40.

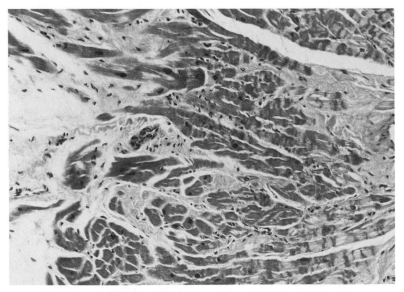

Fig. 7. Higher magnification of specimen from patient no. 18 revealed marked fibrosis and diffuse infiltration of inflammatory cells, mostly lymphocytes. Hematoxylin-eosin stain, × 200.

DISCUSSION

Few patients with nonischemic chronic sustained VT have been regarded as having a good prognosis, and VT has been accepted to be dangerous and life-threatening, when, for example, compared with supraventricular tachycardias. The major indication for surgical intervention in VT is refractoriness to drug treatment and/or intolerable sub-

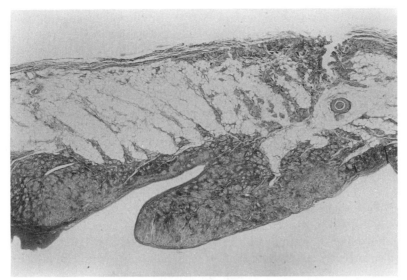

Fig. 8. Patient no. 5, 15 years old, male, ARVD. Specimen taken from the right ventricle. There was a marked decrease in myocytes and abundant fatty tissue. Some of the residual myocardial fibers showed coarse arrangement. Proliferation of media of the peripheral coronary arteries was found. Both the epi- and endocardium were thickened. No inflammatory cells were found in any serial section. Elastica-Van Gieson stain, × 20.

jective symptoms of the patients. Four patients in the present series were referred to us as real emergencies by helicopter or commercial flight while receiving intravenous infusion by the attending doctor and with direct current countershock apparatus. It is believed that there is no other method than surgery to cure VT.

Detailed epicardial mapping is essential for surgery of VT, and the examination must be completed promptly as VT aggravates the hemodynamic condition of patients. Thus, it is inappropriate to measure potential point by point, as for example in mapping of Wolff-Parkinson-White (WPW) syndrome. For this reason, efforts have been made to take concomitant measurement and map potentials at 60–160 points over the entire heart.[11,12] Our 15-point bipolar electrode mat, commercially available 16-channel recorder, and personal computer are less costly and sufficient for epicardial mapping of VT.

VT must be induced and terminated by programmed electrical stimulation during surgery; otherwise it is impossible to determine the origin or earliest excitation site of VT by epicardial mapping. However, many of our VT patients had only PVCs spontaneously or upon electrical stimulation at the time of surgery or admission after long-term high-dose drug therapy at previous hospitals in spite of the fact that they had definite sustained VTs repeatedly during the course of their disease. When their ECGs are carefully studied, however, the pattern of the QRS complex of PVC and VT is the same, indicating a common origin. Our 15-channel bipolar mat electrode and automatic display of data by a computer yielded an epicardial map indicating the operation site after short-term tachycardia or even a single PVC. After completion of this mapping system and introduction of a test anesthesia that does not induce provocation of tachycardia,[9] we confirmed that surgery, previously performed only for reentry and electrically inducible VT, is also applicable to PVC.

Because there is a significant gap in location between the earliest excitation site in epi- and endocardial mapping in ischemic VT, the endocardium must be studied. This is probably due to ischemic fibrous tissue. Such a discrepancy does not exist in non-ischemic hearts. The earliest excitation site of the epicardium always indicates the earliest point of the endocardium. The only exception occurs when VT is of septal origin. We saw 2 patients with left septal origin VT who were diagnosed by preoperative ECG and electrophysiologic studies. In such cases, endocardial mapping was necessary after an incision was made in the left ventricular apex. At the time of surgery, endocardial mapping using a pencil type or catheter electrode was done after making the incision. Complex endocardial mapping advocated for ischemic VT is not practical for nonischemic VT.

Delayed potential was first found in ARVD by Fontaine in 12-lead ECGs during sinus rhythm.[14] Later, it was also found in ischemic heart disease. Much has been written regarding the possibility of a relation between delayed potentials and reentrant VT.[14,15] We proved a macroreentrant circuit existed by epicardial mapping in one ARVD patient.[10] In the other 4 patients studied by 15-point electrode simultaneous epicardial mapping, macroreentry was proved. In those 5 patients, delayed potentials existed during VT and formed diastolic bridging through the cardiac cycle.

VT without accompanying demonstrable organic cardiac diseases used to be called idiopathic VT.[16] Most of the patients reported here, except those with ARVD, were referred to us as idiopathic VT. However, a surgical specimen of the myocardium taken from the origin of VT in a patient in the beginning of the present series revealed myocarditis.[5] Since then we have found myocarditis in 17 of 28 cases (60.7%) studied pathologically. We believe now that myocarditis is the most common cause of nonischemic VT unrelated to organic heart disease. In several recently published reports[16–21] concerning endomyocardial biopsy in patients with nonischemic VT of unknown origin, myocarditis was often found rather unexpectedly. Since we almost always found specific diseases in the myocardium among which myocarditis was most common, so-called idiopathic VT is unlikely to exist.

Several surgical methods have been advocated for treatment of VT, and are listed below divided into methods for ischemic and nonischemic VT. The fact that ischemic VT and nonischemic VT have completely different cardiac pathology, means that the surgical procedure to be employed must be adjusted accordingly. The surgical procedure for the former cannot be used in the latter, and vice versa.

For ischemic VT, Guiraudon[1] reported using an encircling endomyocardial incision. Harken[2] reported endocardial excision. This latter method, which is electrophysiologically guided, has been accepted worldwide with satisfactory results. Cox[3] reported combined use of endocardial excision and cryocoagulation.

For nonischemic VT, several surgical methods have been reported, but are few compared to those for ischemic VT. Simple ventriculotomy was used by Guiraudon.[4] Gallagher[23] and Camm[24] introduced cryocoagulation. We reported myocardial incision plus cryocoagulation.[5,7,25] Guiraudon[26] reported isolation of the entire free wall of the right ventricle for ARVD.

REFERENCES

1. Guiraudon, G., Fontaine, G., Frank, R., Escand, G., Etievent, P., and Cabrol, C. Encircling endocardial ventriculotomy. A new surgical treatment for life-threatening ventricular tachycardias resistant to medical treatment following myocardial infarction. *Ann. Thorac. Surg.* **26**: 438–444, 1978.

2. Harken, A.H., Josephson, M.E., and Horowitz, L. Surgical endocardial resection for the treatment of malignant ventricular tachycardia. *Ann. Surg.* **190**: 456–460, 1979.

3. Cox, J.L., Gallagher, J.J., and Ungerleider, R.M. Encircling endocardial ventriculotomy for refractory ischemic ventricular tachycardia. IV. Clinical indications, surgical technique, mechanism of action and results. *J. Thorac. Cardiovasc. Surg.* **83**: 865–872, 1982.

4. Guiraudon, G. Frank, R., and Fontaine, G. Interet des cartographies dans le traitement chirurgical des tachycardies ventriculaires rebelles recidivantes. *Nour Presse Med.* **3**: 321–327, 1974.

5. Iwa, T., Kobayashi, H., Sato, H., Mukai, K., Hirano, M. Tsuchiya, K., Naganuma, M., and Koike, K. Successful surgical treatment of idiopathic ventricular tachycardia. *Shinzo* **13**: 478–484, 1981. (in Japanese)

6. Guiraudon, G., Fontaine, G., Frank, R., Leandri, R., Barra, J., and Cabrol, C. Surgical treatment of ventricular tachycardia guided by ventricular mapping in 23 patients without coronary artery disease. *Ann. Thorac. Surg.* **32**: 439–450, 1981.

7. Iwa, T., Misaki, T., Kamata, E., Mitsui, T., Hashizume, Y., and Kawasuji, M. Surgical experiences of non-ischemic ventricular tachycardia. *Jpn. Ann. Thorac. Surg.* **3**: 31–38, 1983.

8. Marcus, F.I., Fontaine, G., Guiraudon, G., Frank, R., Laurenceau, J.L., Malergue, C., and Grosgogeat, Y. Right ventricular dysplasia: A report of 24 cases. *Circulation* **65**: 384–398, 1982.

9. Iwa, T., Misaki, T., Mukai, K., Kamata, E., and Ishida, K. Surgical management of non-ischemic ventricular tachycardia. In: Cardiac Arrhythmias. Iwa, T. and Fontaine, G. (eds.), Elsevier, Amsterdam, 1988, pp. 271–292.

10. Iwa, T., Kamata, E., and Misaki, T. Macrorcentry proved by epicardial mapping in chronic non-ischemic ventricular tachycardia. In: Proceedings of the XIth International Congress on Electrocardiology. d'Alche, P. (ed.), Caen, Universite de Caen, 1985, pp. 389–391.

11. Harrison, L., Ideker, R.E., Smith, W.M., Klein, G.J., Kasel, J., Wallace, A.G. and Gallagher, J.J. The Sock electrode array: A tool for determining global epicardial activation during unstable arrhythmias. *PACE* **3**: 531–540, 1980.

12. Cox, J.L. Intraoperative computerized mapping techniques: Do they help us to treat our patients better surgically? In: Cardiac Arrhythmias: Where to Go From Here? Brugada, P. and Wellens, H.J.J. (eds.), Mount Kisco, N.Y., Futura Publishing Company, 1987, pp. 613–637.

13. Fontaine, G., Frank, R., Gallais Hamonno, F., Allali, I., Phan Thuc, H., and Grosgogeat, Y. Electrocardiographie des potentiels tardifs du syndrome de post-excitation. *Arch. Mal. Coeur* **71**: 854–864, 1978.

14. Fontaine, G., Guiraudon, G., Frank, R, Vedel, J., Grosgogeat, Y., and Cabrol, C. Modern concepts of ventricular tachycardia. The value of electrocardiological investigations and delayed potentials in ventricular tachycardia of ischemic and nonischemic aetiology. 31 operated cases. *Eur. J. Cardiolol.* **8**: 565– , 1978.

15. Fontaine, G., Guiraudon, G., Frank, R., Fillette, F., Tonet, J., and Grosgogeat, Y. Correlations between latest delayed potentials in sinus rhythm and earliest activation during chronic ventricular tachycardia. In: Medical and Surgical Management of Tachyarrhythmias. Bricks, W., Loogen, F., Schulte, H.D., and Seipel, L .(eds.), Springer Verlag, 1980, pp. 138–154.

16. Chapman, J.H., Schank, J.P., and Crampton, R.S. Idiopathic ventricular tachycardia: An intracardiac electrical, hemodynamic and angiographic assessment of six patients. *Am. J. Med.* **59**: 470–480, 1975.

17. Edwards, W.D., Holmes, D.R., Jr. and Reeder, G.S. Diagnosis of active lymphocytic myocarditis by endomyocardial biopsy. Quantitative criteria for light microscopy. *Mayo Clin. Proc.* **57**: 419–425, 1982.

18. Strain, J.E., Grose, R.M., Factor, S.M., and Fisher, J.D. Results of endomyocardial biopsy in patients with spontaneous ventricular tachycardia but without apparent structural heart disease. *Circulation* **68**: 1171–1181, 1983.

19. Zee-Cheng, C., Tsai, C.C., Palmer, D.C., Codd, J.E., Pennington, D.G., and Wialilms, G.A. High incidence of myocarditis by endomyocardial biopsy in patients with idiopathic congestive cardiomyopathy. *J. Am. Coll. Cardiol.* **3**: 63–70, 1984.

20. Vignola, P.A., Nonuma, K., Swaye, P.S., Roanski, J.J., Blankstein, R.L., Benson, J., Gosselin, A.J., and Lister, J.W. Lymphocytic myocarditis presenting as unexplained ventricular arrhythmias: Diagnosis with endomyocardial biopsy and response to immunosuppression. *J. Am. Coll. Cardiol.* **4**: 812–819, 1984.

21. Sugrue, D.D., Holmes, D.R., Jr., Gersh, B.J., Edwards, W.D., McLaran, C.J., Wood, D.L., Osborn, M.J., and Hammill, S.C. Cardiac histologic findings in patients with life-threatening ventricular arrhythmias of unknown origin. *J. Am. Coll. Cardiol.* **4**: 952–957, 1984.

22. Hosenpud, J.D., McAnulty, J.H., and Nlles, N.R. Unexpected myocardial disease in patients with life threatening arrhythmias. *Br. Heart J.* **56**: 55–61, 1986.

23. Gallagher, J.J., Aderson, R.W., Kasel, J., Rice, J.R., Pritchett, L.C., Gault, J.H., Harrison, L., and Wallace, A.G. Cryoablation of drug-resistant ventricular tachycardia in a patient with a variant of scleroderma. *Circulation* **57**: 190–197, 1978.

24. Camm, J., Ward, D.E., Cory-Pearce, R., Rees, G.M., and Spurrell, R.A.J. The successful cryosurgical treatment of paroxysmal ventricular tachycardia. *Chest* **75**: 621–624, 1979.

25. Iwa, T., Misaki, T., and Iida, S. Cryocoagulation in the surgical treatment for tachyarrhythmias. *J. Cardiovasc. Surg.* **24**: 447, 1983.

26. Guiraudon, G.M., Klein, G.L., Gulamhusein, S.S., Painvin, G.A., DelCampo, C., Gonzales, J.C., and Ko, P.T. Total disconnection of the right ventricular free wall: Surgical treatment of right ventricular tachycardia associated with right ventricular dysplasia. *Circulation* **67**: 463–470, 1983.

Arrhythmias and Conduction Disturbances in Viral and Idiopathic Myocarditis: A Multicenter Survey in Japan

Keishiro Kawamura, Masahiro Kotaka, Yasushi Kitaura, and Hirofumi Deguchi

Third Division, Department of Internal Medicine, Osaka Medical College, Osaka, Japan

ABSTRACT

In our multicenter surveys of patients with viral or idiopathic myocarditis in Japan, arrhythmias and conduction disturbances were analyzed with reference to incidence, biopsy findings, therapeutic profiles, and outcome of disease. Complete AV block was reported in 45% of 42 patients with biopsy-proven myocarditis, the most common arrhythmia in the acute stage of the disease. Some pathogenetic implications of the high incidence of complete heart block in Japanese patients with acute myocarditis are discussed.

INTRODUCTION

In order to study the clinical status of viral and idiopathic acute myocarditis in Japan, we conducted a nationwide questionnaire survey in 1982 and collected data on 218 patients from 62 institutions. The clinical manifestations, laboratory findings, diagnostic features, and outcome were analyzed with reference to endomyocardial biopsies and serologic studies of virus titers.[1] In that survey, the electrocardiographic findings were reported from 214 patients and only briefly tabulated in the total series. The purpose of this presentation is to analyze the electrocardiograms in more detail with special reference to endomyocardial biopsies and arrhythmias, and in particular complete AV block, which was the most common arrhythmia documented in the acute phase of myocarditis in our survey.

PATIENTS AND METHODS

The design and method of the questionnaire survey and the patient population have been reported previously.[1] Of the total number of 214 patients (group 1) from whom ECG findings were recorded, endomyocardial biopsies were obtained from 82. Cellular infiltration and necrotic foci were noted in 42 patients (group 2) and not identified in 40 patients (group 3). No endomyocardial biopsy data were available in the remaining 132 patients (group 4). In patients with negative biopsy findings or no available biopsy data, myocarditis was diagnosed on the basis of clinical manifestations and laboratory data or autopsy (6 patients) as documented in our previous report.[1]

RESULTS

Frequency of Major Arrhythmias
  Group 1 (Fig. 1, G1). In the acute phase of the disease, a variety of electrocardio-

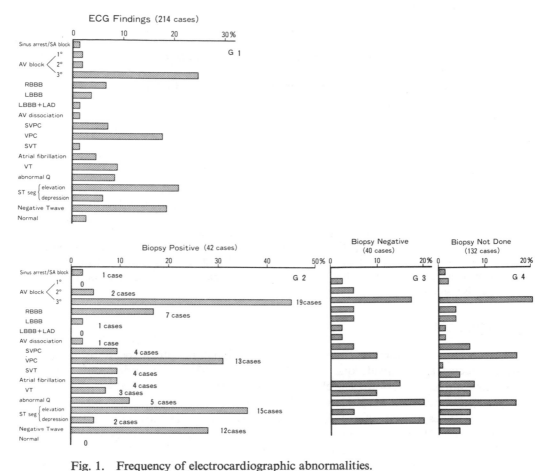

Fig. 1. Frequency of electrocardiographic abnormalities.
     AV: atrioventricular, G: Group, LAD: left-axis deviation, LBBB: left bundle
branch block, RBBB: right bundle branch block, SA: sinoatrial, SVPC: supraventricular premature complex, VPC: ventricular premature complex, VT:
ventricular tachycardia.

graphic abnormalities were documented in all but 3% of the 214 patients in group 1.
Conduction disturbances were quite common, occurring in 43% of patients, including
25% with complete AV block. Sinus arrest and SA block, however, occurred in only
1.4%. Premature contractions occurred in 25% of patients, including 18% with ventricular premature contractions. Ventricular tachycardia occurred in 9%.

     Group 2 (Fig. 1, G2). In 42 patients with endomyocardial biopsy-proven active myo-
carditis, the incidence of complete AV block and ventricular premature contractions
was 45% and 31%, respectively, which was much higher than in their counterparts in
the other groups, whereas the incidence of ventricular tachycardia was only 7%.

     Group 3 (Fig. 1, G3). In 40 patients (with no cellular infiltration or necrotic foci)
complete AV block (18%) and ventricular premature complexes (10%) were much less
frequent but ventricular tachycardia (15%) was more common than in the biopsy-positive group.

Group 4 (Fig. 1, G4). In 132 patients with no available biopsy data, complete AV block (20%) and ventricular premature complexes (17%) were less common than in the biopsy-positive group, but the incidence was still high.

Clinical, Therapeutic, and Prognostic Profiles of Patients with Complete AV Block

Since complete AV block was quite common in the acute clinical phase of viral or idiopathic myocarditis in our survey, more detailed clinical, therapeutic, and prognostic profiles of this crucial complication were retrospectively analyzed. Of 53 patients with complete heart block, 14 (27%) had completely recovered, 32 (60%) were improved with sequelae, and 7 (13%) died.

In this study, complete improvement signified recovery with no electrocardiographic abnormality and no other sequelae. The age of the 14 completely improved patients averaged 29 years. The male/female ratio was 1.8:1. Only 4 patients, or 29%, had had steroid therapy. Of the completely recovered, 43% had biopsies showing active myocarditis, 36% had not had biopsy, and 21% had no cellular infiltration in their biopsies.

In this study, improvement with sequelae signified recovery with some persisting abnormalities in electrocardiograms and other clinical manifestations. The age of the patients with sequelae averaged 32 years. The male/female ratio was 1.5:1. Steroid administration was documented in 12 patients (38%). Of the patients with sequelae, 38% had a permanent pacemaker implanted, 31% had complete right bundle branch block, and 9%, left or right axis deviation. In our survey, it was not clear how many patients among those who had a permanent pacemaker implanted really needed it. In some patients complete AV block might have been transient in nature and spontaneously recovered sometime after pacemaker implantation. Of the patients with sequelae, 41% had biopsy-proven myocarditis, 47% had not had biopsies, and 12% had no cellular infiltration in their biopsies.

None of the 7 dead patients had had a biopsy, but 6 of them underwent autopsies which proved overt myocarditis. The age of the 7 dead patients averaged 35 years. The male/female ratio was 1.3:1. Six of these 7 patients died within 20 days after the clinical onset of the disease; 2 of them had recovered from heart block, but died of shock or heart failure. The other 4 patients did not respond to temporary pacing and died of heart failure or shock. The remaining one patient survived for almost 2 years with permanent pacing and finally died of stroke.

Analysis of the protocols of steroid administration was beyond the scope of this survey. Of a variety of steroid drugs, prednisone was the most commonly used. The initial dosage varied from 20 to 60 mg, most commonly 30 mg a day. The duration of administration also varied markedly, from only 9 days to 4 months with tapering off. It should be noted that the dose of steroids is usually much smaller in Japan than in the West. The percentage of patients who were placed on steroid therapy was 29% in both the improved and the dead groups; this percentage was a little smaller than that (38%) in the group with sequelae. The small number of patients and the variety of treatment protocols made it difficult to evaluate the efficacy of steroids. In this survey there was no report of immunosuppressive therapy with cyclosporine or azathioprine.

SEROLOGIC TESTS FOR VIRUSES

Regarding etiology, of 53 patients with complete AV block, serological tests for viruses were positive in 21% or 11 patients, including Coxsackie B group virus in 7 patients, herpes simplex virus in 2, and mumps and parainfluenza virus in one each. A positive test was defined as a four-fold rise or more in virus titer. In our survey, therefore, at least 20% of patients with complete AV block might have had an associated viral infection. The etiology was unknown in the other 80%.

DISCUSSION

In our previous report, a total of 218 patients (group 1) were diagnosed as having myocarditis. They were categorized into 3 other groups depending upon positive (group 2) or negative findings of myocarditis (group 3) upon endomyocardial biopsies or unavailability of biopsy samples (group 4). Negative biopsy findings did not exclude the clinical diagnosis of myocarditis because of possible sampling error and the small number of the biopsy specimens. It was found that the symptomatology, laboratory features, and incidence of positive serologic tests for virus titers were surprisingly similar in groups 1 to 4 regardless of biopsy findings.[1] Of those 218 patients, 214 had electrocardiographic documentation. In this report, those 214 patients were similarly categorized into groups 1–4 as in the previous study (Fig. 1). In all groups, a variety of arrhythmias and conduction disturbances were common, among which complete AV block and premature ventricular contraction were most frequent, except in group 3 in which ventricular tachycardia was intermediate in incidence between complete AV block and premature ventricular complex (Fig. 1). The incidence of complete AV block varied: 25% in group 1 (total 214 cases), 45% in group 2 (biopsy positive, 42 cases), 18% in group 3 (biopsy negative, 40 cases), and 21% in group 4 (biopsy not done, 132 cases), being the highest in the group of the patients with biopsy-proven myocarditis. Recently Sekiguchi and colleagues studied retrospectively the natural history of 25 patients with biopsy-proven acute myocarditis and 5 autopsy cases of myocarditis, and reported that the incidence of complete AV block was 50%.[2] In our own experience with 21 patients with acute myocarditis of viral or unknown etiology, 7 patients (30%) had complete AV block in the acute phase of the disease. It seems, therefore, that complete AV block is quite common in the acute phase of viral or idiopathic myocarditis in Japan.

In his review article "Viral myocarditis and its sequelae," Abelmann[3] in Boston noted that atrial premature beats and tachyarrhythmias appeared to be remarkably infrequent in human viral myocarditis, while ventricular premature beats were not infrequent. Although he referred to partial and complete heart block as well as bundle branch block in patients with various types of viral myocarditis, he did not mention the incidence of these arrhythmias, particularly complete AV block. Recently Kopechy and Gersh from the Mayo Clinic reviewed the natural history and clinical manifestations of myocarditis, and reported that "atrial and ventricular arrythmias were common, along with variable degrees of heart block, which were usually transient but may require permanent pacing."[4] These authors did not mention, however, how common those arrhythmias and conduction disturbances were in patients with acute myocarditis. Gardiner and Short[5] in Scotland studied 60 patients with acute myocarditis or pericarditis or a combination of the 2 conditions of whom 48 patients were admitted directly to hospital as emergencies and the remaining 12 were seen initially in their homes or in urgent outpatient consultations. Electrocardiograms were abnormal at some time in the course of the illness in every patient except one. The electrocardiographic abnormalities during the acute stage were classified into 3 types: ST elevation (21 patients), ST/T depression (35 patients), and left bundle branch block (2 patients). No other conduction disturbance or arrhythmia was described in their report. Lim *et al.*[6] in

Singapore described 10 patients with acute nonspecific myocarditis who developed Stokes-Adams syndrome due to complete heart block who were managed at the coronary care unit. The patients were all below 30 years of age and comprised 8 females and 2 males. Only one patient was not of Chinese descent. The electrocardiograms returned to normal in 6 patients and all 10 patients survived their acute illness. Reviewing 8 English articles on myocarditis, Lim et al.[6] found only 16 cases of acute myocarditis producing Stokes-Adams syndrome due to complete heart block, and commented that this clinical heart condition was uncommon. The majority of the reported cases were in male adults over 30 years old.

In our survey on the patients with viral or idiopathic myocarditis in Japan, complete AV block was quite common in the acute stage of the disease; the age of those who developed complete AV block was often more than 30 years and the male/female ratio was 1.3–1.8:1. If acute complete AV block is the most common of all the arrhythmias and its incidence is much higher in Japanese patients than in other populations, several factors may be involved.

1. Etiological Considerations

In our survey, the etiological diagnosis of viral myocarditis was substantiated by elevated viral titers and at least 20% of patients with complete AV block had positive serologic tests for viruses of the Coxsackie B group, herpes simplex, mumps, and parainfluenza. These serologic features appeared to be similar to those in other industrialized countries.[5,7] The etiology was unknown in the remaining patients and rheumatic fever and diphtheria were unlikely.

2. Possible Underestimation of Arrhythmias and Conduction Disturbances

The source and selection of patients for surveys may be different in Japan compared to other countries. Our survey in Japan included a number of acute patients who had transient complete AV block whereas in other countries patients with more chronic forms of the disease might have been selected, so that complete AV block might not appear to be as prevalent as in Japan. Complete AV block, even transient, is a serious complication that usually requires emergency care including temporary cardiac pacing, and is rarely overlooked by careful physicians. In contrast, first- or second-degree AV block, bundle branch block, and sinus or atrial arrhythmias may remain unrecognized or overlooked unless patients have clinical manifestations which lead to the suspicion and the correct diagnosis of myocarditis. Electrocardiograms are rarely recorded from patients who present only flu-like syndromes. This may cause underestimation of the incidence of minor arrhythmias and conduction disturbances in the atria and ventricles.

3. Variations in Susceptibility

The high incidence of complete AV block in our survey might reflect racial or genetic variation of susceptibility to the disease. When complete AV block complicates the disease, the block is often transient. It seems, therefore, unlikely that specialized tissues undergo irreversible damage. Instead, the block may be caused by interstitial edema, ionic imbalance, and/or nerve injury which occur in association with acute inflammatory reactions and are reversible in the AV junctional tissue. Despite lack of evidence, the cytotoxic effect of interleukin 1 and other cytokines may also be involved in the transient disturbance of excitation conduction in the AV junctional tissue. Recent studies on multiple murine strains with experimental Coxsackie B virus myocarditis has demonstrated that variability in antibody formation to myocyte antigens and cellular infiltration of the myocardium is genetically determined.[8] In order to study this issue in the conduction system of the human heart, the criteria for not only morphologic but also etiologic diagnosis should be established. An immunohereditary approach in patients and study in animal models[9] will also be necessary.

ACKNOWLEDGMENT

This study was supported in part by a Research Grant for Intractable Diseases from the Ministry of Health and Welfare, Japan.

REFERENCES

1. Kawamura, K., Kitaura, Y., Morita, H., Deguchi, H., and Kotaka, M. Viral and idiopathic myocarditis in Japan: A questionnaire survey. *Heart Vessels* **1**: Suppl. 18–22, 1985.
2. Sekiguchi, M., Hiroe, M., Inami, M., Hirakou, S., Morimoto, S., and Izumi, T. Long-term prognosis of acute myocarditis. Presented at the Meeting of the Idiopathic Cardiomyopathy Research Committee of the Ministry of Health and Welfare of the Japanese Government, August 20, 1988. (in Japanese)
3. Abelmann, W.H. Viral myocarditis and its sequelae. *Annu. Rev. Med.* **24**: 145–152, 1973.
4. Kopecky, S.L. and Gersh, B.J. Dilated cardiomyopathy and myocarditis: Natural history, etiology, clinical manifestations, and management. *Curr. Probl. Cardiol.* **12**: 569–647, 1987.
5. Gardiner, A.J.S. and Short, D. Four faces of acute myopericarditis. *Br. Heart J.* **35**: 433–442, 1973.
6. Lim, C.-H., Toh, C.C.S., Chia, B.-L., and Low, L.-P. Stokes-Adams attacks due to acute nonspecific myocarditis. *Am. Heart J.* **90**: 172–178, 1975.
7. Daly, K., Richardson, P.J., Olsen, E.G.J., Morgan-Capner, P., McSorley, C., Jackson, G., and Jewitt, D.E. Acute myocarditis: Role of histological and virological examination in the diagnosis and assessment of immunosuppressive treatment. *Br. Heart J.* **51**: 30–35, 1984.
8. Wolgram, L.J., Beisel, K.W., Herskowitz, A., and Rose, N.R. Variations in susceptibility to Coxsackie virus B_3-induced myocarditis among different strains in mice. *J. Immunol.* **136**: 1846–1858, 1986.
9. Terasaki, F., Kitaura, Y., Hayashi, T., Nakayama, Y., Deguchi, H., and Kawamura, K. Arrhythmias in Coxsackie B_3 virus myocarditis. Continuous electrocardiography in conscious mice and histopathology of the heart with special reference to the conduction system. *Heart Vessels* (Suppl.), 1989. (in press)

Clinical Aspects of Long-Term Follow-Up of Myocarditis: Arrhythmias and Conduction Disturbances

Peter J. Richardson and Dylmitr Rittoo

Cardiac Department, King's College Hospital, London, U.K.

ABSTRACT

Myocarditis is often a subclinical condition with transient electrocardiographic abnormalities, but significant arrhythmias may also occur. The specific diagnosis of myocarditis can be confirmed by myocardial biopsy. The case report of a 16-year-old boy is presented to illustrate the arrhythmias that may be encountered and the progression to dilated cardiomyopathy (postmyocarditic). Ventricular arrhythmias are common. The prognostic significance of ventricular tachycardia is controversial. The pathogenesis of arrhythmias is multifactorial and includes myocardial inflammation, subsequent fibrosis, ventricular dilatation with reduced contractility, and activation of the neurohumoral responses. Treatment therefore may include ACE inhibitors, specific antiarrhythmic drugs, and pacing.

INTRODUCTION

The clinical diagnosis of myocarditis is not always easy. Even those patients who may have significant arrhythmias are often asymptomatic. Indeed, myocarditis may only be suspected because of unexplained changes in the electrocardiogram or the detection of arrhythmias. Until the advent of endomyocardial biopsy the diagnosis of myocarditis was by either viral culture or the detection of a four-fold rise in viral neutralization antibody titers. Noninvasive methods of diagnosis of myocarditis such as thallium scanning have not proved reliable. Endomyocardial biopsy therefore remains the best way of proving the diagnosis. However, in the context of arrhythmias and conduction disturbances, there have been no serial studies with systematic documentation of arrhythmias by means of 24-hr tape monitoring. The precise relationship of arrhythmias and conduction disturbance to the natural history of myocarditis is thus difficult to determine in many cases. The majority of studies that have been performed relate to patients with clinically diagnosed dilated cardiomyopathy.

CASE REPORT

A 16-year-old boy who had been previously well presented with an 8-week history of increasing shortness of breath on exertion (NYHA III). A diagnosis of possible glandular fever had been made a year previously, but not confirmed. There was no recent history to suggest a viral illness. On examination his pulse was 110/min and regular; blood pressure was 80/50 mmHg. The JVP was raised 3 cm above the sternal angle and a pansystolic murmur was audible at the apex.

Investigations revealed the following findings: The electrocardiogram showed sinus

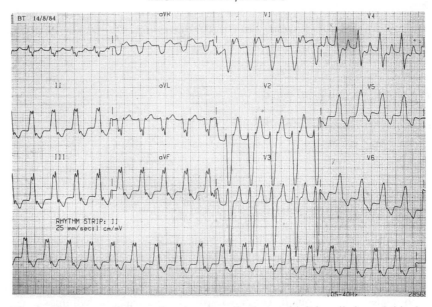

Fig. 1.   Electrocardiogram showing sinus rhythm and left bundle branch block.

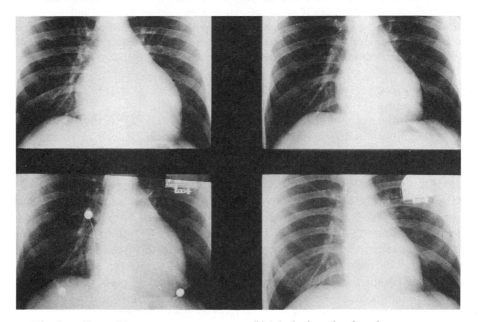

Fig. 2.   Chest X-ray:

(a) Marked cardiomegaly with clear lung fields.

(b) Marked reduction in transverse cardiac diameter after one-month treatment.

(c) Marked increase in heart size at 3-month follow-up; pacemaker in situ.

(d) Reduced heart size at 6-month follow-up.

rhythm and left bundle branch block (Fig. 1). Chest X-ray showed marked cardiomegaly but the lung fields were clear (Fig. 2a). The echocardiogram showed a dilated left ventricle (LVed 8 cm, LVes 6.9 cm). Left ventricular contraction was reduced. The findings were consistent with a dilated cardiomyopathy. Right ventricular endomyocardial biopsy was performed and histopathologic evaluation by Dr. E.G.J. Olsen (National Heart Hospital, London) showed myocarditis, compatible with the healing phase.

In view of the fact that the endomyocardial biopsy showed a healing myocarditis with relatively few foci of activity it was clinically decided not to treat him with immunosuppressive therapy. He therefore was continued on antifailure therapy with diuretics to which he responded satisfactorily.

Follow-up

Clinical follow-up after one month's treatment on antifailure therapy revealed that the patient was well. The chest X-ray performed at that time showed marked reduction in the transverse cardiac diameter. The lung fields remained clear (Fig. 2b). The electrocardiogram now revealed sinus rhythm with T wave inversion in leads AVL and V1-V4. The left bundle branch block had disappeared (Fig. 3). Echocardiography revealed an improvement in the left ventricular cavity dimensions. The LVed previously 8 cm was reduced to 5.5 cm.

Two months later, although the patient remained clinically asymptomatic, routine follow-up investigations indicated deterioration. There was a marked increase in heart size as seen on chest X-ray (Fig. 2c) and on echocardiography. Coincident with this his electrocardiogram again showed left bundle branch block. A left ventricular endomyocardial biopsy was performed, and showed changes of a healed myocarditis. There was thickening of the endocardium with a prominent smooth muscle component, and focal subendocardial fibrosis. A few chronic inflammatory cells were visible, but there was no evidence of active myocyte necrosis.

The patient then reported 3 episodes of syncope. Twenty-four hour ambulatory monitoring revealed episodes of repetitive ventricular couplets and an atrioventricular tachycardia with retrograde conduction. Intermittent third-degree A-V block was also documented.

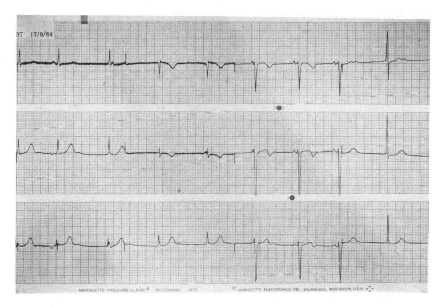

Fig. 3. Electrocardiogram showing sinus rhythm with T wave inversion in leads AVL, V1-V4. No bundle branch block.

In view of the ambulatory monitoring findings a permanent dual-chamber pacemaker was inserted and amiodarone commenced. The patient had no further syncopal episodes and 6 months later his chest X-ray (Fig. 2d) and echocardiographic left ventricular dimensions were at the upper limits of normal. Long-term review 3.5 years after his initial presentation revealed an aysmptomatic patient who was in active employment. His echocardiogram, however, showed a hypocontractile dilated left ventricle (LVed 8 cm, LVes 6 cm) with dilatation of the left atrium. Doppler color-flow mapping demonstrated functional mitral and tricuspid regurgitation. The findings are consistent with a diagnosis of dilated cardiomyopathy.

The above case history illustrates the often subclinical nature of active myocarditis together with the arrhythmias that may be encountered in the active or healing phase as well as the progression of myocarditis to dilated cardiomyopathy.

ARRHYTHMIAS RELATED TO MYOCARDITIS

The clinical manifestations of myocarditis whether in the active, healed, or healing phase must depend on the extent of the myocardial involvement, which may be focal or diffuse. In the majority of hearts the lesions are randomly distributed. A small single lesion that involves the conducting system may have serious consequences.[1] Life-threatening arrhythmias have been described in both varicella[2] and Coxsackie B$_3$[3] myocarditis. This may explain the etiology of sudden death in children and young adults. The electrocardiographic abnormalities are in the main transient and are more common than the clinical manifestation of myocardial involvement.[4] The most common abnormalities are ST segment and T wave changes. Atrioventricular arrhythmias, atrioventricular and intraventricular conduction defects, and rarely Q waves may be seen.[4]

Kitaura and Morita followed up 11 patients with acute viral myocarditis or myopericarditis between May 1964 and March 1977.[5] The patients were followed up for 1.5 to 13 years, with review of the clinical symptoms, physical signs, chest X-ray, electrocardiogram, echocardiography, and cardiac catheterization. Ventricular endomyocardial biopsies were examined in 10 patients. The electrocardiographic changes in the acute stage were as follows: ST elevation was seen in 5 patients, ventricular tachycardia in one, first-degree A-V block in one, second-degree A-V block in one, and third-degree A-V block in 4. The patients with ST elevation only at presentation had normal electrocardiograms at 10- and 11-year follow-up. One patient with ST elevation had T wave inversion at 3-year follow-up. The one patient with atrial fibrillation remained in this rhythm for 3 years. Patients with third-degree A-V block had the worst prognosis. One died 2 days after presentation. He had had recurrent Stokes-Adams attacks and went into cardiogenic shock in spite of transvenous right ventricular pacing. Third-degree A-V block persisted in one patient for 13 years after the initial diagnosis; the third patient with third-degree A-V block subsequently developed incomplete right bundle branch block and left anterior hemiblock at 18-month follow-up. Sekiguchi et al.[6] followed up 20 patients with biopsy-proven myocarditis for 10 years. The electrocardiogram returned to normal on only 2 patients. The remainder showed intraventricular conduction disturbances. Three patients required permanent pacemakers. Three of the patients progressed from myocarditis to dilated cardiomyopathy.

Insight into postmyocarditic arrhythmias may be gained by selecting patients with arrhythmias and investigating them with endomyocardial biopsy. Vignola et al.[7] studied 65 patients who had either been resuscitated from sudden death, or had ventricular tachycardia resistant to standard arrhythmic therapy and high-grade ventricular arrhythmias (Lown class greater than or equal to IVb) with or without syncope. In 17 patients no cause was identified. Twelve of those 17 patients had right ventricular biopsy and in 6 of them clinically unsuspected lymphocytic myocarditis was diagnosed. Strain et al.[8] studied 18 patients with ventricular tachycardia or fibrillation in whom no structural heart disease was apparent. None of those patients was found to have significant coronary artery lesions or impairment of left ventricular function at catheterization. However, right ventricular biopsy specimens were abnormal in 16 of 18 (89%) patients. Nine (50%) had histologic changes of a nonspecific cardiomyopathy, but in 3 (17%) subacute inflammatory myocarditis was diagnosed. Van Hougenhuyze et al.[9] reported 15 patients with ventricular tachycardia in whom the cause was clinically not apparent. Four of those 15 patients had endomyocardial biopsies consistent with "chronic myocarditis." Reeder et al.[10] also reported 17 patients with unexplained life-threatening arrhythmias. They found 5 patients in whom endomyocardial biopsy showed a myocarditis with lymphocytic infiltration and interstitial edema.

There is mounting evidence that dilated cardiomyopathy represents a culmination of previous viral myocarditis. Data from animal models was provided by Matsumori and Kawai.[11] Fuster et al.[12] studied 104 patients with idiopathic dilated cardiomyopathy, of whom 20% had had severe influenza-like illness prior to presentation. Serologic evidence of a recent Coxsackie viral infection has been demonstrated by Cambridge et al.[13] and also by Daly et al.[14] More recently, Bowles et al.[15] demonstrated the presence of enteroviral RNA in the myocardium of patients with not only myocarditis but also dilated cardiomyopathy. It is therefore justified to think of dilated cardiomyopathy as a postmyocarditic syndrome. Arrhythmias, conduction disturbance, and sudden death are well documented in dilated cardiomyopathy.

Arrhythmias in Dilated Cardiomyopathy

Huang et al.[16] studied 35 patients with idiopathic dilated cardiomyopathy. Holter monitoring revealed atrial fibrillation in 20%, atrial premature beats (more than 30/hr) in 54%, supraventricular tachycardia in 25%, ventricular premature beats (more than 30/hr) in 83%, complex ventricular premature beats (Lown grade III-V) in 93%, and ventricular tachycardia in 60%. No difference was noted in patients with or without ventricular tachycardia with respect to their presenting symptoms, functional classification, electrocardiographic findings, heart size on chest X-ray, cardiac index, left ventricular end-diastolic pressure, or ejection fraction. These patients were followed up for 4 to 74 months. Two patients died suddenly, one with and the other without ventricular tachycardia. A third patient died from congestive heart failure and a fourth from sepsis. It was concluded that the incidence of ventricular arrhythmias in dilated cardiomyopathy was high. Ventricular tachycardia was frequent and nonsustained and there was no correlation of ventricular tachycardia with the clinical or hemodynamic findings. The presence of ventricular tachycardia did not appear to predict the prognosis. However, Van Hougenhuyze et al.[17] performed 24-hr ambulatory electrocardiograms on 60 patients with idiopathic dilated cardiomyopathy. All those patients had left ventricular ejection fractions of less than 55%. Every patient had ventricular extrasystoles. In 18% they were rare, although they were moderately frequent (101–100/24 hr) in 40% and frequent (greater than 1000/24 hr) in 42%. Multiform extrasystoles were recorded in 95%, paired ventricular extrasystoles in 78%, and nonsustained ventricular tachycardia (3–19 beats) in 42%. During the follow-up period of 12 ± 5 months 7 patients died, 4 from congestive heart failure and the other 3 from sudden death.

Meinertz et al.[19] presented similar data on 74 patients with idiopathic dilated cardiomyopathy. They concluded that patients with reduced left ventricular ejection fractions (less than 40%) and frequent episodes of ventricular tachycardia or ventricular pairs were at risk of sudden death.

Supraventricular arrhythmias are not uncommon in patients with dilated cardiomyopathy. Haissaguerre et al.[19] studied 236 patients in whom atrial fibrillation was found in 27%. In 13 patients atrial fibrillation was the mode of presentation. Embolic complications were observed in 25% of cases with atrial fibrillation. The latter was found in 50% of patients with embolic phenomena. The authors concluded that the prognosis of patients with or without atrial fibrillation was not significantly different.

PATHOGENESIS OF ARRHYTHMIAS

There are a number of factors responsible for arrhythmias in postmyocarditic patients. Initially diffuse or focal acute inflammation may be the main factor. Arrhythmias and conduction disturbances are then perpetuated by the onset of myocardial fibrosis subsequent upon the initial acute myocardial inflammation. It should be remembered that it is not only in Chagas's disease but also in focal myocarditis that small ventricular aneurysms may develop which can be the source of arrhythmias. Hoshino et al.[20] demonstrated the relationship between ventricular aneurysms and ventricular arrhythmias in Coxsackie B_1-induced myocarditis in Syrian golden hamsters.

When the myocardium begins to fail other factors may be responsible for either the initiation or maintenance of arrhythmias. The sympathetic nervous system and the renin-angiotensin systems may also be activated. This results in elevation of the circulating levels of catecholamine, renin, and angiotensin. This may be arrhythmogenic. Drugs such as digitalis, diuretics, and antiarrhythmic therapy may all produce or aggravate arrhythmias.

TREATMENT ASPECTS

Patients with a postmyocarditic syndrome are frequently asymptomatic but commonly have supraventricular and ventricular arrhythmias and unexpected sudden death may occur. In spite of these facts, there is no current consensus on whether ventricular arrhythmias represent an independent predictor of death. In fact there has been no randomized, controlled study of the efficacy of antiarrhythmic therapy in patients with myocarditis, whether healing or healed.

REFERENCES

1. James, T.N., Schlant, R.C., and Marshall, T.K. Randomly distributed focal myocardial lesions causing destruction in the His bundle or a narrow origin left bundle branch. *Circulation* **57**: 816, 1978.
2. Woolf, P.K., Chung, T.S., Stewart, J., Lialios, M., Davidian, M., and Gewitz, M.H. Life threatening dysrhythmias in varicella myocarditis. *Clin. Pediatr.* **26**: 480–482, 1987.
3. Sareli, P., Schamroth, C.L., Passias, J., and Schamrote, L. Torsade de pointes due to Coxsackie B_3 myocarditis. *Clin. Cardiol.* **10**: 361–362, 1987.
4. Reyes, M.P. and Lerner, A.M. Coxsackie myocarditis—with specific reference to acute and chronic effects. *Prog. Cardiovasc. Dis.* **27**: 373, 1985.
5. Kitaura, Y. and Morita, H. Secondary myocardial disease—virus myocarditis and cardiomyopathy. *Jpn. Circ. J.* **43**: 1017–1031, 1979.
6. Sekiguchi, M., Hiroe, M., Kaneko, M., and Kusakabe, K. Natural history of 20 patients

with biopsy proven acute myocarditis. A 10-year follow-up (abstr). *Circulation* **72** (Suppl. 111): 109.

7. Vignola, P.A., Kazutaka, A., Pauls, S., Rozanski, J., Blankstein, R., Benson, J., Gosselin, A., and Lister, J. Lymphocytic myocarditis presenting as unexplained ventricular tachycardia: Diagnosis with endomyocardial biopsy and response to immunosuppression. *JACC*, **4**: 812–819, 1984.

8. Strain, J., Grose, R., Factor, S., and Fisher, J. Results of endomyocardial biopsy in patients with spontaneous ventricular tachycardia but without apparent structural heart disease. *Circulation* **68**: 1171–1181, 1983.

9. Van Hougenhuyze, D., Olsen, E., Crook, B., and Van de Brand, M. Myocardial biopsy in patients with ventricular tachycardia (abstr.). *Am. J. Cardiol.* **47**: 409, 1981.

10. Reeder, G.P., Holmes, D.R., Hartzier, G.O., and Edward, W.D. Endomyocardial biopsy in patients with life threatening dysrhythmia (abstr.). *Am. J. Cardiol.* **47**: 499, 1981.

11. Matsumori, A. and Kawai, C. An animal model of congestive (dilated) cardiomyopathy: Dilatation and hypertrophy of the heart in the chronic stage in DBA/s mice with myocarditis caused by encephalomyocarditis virus. *Circulation* **66**: 355–360, 1962.

12. Fuster, V., Gersh, B., Guiliani, E., Tatch, A., Brandenburg, R., and Frye, R. The natural history of idiopathic dilated cardiomyopathy. *Am. J. Cardiol.* **47**: 525–531, 1981.

13. Cambridge, C., MacArthur, C.G.C., Waterson, A.B., Goodwin, J.F., and Oakley, C.M. *Br. Heart J.* **41**: 692–696, 1979.

14. Daly, K., Richardson, P.J., Olsen, E.G.J., Morgan-Capner, P., McSorley, C., Jackson, G., and Jewitt, D.E. Acute myocarditis: Role of histological and virological examinatinn in the diagnosis and assessment of immunosuppressive treatment. *Br. Heart J.* **51**: 30–35, 1984.

15. Bowles, N.E., Olsen, E.G., Richardson, P.J., and Archard, L.C. Detection of Coxsackie B virus-specific RNA sequences in myocardial biopsy samples from patients with myocarditis and dilated cardiomyopathy. *Lancet* **1**: 1120, 1986.

16. Huang, S.K., Messer, J.V., and Denes, P. Significance of ventricular tachycardia in idiopathic cardiomyopathy: Observations in 35 patients. *Am. J. Cardiol.* **51**: 507–512, 1983.

17. Von Olshausen, R., Schater, A., Mehmet, H.C., Schwartz, F., Senges, J., and Kubler, W. Ventricular arrhythmia in idiopathic dilated cardiomyopathy. *Br. Heart J.* **51**: 195–201, 1984.

18. Meinertz, T., Hoffmann, T., Wolfgang, K., *et al*. Significance of ventricular arrhythmia in idiopathic dilated cardiomyopathy. *Am. J. Cardiol.* **53**: 902–907, 1984.

19. Haissaguerre, J., Bonnet, M.A., Billes, G. *et al. Arch. Mal. Coeur* **4**: 536–541, 1985.

20. Hoshino, T., Matsumori, A., Kawai, C., and Imai, J. Ventricular aneurysm, and ventricular arrhythmias complicating Coxsackie virus B_1 myocarditis of Syrian golden hamsters. *Cardiovasc. Res.* **18**: 24–29, 1984.

Morphologic Features and Electric Disturbances in Experimental Viral Myocarditis

Akira Matsumori, Tatsuo Hoshino, Chiharu Kishimoto, and Chuichi Kawai

The Third Division Department of Internal Medicine, Kyoto University, Kyoto, Japan

ABSTRACT

Various morphologic abnormalities and electric disturbances were seen in animal models of viral myocarditis induced by encephalomyocarditis (EMC) virus and coxsackievirus. Congestive heart failure developed in the acute stage, and dilatation and hypertrophy of the heart were seen in the chronic stage of EMC virus myocarditis in mice. Ventricular aneurysms were noted in the acute and chronic stages. Severe myocardial fibrosis, which predominated on the endocardial side of the ventricle, was seen in some mice. These findings suggest a pathogenetic role of viral infection in ventricular aneurysm, ventricular dysplasia, or restrictive cardiomyopathy. Atrial and ventricular premature complexes, atrioventricular block, and ventricular tachycardia were seen in the acute stage of EMC virus myocarditis, and atrial premature contraction (APC) and/or ventricular premature contraction (VPC) persisted in the chronic stage. Similar changes were also noted in the acute stage of coxsackievirus B_1 myocarditis in hamsters. VPC persisted in the chronic stage in hamsters, in which ventricular aneurysms were seen. The presence of arrhythmias in the chronic stage of myocarditis suggests that some patients with arrhythmias who have no other clinical manifestations have had previous viral myocarditis.

INTRODUCTION

Since endomyocardial biopsy has been widely used for the diagnosis of myocardial diseases,[1] active myocarditis has been documented histologically in a significantly large number of patients with unexplained arrhythmias, especially ventricular arrhythmia such as ventricular tachycardia.[2] Various morphologic abnormalities, conduction disturbances, and arrhythmias are seen in animal models of viral myocarditis induced by Coxsackie B viruses[3,4] and encephalomyocarditis (EMC) virus.[5] We studied serial changes of electrocardiographic (EKG) abnormalities in animal models of viral myocarditis in order to clarify the relationship between EKG changes and pathologic findings.

ARRHYTHMIAS AND CONDUCTION DISTURBANCE IN VIRAL MYOCARDITIS IN MICE

1. Animal Models of EMC Virus Myocarditis in Mice

We found severe myocarditis in inbred strains of BALB/c mice inoculated with the M variant of EMC virus. Congestive heart failure developed in the acute stage.[6] Following that study, we found severe myocarditis in an inbred strain of DBA/2 mice inoculated with the M variant of EMC virus. Mice with severe myocarditis died of

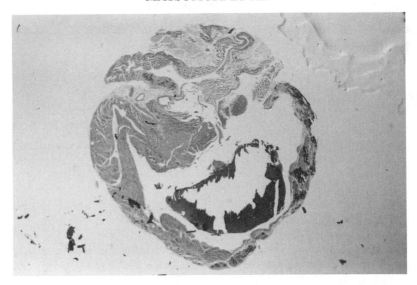

Fig. 1.   DBA/2 mouse 5 months after inoculation with EMC virus. Left ventricular aneurysm and transmural fibrosis are seen. Hematoxylin and eosin stain, × 8.

congestive heart failure in the acute stage. In the surviving mice with myocarditis, on day 90 both the heart weight and the heart weight/body weight ratio were significantly increased and the cavity dimension of the left ventricle was enlarged. Myocardial fibrosis was prominent and hypertrophy of myocardial fibers was evident. There was no mononuclear cell infiltration at this stage. Congestion of the lungs and liver was observed in both the acute and chronic stage.[7]

These findings suggest that congestive cardiomyopathy may develop as early as 3 months after virus infection. Dilatation and hypertrophy of the heart persisted up to the 8th month after inoculation with EMC virus in C3H/He and DBA/2 mice.[8] In these mice, atrial muscle was also involved in the disease process.[8] In the acute to chronic stage, myocardial cells were destroyed transmurally and ventricular aneurysms were seen in the right[9] and also in the left ventricles (Fig. 1). In some mice, fibrosis predominated on the subendocardial side of the left ventricle. These mice may show restrictive physiology (Fig. 2).

2. Arrhythmias and Conduction Disturbance in EMC Virus Myocarditis

Electrocardiographic changes were studied using these murine models. For the control recordings, mice were anesthetized by intraperitoneal administration of sodium pentobarbital. After inoculation with the virus, the recordings could be performed without anesthesia because the mice moved less actively. Electrocardiograms were taken using a direct ink-writing 3-channel Mingograph. Electrocardiograms were recorded at a paper speed of 100 mm/sec. The 3 waveforms, the P wave, the QRS complex, and the T wave, could be distinguished in the baseline electrocardiograms. Many kinds of electrocardiographic abnormalities appeared after day 4, including atrial and ventricular premature complexes (APCs, VPCs) and various degrees of atrioventricular block (Fig. 3). In the acute stage, the most frequent conduction disturbance was complete

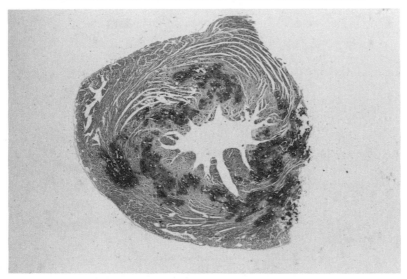

Fig. 2.   C3H/He mouse 6 months after inoculation with EMC virus. Prominent fibrosis is seen on the subendocardial side of the left ventricle. Hematoxylin and eosin stain, × 8.

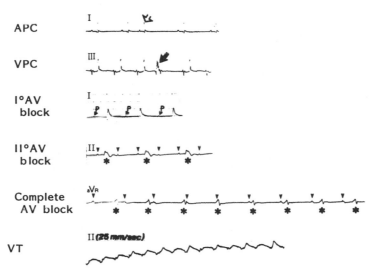

Fig. 3.   EKG abnormality in EMC virus myocarditis in mice. APC, VPC, various degrees of AV blocks (arrowheads indicate the P waves and asterisks indicate QRS complexes), and ventricular tachycardia (VT) are seen.

AV block. In the subacute stage, the most prominent EKG changes were low voltage of the QRS complex and increased heart rate. In the chronic stage, APCs and VPCs remained (Fig. 4).

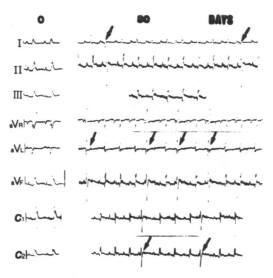

Fig. 4.   Ectopic complexes remain, even in the chronic stage of viral myocarditis.

ARRHYTHMIAS AND CONDUCTION DISTURBANCE IN COXSACKIEVIRUS B_1 MYOCARDITIS IN HAMSTERS

1. Electrocardiographic Abnormalities in Syrian Golden Hamsters with Coxsackievirus B_1 Myocarditis

Two-week-old Syrian golden hamsters were inoculated with coxsackievirus B_1 (CVB_1) which was propagated 7 times in an *in vivo* hamster heart before experimental use. Sixty-two hamsters were inoculated with CVB_1, and 39 of them were examined electrocardiographically and histopathologically. Of the 39 CVB_1-infected hamsters, EKG abnormalities and histologic evidence of myocarditis were found in 31, but neither could be detected in 2. In the remaining 6, myocarditis, with a few small patchy lesions, was proved histologically. EKGs did not reveal significant changes. Multiple abnormalities were recorded in 4 hamsters: 3 showed ST-T change followed by first-degree AV block, complete AV block, and transient second-degree AV block with supraven-

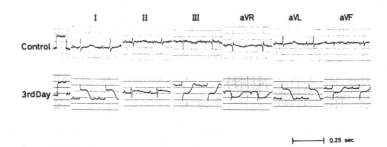

Fig. 5.   Three days after inoculation of coxsackievirus B_1 in a Syrian golden hamster. Marked ST displacement, without abnormal Q waves, is seen.

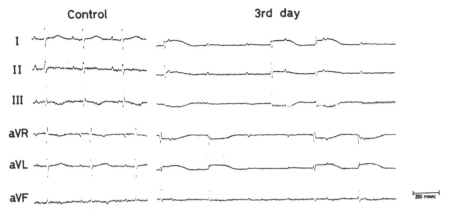

Fig. 6. Complete AV block recorded in a hamster 3 days after inoculation with coxsackievirus B_1.

tricular extrasystoles, respectively; one showed first-degree AV block and left bundle branch block (LBBB) pattern simultaneously. Eighty percent of the 31 hamsters showed ST-T change either as the sole EKG abnormality or as the first among other abnormalities (Fig. 5). The ST was displaced in various manners. Usually, the T waves flattened transiently from most of the leads in the recovery phase, and then they gradually became normal. The occurrence of conduction disturbances on the EKG closely corresponded with the histologic location of myocarditis: basal IVS was always injured by myocarditis in the cases with AV blocks. Complete AV block was recorded on the third day (Fig.6).

2. Ventricular Aneurysms and Ventricular Arrhythmias Complicating Coxsackievirus B₁ Myocarditis of Syrian Golden Hamsters

Serial EKGs were recorded from 10 hamsters which survived the acute and electrocardiographically manifested myocarditis. In a mean 17.8-week (range 9 to 31 weeks) follow-up period, chronic VPCs followed the acute EKG changes in 3 of the animals.

In one hamster, acute EKG abnormality, intraventricular conduction disturbance with flat T waves, and deviation of the electrical axis to the left were recorded on the 4th day. A few VPCs of uniform contour were detected for the first time in the hamster on day 63, and were recorded in bigeminy from day 70 until the death of the animal on day 217. Ventricular bigeminy was seen on day 168 (Fig. 7). Pathologic examination of the heart disclosed thick fibrosis in the inner layers of the anterior wall of the left ventricle, and protrusion of that part of the ventricular wall. Lesions of thin fibrosis were also found in both ventricles, mostly on the left side of the interventricular septum. VPCs had 2 kinds of contour in the other 2 hamsters, each of which had 2 ventricular aneurysms. No VPC was recorded from the other 7 hamsters, which had no aneurysms in the heart. None of the inoculated animals died during the follow-up period, irrespective of the existence of ventricular aneurysm, after surviving the first 2 weeks postinfection. The results demonstrate a close relationship between chronic VPC of uniform contours following CVB_1 myocarditis and the formation of ventricular aneurysms in Syrian golden hamsters. The hamsters were able to live for a considerably long period with the aneurysms. Ventricular aneurysms following CVB_1 myocarditis in Syrian golden hamsters may be an experimental model of human ventricular aneurysms of unknown etiology.

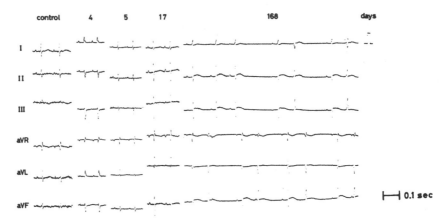

Fig. 7.   Coxsackievirus B_1 myocarditis in a hamster. Intraventricular conduction disturbance with flat T waves and deviation of the electrical axis to the left were seen on day 4. Ventricular bigeminy was seen on day 168.

ACKNOWLEDGMENTS

This work was supported in part by a research grant from the Ministry of Health and Welfare, and by Grants-in-Aid for Scientific Research on Priority Areas and for General Scientific Research from the Ministry of Education, Science and Culture, Japan, and the Kanazawa Research Fund.

REFERENCES

1. Kawai, C., Matsumori, A., and Fujiwara, H. Myocarditis and dilated cardiomyopathy. *Ann. Rev. Med.* **38**: 221–239, 1987.
2. Nippoldt, T.B., Edwards, W.D., Holmes, D.R., Jr., Reeder, G.S., Hartzler, G.O., and Smith, H.C. Right ventricular endomyocardial biopsy. Clinicopathologic correlates in 100 consecutive patients. *Mayo Clin. Proc.* **57**: 407–418, 1982.
3. Hoshino, T., Matsumori, A., Kawai, C., and Imai, J. Electrocardiographic abnormalities in Syrian golden hamsters with coxsackievirus B_1 myocarditis. *Jpn. Circ. J.* **46**: 1305–1312, 1982
4. Hoshino, T., Matsumori, A., Kawai, C., and Imai, J. Ventricular aneurysms and ventricular arrhythmias complicating coxsackievirus B_1 myocarditis of Syrian golden hamsters. *Cardiovasc. Res.* **18**: 24–29, 1984.
5. Kishimoto, C., Matsumori, A., Ohmae, M., Tomioka, N., and Kawai, C. Electrocardiographic findings in experimental myocarditis in DBA/2 mice: Complete atrioventricular block in the acute stage, low voltage of the QRS complex in the subacute stage and arrhythmias in the chronic stage. *J. Am. Coll. Cardiol.* **3**: 1461–1468, 1984.
6. Matsumori, A. and Kawai, C. An experimental model for congestive heart failure after encephalomyocarditis virus myocarditis in mice. *Circulation* **65**: 1230–1235, 1982.
7. Matsumori, A. and Kawai, C. An animal model of congestive (dilated) cardiomyopathy: Dilatation and hypertrophy of the heart in the chronic stage in DBA/2 mice with myocarditis caused by encephalomyocarditis virus. *Circulation* **66**: 355–360, 1982.
8. Matsumori, A., Kawai, C., and Sawada, S. Encephalomyocarditis virus myocarditis in inbred strains of mice: Chronic stage. *Jpn. Circ. J.* **46**: 1192–1196, 1982.
9. Matsumori, A., Kishimoto, C., Kawai, C., and Sawada, S. Right ventricular aneurysms complicating encephalomyocarditis virus myocarditis in mice. *Jpn. Circ. J.* **47**: 1322–1324, 1983.

Immunologic Aspects in Arrhythmias and Cardiac Conduction Disturbances

Bernhard Maisch,* Ulrich Lotze,** Andreas Schuster,*** and Jakob Schneider†

* University Hospital of Internal Medicine, Marburg, FRG
** University Hospital of Internal Medicine, Homburg, FRG
*** University Hospital of Internal Medicine, Würzburg, FRG
† University Institute of Pathology, Zürich, Switzerland

ABSTRACT

Immunologic investigations in cardiac conduction disturbances and arrhythmias have previously focused on the demonstration of antibodies to heterologous Purkinje fibers with ox false tendons as antigen in patients with left bundle branch block (positive in only 5%). This has also been undertaken in patients with right bundle branch block (positive in 38% of patients with rheumatoid arthritis) and in congenital AV block (SSA/Ro and SSB/La antibodies). Only recently anti-(human) sinus node, anti-(human) AV node, and anti-His antibodies were investigated in sick sinus syndrome (SSS) and AV block of elderly patients with pacemakers. This overview will focus on a study of 55 patients with pacemakers with first- to third-degree AV block and of 62 patients with SSS in whom the presence of predisposing inflammatory heart disease and the coexistence of anti-sinus node, of anti-AV node and anti-His antibodies was examined. Anti-sinus node antibodies were found in 29% of patients with SSS and in 20% of patients with AV block. Circulating anti-AV node antibodies were present in 18% of patients with SSS and in 20% of patients with AV block, whereas the incidence in age-matched controls was 3% and 10%, respectively. Anti-sinus node antibodies, anti-AV node antibodies, and also anti-myolemmal antibodies were predominantly found in patients with previous myocarditis or rheumatic fever. For patients with anti-sinus node antibodies therefore a ten-fold risk of developing SSS and for patients with anti-AV node antibodies a 2.2-fold risk of developing AV block can be calculated from this population and age-matched controls. Myocarditis and rheumatic fever appear to predispose for anti-sinus node and anti-AV node antibodies. These in turn seem to be diagnostic and prognostic markers of SSS and AV block.

INTRODUCTION

For the cardiologist, a number of questions arise in cardiac conduction and automaticity disturbances, the answers for which immunologic investigations may contribute. Those questions include the following:

1. What are the different etiologies in cardiac conduction and automaticity disturbances?

2. Is there a rationale for an etiologically or pathophysiologically based treatment of SSS, AV block, or arrhythmias?

3. Can risk groups of patients be identified by clinical or serologic methods?

For the immunologist interested in electric disturbances of the heart, the following problems are of interest:

1. Which etiologies of conduction or automaticity disturbances are autoreactive?

223

2. Which clinical manifestations are associated with such immunological abnormalities?

3. Are there diagnostic markers in left bundle branch block, right bundle branch block, SSS, AV block, bradyarrhythmia, ventricular extrasystoles, tachycardia, or fibrillation that can be determined by immunologic methods?

4. Can risk groups for these diseases or of sudden death be identified by immunologic markers?

ETIOLOGIES OF ARRHYTHMIAS AND CARDIAC CONDUCTION DISTURBANCES

The clinical disorders in which cardiac conduction disturbances and arrhythmias are observed vary considerably. Sudden death, which is most often due to ventricular tachycardia, flutter, or fibrillation, has been described repeatedly in coronary artery disease and after infarction, in dilated cardiomyopathy, in secondary heart muscle diseases, in myocarditis, and after the administration of toxic substances like alcohol and several drugs, even after antiarrhythmics which may have proarrhythmic effects. SSS and AV block have also been associated with a wide range of cardiac or systemic diseases,[1] *e.g.*, coronary artery disease (more often with inferior than with anterior infarction),[2,3] dilated cardiomyopathy,[2,4] active or healed myocarditis,[5-8] rheumatic fever,[2] chronic chagasic heart muscle disease,[9] previous diphtheria,[10] collagen diseases,[2] particularly sacroileitis,[11,12] polymyositis,[13] systemic sclerosis,[14] rheumatoid arthritis,[15,16] rarely Reiter's syndrome,[17] lupus erythematosus,[18] mixed connective tissue disease,[19] mastocytosis,[20] hypertrophic cardiomyopathy,[21] and muscular dystrophy,[22] and after aortic and mitral valve surgery.[23] In patients with diabetes mellitus or with hypertension, these disorders may be overrepresented, although the pathophysiologic cause-consequence relationship remains speculative.

SSS presents clinically with different manifestations,[24-26] *e.g.*, with sinuatrial (SA) block, tachycardia-bradycardia syndrome, and pathologic sinus bradycardia. Its histopathology has 3 anatomical features in common: there are destructive lesions of the SA node,[27] dilation of the atria,[28] and pathologic changes of the atrial muscle. Idiopathic fibrosis of the sinus node has also been described[29-31] and has been attributed most often to aging.[32] It may include the deposition of an amyloid-like substance[32] or its replacement by fat.[32] Lymphocytic infiltrations may occur in some cases.[30-36] It is still controversial whether coronary artery disease is the main etiology responsible for SSS,[24,35] since SSS can occur without significant stenosis of the sinus node artery or the proximal right coronary artery[35] in elderly patients.

A similar list with almost the identical spectrum of cardiac or systemic disorders can be compiled for the different possible pathologies of AV block, and left bundle or right bundle branch block. In AV block as in SSS degenerative lesions predominate in the pathohistologic analysis according to extensive studies by Lenègre,[4,36-38] Lev,[33,39-41] and Davies.[2,29,42]

IMMUNOLOGIC FEATURES AND POSSIBLE IMMUNOPATHOGENESIS IN CONDUCTION DISTURBANCES

Previous immunological investigations of the cardiac conduction system have been limited in number (Table 1). Antibodies against bovine cardiac Purkinje cells

TABLE 1.   Autoantibodies in Arrhythmias and Cardiac Conduction Disturbances—Review of Literature

Electrical disturbance	Reference	Antibody type	% positive
Heart block	Fairfax & Doniach 1976[43]	ACPCab	8.6
Right bundle branch block (rheum. arth.)	Villeco et al. 1983[16]	ACPAab	38.0
"Congenital" AV block	Reed et al. 1983[46] Scott et al. 1983[45] Lee and Weston 1984[48]	SS-A/Ro & SS-B/La	88.3– 100.0
SSS	Lotze et al. 1984[49] Maisch et al. 1986[50] and 1987[51]	ASNab	29
AV block	Maisch et al. 1988[53]	AAVNab	18

ASANab: anti-sinus node antibodies, AAVNab: anti-AV node antibodies, CPCab: anti-cardiac Purkinje cell antibodies, SS–A/Ro and SS–B/La: ribonuclein antibodies (markers in SLE).

(CPC) were first reported to occur in 8.6% of patients with heart block by Fairfax and Doniach[43] and recently reexamined by Obbiassi et al.,[44] who found a comparable proportion of positive patients. In patients with rheumatoid arthritis and right bundle branch block this antibody was also noted but with a much greater incidence.[16] Recently, SS-A/Ro and SS-B/La antibodies, a diagnostic marker of lupus erythematosus, were demonstrated in the mothers and intermittently in the newborns themselves with congenital heart block.[45–48]

Apart from our own reports on SSS[49–51] and AV block,[51,52] antibodies directed to human conducting tissue in conduction or automaticity disturbances have not been investigated.

This overview is primarily based on our clinical and immunologic data from pacemaker patients with conduction and automaticity disturbances, as previously described.[49–52]

PATIENT GROUPS

1. SSS

Sixty-two patients (35 males, 27 females, mean age 68.7 ± 9.3 years) with atrial conduction or automaticity disturbances, who had undergone pacemaker implantation were studied. Twenty-two patients had a second- or third-degree SA block (7 males, 15 females, mean age 68.3 ± 10.5 years); 8 patients had the tachycardia-bradycardia syndrome (4 males, 4 females, mean age 66.1 ± 14.5 years). Sinus bradycardia was present in 15 patients (11 males, 4 females, mean age 67.0 ± 9 years). All 3 subgroups together constitute the group of patients with classic SSS (22 males, 23 females, mean age 67.5 ± 10.6 years). A group of 17 patients with bradyarrhythmia consisted of 13 male and 4 female patients (mean age 71.0 ± 8.5 years).

2. AV Block

Fifty-five pacemaker patients (32 males and 23 females; mean age 71.7 ± 9.9 years) with AV block of different degrees were included. Binodal disease was present in 16 patients. Thirty-three patients (60%) had third-degree AV block (17 males, 16 females, mean age 72.8 $\pm$ 9.8 years); 12 patients second-degree AV block of Wenckebach or Mobitz type II (9 males, 3 females, mean age 69.1 $\pm$ 11.6 years); 10 patients first-degree AV block (6 males, 4 females, mean age 71.3 $\pm$ 7.8 years) associated with distal bifascular block ($n=4$) or binodal disease ($n=6$).

3. Bradyarrhythmia

A group of 17 patients with bradyarrhythmia was composed of 13 males and 4 females patients (mean age 71.0 $\pm$ 8.5 years).

4. Control Group

The control group was composed of 31 age-matched patients with coronary artery disease, hypertension, cardiomyopathy, and previous myocarditis. A second control group included 23 patients (16 males, 7 females, mean age 65.6 $\pm$ 8.7) in whom previous myocarditis, cardiomyopathies, or symptomatic coronary artery disease were ruled out (noncardiac controls).

PREDISPOSING FACTORS AND ETIOLOGY OF CONDUCTION DISTURBANCES IN OUR PATIENTS

Former inflammatory diseases in SSS were diphtheria in 20 patients; myopericarditis,

TABLE 2. Predisposing Factors in SSS, Bradyarrhythmia and AV Block (reprinted, with permission[50])

Predisposing or etiological factor	Bradyarrhythmia ($n=17$)		SSS ($n=45$)		First- to third-degree AV block ($n=55$)	
	% pos.	Time elapsed (years)**	% pos.	Time elapsed (years)**	% pos.	Time elapsed (years)**
Former diphtheria	29	29–62	20	25–59	15	30–57
Former myocarditis or myopericarditis	12	20–29	13	0–31	16	0–27
Myocardial infarction (recent)	41	0–12	11	0–12	16	0– 7
Former rheumatic fever	18	27–66	9	35–62	16	39–60
Hypertension	18	0–12	20	2–14	18	0–22
Diabetes mellitus	18	0–11	22	0–12	18	0–15
Binodal disease	35	*	20	*	29	*
Hyperthyroidism	0	*	3	*	2	*
Goiter (grade 2)	0	*	5	*	4	*
Heart surgery	6	0– 5	2	0– 6	2	0– 2
Mitral valve prolapse	6	*	9	*	2	*
Dilated cardiomyopathy	11	*	0	*	0	*

* Present at time of investigation.
** Time span in years elapsed from diagnosis of possible underlying disease to pacemaker implantation.

diagnosed by biopsy in 2, and clinically by segmental wall motion abnormality or cardiomegaly with pericardial effusion or rubs in 4, and rheumatic fever in another 4. The time that had elapsed between pacemaker implantation and the acute diseases can be seen in Table 2.[50] Diphtheria could be dated from childhood, often more than 60 years previously, as could rheumatic fever. Myocarditis had been diagnosed at some time before pacemaker implantation by biopsy, or many years before.

In bradyarrhythmia, the incidence of former infarction was highest; in 41 % of patients diphtheria followed in frequency with 29 %, and rheumatic fever in 18 %, with variable time spans having elapsed before onset of bradyarrhythmia (Table 2). The etiology of AV block was often unknown; the incidence of former diphtheria, myopericarditis, and rheumatic fever ranged between 15 % to 16 %.

METHODOLOGICAL CONSIDERATIONS

Since methodology is important in avoiding false positive results due to nonspecific reactions and also in interpreting humoral reactions to human cardiac conducting tissue correctly, our method will be briefly outlined. The indirect immunofluorescence or immunoperoxidase technique test using human and heterologous cardiac tissue (blood group O donors only) was employed[52-56] with cryostat sections of fresh human and rat myocardium, skeletal muscle, kidney, and liver to test for anti-myocardial and nonorgan-specific antibodies. Heterophilic antibodies were assumed when anti-endothelial and anti-sarcolemmal antibodies from the rat only were positive[57] and therefore excluded. Antibodies against Purkinje fibers were tested with the ox false tendon prepared according to the method of Fairfax and Doniach.[43] To assess circulating anti-conducting tissue antibodies, human sinus node, AV node, and His bundle were prepared from young cases having died of noncardiac causes according to the method of Davies[2] and Schneider et al.[31] within 2 to 6 hr after death and checked for irregularities by hematoxylin-eosin (HE) staining, before being used to prepare 5-μm cryostat sections. First, patients' sera were used unabsorbed, to check for anti-muscle and other nonorgan-specific antibodies and all patients were checked for conducting tissue antibodies. Sera positive for any of the conducting tissue antibodies were then absorbed with human ventricular myocardium[50-52] and used again. Antibodies directed against the myolemma of isolated myocytes were demonstrated on isolated adult rat cardiocytes[58] or adult human atrial myocytes.[58] The staining of the antibodies was performed with polyspecific FITC- or peroxidase-labeled anti-human immunoglobulins, (F (ab)$_2$ fragments, affipure, H- and L-chain-specific, Behring, dilution 1:10 or 1:50). Positive samples were tested for immunoglobulin subclasses by polyspecific antisera (Behring, F (ab)$_2$ fragments, dilution 1:10) and complement (C$_3$, Behring). Sera positive for anti-nuclear antibodies were tested for single- and double-stranded DNA, the latter radioimmunologically (DNA 125 J-Antibody Kit; Amersham), and for SS-A/Ro and SS-B/La antibodies. The immunofluorescence test was evaluated by 2 independent observers in a blinded fashion. Interobserver variability was <9 % for grading ($n = 124$). Intraassay variance was <5 % ($n = 10$) and interassay variance ($n = 10$) was 0 for 2 standard positive sera tested in each assay.

Autofluorescence may interfere with staining by antibodies, and is observed more frequently in the sinus node and in the central fibrous body of the AV node than in the His region. The bundle of His itself is free of autofluorescence. The problem was solved by 2 approaches:

1. Autofluorescence was assumed only when fluorescence signals were seen by both filter blocks I_2 (blue light) and N_2 (green light). FITC-positive labeling was seen with filter block I_2 (blue light) only.

2. Since autofluorescence was seen regionally and sparsely only, the fluorescence derived from FITC-labeled antisera was to be seen on all structures of the same morphology.

BIOCHEMICAL AND HISTOLOGICAL ASPECTS OF THE CONDUCTION SYSTEM AND CHARACTERISTIC STAINING PATTERNS

1. Sinus Node and Anti-Sinus Node Antibodies

Histologically the sinus node is located at the sinus node artery. It is made up of more peripheral conducting and more centrally located, glycogen-rich pacemaker cells. Autoreactive antibodies are directed primarily to the membrane of cells. Cross-reactive antibodies to regular ventricular heart cells have been demonstrated, as have sinus node-specific antibodies, that could not be absorbed by ventricular myocardium. On cryostat sections it cannot be distinguished whether the antibody is directed to the interstitial tissue, the extracellular matrix, or specific surface determinants of the cells of the sinus node. A positive staining for ASN antibodies is shown in Fig. 1 of a patient with SSS due to previous myocarditis. It is positive for the membrane of the cells in the sinus node area. The sinus node was identified histologically in a first section, which was stained with HE. This section was then compared to the immunofluorescence in the subsequent sections. A differentiation of more central pacemaker cells to peripheral cells was not possible, however, although identification of the conducting tissue was easy.

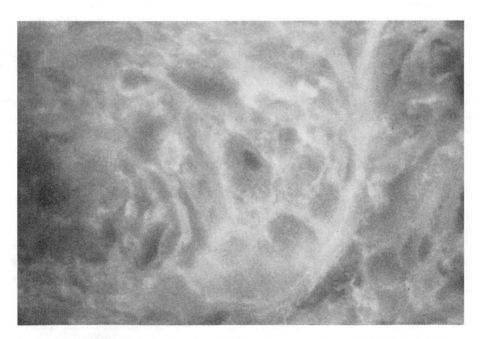

Fig. 1.   Demonstration of antibodies (IgG class, titer 1:80) binding to the human sinus node in a patient with SSS in former rheumatic fever (peroxidase-labeled second antibody). (Reprinted, with permission.[50])

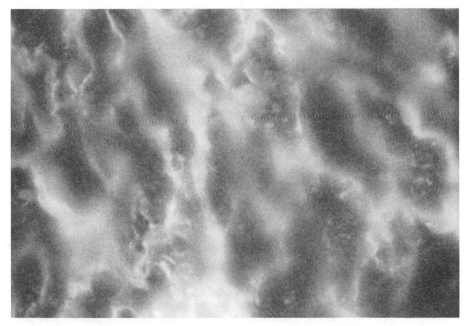

Fig. 2. Antibodies (IgG class, titer 1:40) directed against the AV node in a 42-year-old female patient with biopsy-proven myocarditis and acute third-degree AV block requiring pacemaker implantation. The patient died 10 years after the first episode of myocarditis from a recurrent necrotizing inflammatory cardiac process.

2. AV Node and Anti-AV Node Antibodies

Its well-known location makes the AV node easily identifiable in tissue sections. The humoral autoreactive response is directed to the membrane and the interstitial tissue. Antibodies to the human AV node have been identified using the same approach as ASN antibodies by comparing HE staining of the cryostat section with immunochemistry (POD) or IFT staining. A positive staining from a 39-year-old female patient with long-standing, biopsy-proven, active, recurring myocarditis is again directed to the membrane (Fig. 2). This patient was also positive for antimyolemmal antibodies characterized by adult human myocytes. The staining was specific for the AV node, since it could not be absorbed with human ventricular myocardium, which abolished the anti-sarcolemmal staining of the rest of the myocardium.

3. Anti-His Antibodies

After localization of the bundle of His close to the central fibrosus body by HE staining, anti-His antibodies, which occurred rarely, were identified based on their diffuse or membrane staining pattern (Fig. 3).

4. Anti-Purkinje Cell Antibodies

Central parts of the ox false tendon contain Purkinje cells. Heterologous anti-Purkinje cell (APC) staining was observed frequently in patients, but also occasionally in controls. An example of the mostly diffuse cytoplasmic, sometimes also seen upon membrane-associated staining, is shown in Fig. 4. With sera containing anti-myosin or anti-mitochondrial antibodies a positive staining was also obtained. Thus a specific diagnosis

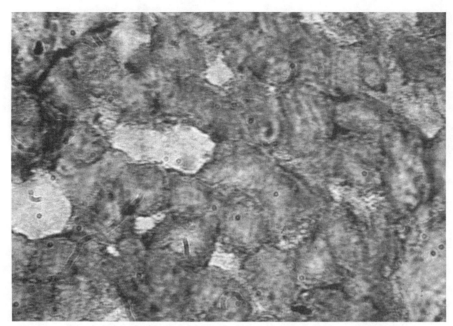

Fig. 3. Anti-His antibodies (IgG class, titer 1:20) in a 67-year-old patient with binodal disease (intermittent sinus bradyarrhythmia and second-degree AV block of the Wenckebach type).

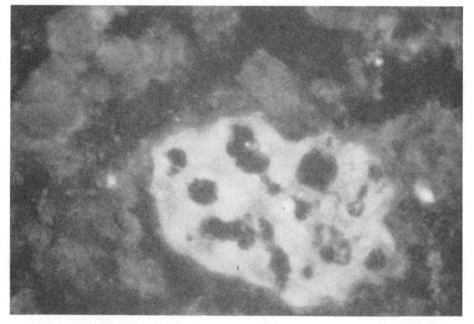

Fig. 4. Anti-Purkinje fiber antibodies homogenously stain the ox false tendon.

in the IFT for a specific conducting tissue antibody must exclude anti-muscle or anti-mitochondrial antibodies; the first appears as a cross-striated, and the latter as a diffuse cytoplasmic pattern upon staining.

ASSOCIATION OF CONDUCTING TISSUE ANTIBODIES WITH CARDIAC DISEASES

1. Anti-Sinus Node Antibodies

Antibodies against the SA node, primarily of the IgG (rarely of the IgM or IgA) class, were demonstrated in 29% of the sera of patients with SSS (Table 3). The incidence differed significantly from that in age-matched controls (including those with cardiac diseases) ($X^2 = 8.04$, $2P < 0.001$). When compared to noncardiac controls, the difference was even more pronounced ($X^2 = 8.21$, $2P < 0.01$), since in age-matched controls with cardiac diseases, only 3% of patients demonstrated ASN antibodies. In age-matched controls without cardiac diseases (noncardiac controls), no ASN antibodies were detected at all. In first- to third-degree AV-block ASN antibodies occurred in 24%, when compared to either of the control groups ($X^2 = 6.2$, $2P < 0.05$, or $X^2 = 10.4$ $2P < 0.05$, respectively; Table 3). Seven of the positive patients had binodal disease, however. In bradyarrhythmia, ASN antibodies were also found more often than in controls ($X^2 = 4.85$; $2P < 0.05$). Two of the sera (11.8%) stained positive, even after they were absorbed with ventricular myocardium ($X^2 = 3.81$; $P < 0.05$), so a monospecific antibody to the sinus node can be postulated.

From these data a ten-fold risk for patients with the ASN antibody to develop SSS can be calculated.

TABLE 3. Anti-conducting Tissue Antibodies in Cardiac Conduction and Automaticity Disturbances (Reprinted, with permission[50])

Antibody type	SSS ($n=45$) % pos.	Bradyarrhythmia ($n=17$) % pos.	AV block ($n=65$) % pos.	Age-matched controls ($n=31$) % pos.	Noncardiac controls ($n=23$) % pos.
Anti-sinoatrial-node (human)	29[a,b]	24[a]	22[a]	3	0
Anti-AV-node (human)	18[a]	29[a]	24[a,b]	10	0
Anti-His-node (human)	21[a]	6	13[a]	10	0
Anti-Purkinje fibers (bovine)	11[a]	35[a]	27	19	4
AMLAs (homologous)	44[a]	82[a]	68[a,b]	35	22
AMLAs (heterologous)	24	53	62	42	43
ASAs (antisarcolemmal)					
homologous type	30	18	61[a,b]	29	26
heterologous type	41	59	70	74	70
IFAs (antiinterfibrillary)	16	24	15	3	0
IFAs (antifibrillary)	9	56	7	23	26
AEAs (antiendothelial)	33	47	52	42	39
ANAs (antinuclear)	47	24	54	29	30
dsDNA 25 U/ml	11	0	12	0	0
ss-DNA	7	0	0	0	0
SMA (smooth muscle)	7	0	4	0	0

[a] $2p < 0.05$ by chi-square analysis when compared to noncardiac controls ($n=23$).
[b] $2p < 0.05$ by chi-square analysis when compared to age-matched controls ($n=31$).
SS-Ro and SS-La antibodies were all negative in controls with heart disease ($n=31$).

2. Anti-AV Node Antibodies

Anti-AV node (AAVN) antibodies were found in patients with SSS (18%) significantly more often than in the noncardiac controls (0%) (Table 3).

In bradyarrhythmia 5 sera before and 1 after absorption were positive for the AV node. Two of the 5 patients also had binodal disease with third-degree AV block. AAVN antibodies were demonstrated in 24% of patients with third-degree AV block, in 8% of patients with second-degree AV block, and in 30% of patients with first-degree AV block. They were primarily of the IgG class and less frequently of the IgA ($n=3$) or the IgM type ($n=2$). Complement fixation (C_3) could be demonstrated in 27% to 35% of cases with SSS or AV block, which were already positive for immunoglobulin binding. Only 10% of all age-matched controls ($n=31$), including those with heart disease, were positive for AAVN antibodies. In noncardiac controls, no AAVN antibodies could be found. Differences between the 2 control groups and all the patients with different degrees of AV block are outlined in Table 3.

From these data for patients with AAVN antibodies, a two- to three-fold risk for AV conduction disturbances can be derived when compared with age-matched controls. If compared with noncardiac controls, the calculated risk is much higher.

When sera preabsorbed with ventricular myocardium were used for staining, AAVN antibodies were still detected in one patient. A microheterogeneity of at least 2 AAVN antibodies can therefore be defined: one is cross-reactive with ventricular myocardium and one is an AV node-specific antibody.

3. Antibodies Against the Human His Bundle

Antibodies against the human His bundle were found in 22% of patients with SSS ($P<0.05$, when compared to noncardiac controls), in 6% of patients with bradyarrhythmia, and in 13% of patients with AV block (Table 3).

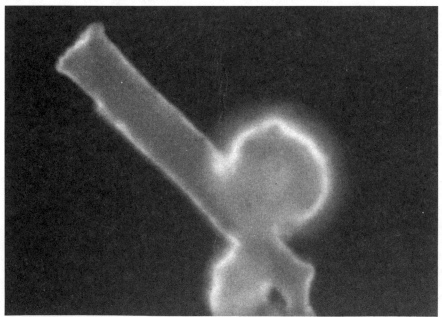

Fig. 5. Demonstration of anti-myolemmal antibodies (AMLAs) in a patient with third-degree AV block and biopsy-proven active myocarditis (titer 1:320; IgG-, IgM-, and C_3-positive).

4. Anti-Purkinje Cell Antibodies

Antibodies directed against bovine Purkinje cells were found more frequently in patients than in controls and significantly more often in patients with heart block than in noncardiac controls. Data can be derived from Table 3.

5. Anti-myolemmal Antibodies

Anti-myolemmal antibodies (AMLAs) of the homologous type were tested with

TABLE 4. Etiology of Conduction Disturbances and Incidence of Anti-conducting Tissue Antibodies (Reprinted, with permission[50])

Antibody type in Nonabsorbed sera SSS (n=55)	Diphtheria		Myocarditis		Rheumatic fever		Myocardial infarction	
	pos. (n=9) %	neg. (n=36) %	pos. (n=6) %	neg. (n=39) %	pos. (n=4) %	neg. (n=41) %	pos. (n=5) %	neg. (n=40) %
Anti-sinus node	11	33	67[b]	23	50	27	25	30
Anti-AV node	22	17	34	15	50[a]	15	25	18
Anti-His bundle	11	25	17	23	0	24	60[b]	18
Anti-Purkinje fibers	11	11	17	10	25	10	0	10
AMLAs[4] (heterologous)	33	22	34	23	25	25	0	28
AMLAs (homologous/ human)	22	50	50	44	25	46	20	48
ASAs[5]	44	53	50	52	50	49	80	48

Bradyarrhythmia (n=17)	Diphtheria		Myocarditis		Rheumatic fever		Myocardial infarction	
	pos. (n=5) %	neg. (n=12) %	pos. (n=2) %	neg. (n=15) %	pos. (n=3) %	neg. (n=14) %	pos. (n=7) %	neg. (n=10) %
Anti-sinus node	40	17	50	20	33	21	29	20
Anti-AV node	20	39	50	27	67	21	29	30
Anti-His bundle	0	8	0	7	0	7	0	10
Anti-Purkinje fibers	60	25	50	33	33	38	14	50
AMLAs[4] (heterologous)	20	67[a]	50	53	67	50	57	50
AMLAs (human/ homologous)	100	75	100	80	100	79	86	80
ASAs[5]	40	67	100	53	100	50	71	50

AV Block (n=5)	Diphtheria		Myocarditis		Rheumatic fever		Myocardial infarction	
	pos. (n=8) %	neg. (n=47) %	pos. (n=9) %	neg. (n=46) %	pos. (n=6) %	neg. (n=49) %	pos. (n=9) %	neg. (n=46) %
Anti-AV node (human)	0	26[b]	44	17[a]	67	17[b]	0	26[a]
Anti-sinoatrial node (human)	38	21	33	22	50	20	33	22
Anti-His (human)	0	15	22	11	17	12	0	15
Anti-Purkinje fiber (bovine)	13	30	11	30	33	27	33	26
AMLAs (heterologous)	50	64	78	59	50	63	89[a]	57
AMLAs (homologous)	50	72	56	72	17	67	50	61
ASAs	75	57	56	61	50	61	44	63

[a] p<0.05. [b] p<0.01.

human atrial heart cells (Fig. 5). They were found significantly more often in all groups of patients when compared to noncardiac controls. They have been demonstrated previously to be a diagnostic marker of inflammatory cardiac processes when they fix complement or include the IgG and IgM subclasses.[53–56,58] Most important, however, is their functional property of lysing vital adult myocytes in the presence of (and, less frequently, as cytotoxic antibodies also in the absence of) complement both in adults[54–56,58,59] and in children.[60]

ARE ANTIBODIES TO CARDIAC CONDUCTING TISSUES A MARKER OF FORMER INFLAMMATORY HEART DISEASE?

The incidence of ASNA or AAVN antibodies in either SSS or AV block were highest in the group of patients with former myocarditis and former rheumatic fever, as shown in Fig. 5a/b and Table 3. Previous infection with diphtheria or myocardial infarction did not induce antibodies directed against human conducting tissue. AMLAs predominated in these 2 groups of patients as well (Table 4). Thus former myocarditis in the past or rheumatic fever may have induced these antibodies directed against sinus or AV node. Their presence defines patients at risk for SSS, AV block, bradyarrhythmia, and binodal disease.

This can also be derived from preliminary data on patients with active myocarditis in whom anticonducting tissue antibodies were found more frequently than in age-matched controls (unpublished). Not all of those patients, however, exhibited significant rhythm disturbances and blocks, although there was suggestive evidence for this in a 39-year-old female patient with recurrent, chronic necrotizing lethal myocarditis. She demonstrated ASN and AAVN antibodies in her early sera when AV block had developed initially.[8]

To substantiate this suggestive hypothesis, follow-up studies over many years are needed and functional assays must be developed to assess the effect of these antibodies on isolated AV node and sinus node cells *in vitro*. Until then the pathogenic role of anticonducting tissue antibodies remains an intriguing but still speculative hypothesis.

ACKNOWLEDGMENT

Support by grants from the Deutsche Forschungsgemeinschaft (Ma 780/1–6) is acknowledged.

REFERENCES

1. Landegren, J. and Bjorck, G. The clinical assessment and treatment of complete heart block and Adams-Stokes attacks. *Medicine* **42**: 171–196, 1963.
2. Davies, M.J. Pathology of Conducting Tissue of the Heart. London, Butterworth & Co, 1971.
3. Johannson, B.W. Complete heart block. A clinical, hemodynamic and pharmacological study in patients with and without an artificial pacemaker. *Acta Med. Scand* **180**: Suppl., **451**: 1, 1966.
4. Lenegre, J. Les lésions du système de His-Tawara dans les blocs auriculoventriculaires de haut degré. *Cardiologia* **46**: 261–267, 1965.
5. Hudson, R.E.B. Cardiovascular Pathology. London, Edward Arnold, 1965.
6. Penton, G.B., Miller, H., and Levine, S.A. Some clinical features of complete heart block. *Circulation* **13**: 810–824, 1956.

7. Cui, G.G. Viral myocarditis associated with complete heart block and Adams-Stokes attacks. *Chung Hua Nei Ko Tsa Chih* **22**: 348–351, 1983.
8. Maisch, B., Mueller-Hermelink, H.K., Ertl, G., and Kochsiek, K. Lethal myocarditis with AV-block and ventricular tachycardia. *Heart Vessels* (submitted).
9. Rosenbaum, M.B. Chagasic myocardiopathy. *Prog. Cardiovasc. Dis.* **7**: 199–225, 1964.
10. Butler, S. and Levine, S.A. Diphtheria as a cause of late heart block. *Am. Heart J.* **5**: 592–598, 1930.
11. Nitter-Hauge, S. and Otterstad, J.E. Characteristics of atrioventricular conduction disturbances in ankylosing spondylitis (M. Bechterew). *Acta Med. Scand.* **210**: 197–200, 1981.
12. Bergfeld, L., Edhag, O., and Vallin, H. Cardiac conduction disturbances, an underestimated manifestation in ankylosing spondylitis. A 25-year-old follow-up study of 68 patients. *Acta Med. Scand.* **212**: 217–233, 1982.
13. Kehoe, R.F., Bauernfeind, R., Rommaso, C., Wyndham, C., and Rosen, K.M. Cardiac conduction defects in polymyositis: Electrophysiologic studies in our patients. *Ann. Intern. Med.* **94**: 41–43, 1981.
14. Botstein, G.R., Leroy, E.C. Primary heart disease in systemic sclerosis (scleroderma): advances in clinical and pathologic features, pathogenesis, and new therapeutic approaches. *Am. Heart J.* **102**: 913–919, 1981.
15. Ahern, M., Lever, J.V., and Cosh, J. Complete heart block in rheumatoid arthritis. *Ann. Rheum. Dis.* **42**: 389–397, 1983.
16. Villecco, A.S., de Liberali, E., Bianchi, F.B., and Pisi, E. Antibodies to cardiac conducting tissue and abnormalities of cardiac conduction in rheumatoid arthritis. *Clin. Exp. Immunol.* **53**: 536–540, 1983.
17. Ruel, M., Haas, C., and Heulin, A. Auriculoventricular block in Fiessinger-Leroy-Reiter's syndrome. *Nouv. Presse Med.* (Paris) **11**: 2786–2787, 1982.
18. Meyniel, D., Beaufils, M., Bochoucha, S., Mayand, C., and Akonn, G. Complete atrioventricular block in a developmental flare-up of acute systemic lupus erythematosus (letter). *Nouv. Presse Med.* (Paris) **11**: 3797–3799, 1982.
19. Rakovec, P., Kenda, M.F., Rozman, B., Zemva, A., and Cibic, B. Panconductional defect in mixed connective tissue disease: Association with Sjögren's syndrome. *Chest* **81**: 257–259, 1981.
20. Thomas, D., Dragodanne, C., Frank, R., Prier, A., Chomette, G., and Grosgogeat, Y. Systemic mastocytosis with myo-pericardial localization and atrioventricular block. *Arch. Mal. Coeur* **74**: 215–221, 1981.
21. Touboul, P., Kirkorian, G., Atallah, G., Cahen, P., de Zuloaga, C., and Moleur, P. Atrioventricular block and preexcitation in hypertrophic cardiomyopathy. *Am. J. Cardiol.* **53**: 961–963, 1984.
22. Pailloncy, M., Citron, B., Hersch, B., Heiligenstein, D., Ponsonnaille, J., and Gras, H. Electrocardiograms of women carriers of Duchenne-type muscular dystrophy: A study of a family with a case of complete atrioventricular heart block. *Ann. Cardiol. Angiol.* (Paris) **31**: 47–50, 1982.
23. Fairfax, A.J. and Doniach, D. Autoantibodies to cardiac conducting tissue and their characterization by immunofluorescence. *Clin. Exp. Immunol.* **23**: 1–8, 1976.
24. Ferrer, J. The sick sinus syndrome in atrial disease. *JAMA* **206**: 645–646, 1968.
25. Ferrer, J. The sick sinus syndrome. *Circulation* **47**: 635–641, 1973.
26. Bloemer, H., Wirtzfeld, A., Delius, W., and Sebening, H. Das Sinusknotensyndrom. *Perimed. Erlangen.* 1977
27. Draper, G. Pulsus irregularis perpetuus with fibrosis of the sinus node. *Heart* **3**: 13–21, 1911.
28. Laas, E. Das Arrhythmie-Herz. *Zentralbl Allg. Pathal.* **103**: 552–555, 1962.
29. Davies, M.J. A histological study of the conduction system in complete heart block. *J. Path.* **94**: 351–358, 1969.

30. Doerr, W. Morphologische Aequivalente bei Rhythmusstoerungen des Herzens. *Verh. Dtsch. Ges. Inn. Med.* **81**: 36–38, 1975.

31. Schneider, J. Der ploetzliche Herztod als Folge einer Reizleitungsstoerung. 1. Teil: Quantitative Pathologie der Reizbildungs- und Reizleitungsstoerungen. *Schweiz. Med. Wochenschr.* **111**: 366–374, 1981.

32. Pomerance, A. Senile cardiac amyloidosis. *Br. Heart J.* **27**: 711–718, 1965.

33. Lev, M. Aging changes in the human sinoatrial node. *J. Geront.* **9**: 1–9, 1954.

34. James, T.N. and Marshall T.K. De subitanibus mortibus: XVII. Multifocal stenoses due to fibromuscular dysplasia of the sinus node artery. *Circulation* **53**: 736–742, 1976.

35. Engel, T.R., Steven, G.M., Gilson, S.F., Fischer, H.A., and Frankl, W.S. Appraisal of sinus node artery disease. *Circulation* **52**: 286–291, 1975.

36. Lenègre, J. Les blocs auriculoventriculaires complets chroniques. Etude des causes et des lesions a propros de 37 cas. *Malattie Cardiovascolari* **3**: 311–343, 1962.

37. Lenègre, J. Etiology and pathology of bilateral branch block in relation to complete heart block. *Prog. Cardiovasc. Dis.* **6**: 409–444, 1964.

38. Lenègre, J. Le bloc auriculo-ventriculaire chronique: Etude anatomique clinique, et histologique. *Archs. Mal. Coeur* **56**: 867–888, 1963.

39. Lev, M. The pathology of complete atrio-ventricular block. *Prog. Cardiovasc. Dis.* **6**: 317–326, 1964.

40. Lev, M. Anatomic basis for atrioventricular block. *Am. J. Med.* **37**: 742–748, 1964.

41. Lev, M. and Unger, P.N. The pathology of the conduction system in acquired heart disease. I. Severe atrioventricular block. *A.M.A Arch. Pathol.* **60**: 502–529, 1955.

42. Davies, M.J. Pathological basis of primary heart block. *Br. Heart J.* **31**: 219–226, 1969.

43. Fairfax, A.J. and Doniach, D. Autoantibodies to cardiac conducting tissue and their characterization by immunofluorescence. *Clin. Exp. Immunol.* **23**: 1–8, 1976.

44. Obbiassi, M., Brucato, A., Meroni, P.L., Vismara, A., Lettino, M., Poloni, F., Finzi, A., Fenini, M.G. and Rossi, L. Antibodies to cardiac Purkinje cells: Further characterization in autoimmune diseases and atrioventricular heart block. *Clin. Exp. Immunol.* **42**: 141–150, 1987.

45. Reed, B.R., Lee, L.A., Harman, C., Wolfe, R., Wiggins, J., Peeblos, C., and Weston, W.L. Autoantibodies to SS-A/Ro in infants with congenital heart block. *J. Pediatr.* **103**: 889–891, 1983.

46. Scott, J.S., Maddison, P.J., Taylor, P.V., Esser, E., Scott, O., and Skinner, P.R. Connective tissue disease, antibodies to ribonucleoprotein, and congenital heart block. *N. Engl. J. Med.* **309**: 209–212, 1983.

47. Lee, L.A. and Weston, W.L. New findings in neonatal lupus syndrome. *Am. J. Dis. Child.* **138**: 233–236, 1984.

48. Vetter, V.I. and Rashlaina, W.J. Congenital heart block and connective tissue disease (editorial). *N. Engl. J. Med.* **309**: 236–238, 1983.

49. Lotze, U., Maisch, B., Schneider, J., and Kochsiek, K. Antibodies against cardiac conducting tissue in sick sinus syndrome (SSS) and hypertensive carotid sinus syndrome (CSS) (abstract). *Eur. Heart J.* **5** (suppl. I): 255, 1984.

50. Maisch, B., Lotze, U., Schneider, J., and Kochsiek, K. Antibodies to human sinus node in sick sinus syndrome. *PACE* **9**: 1101–1109, 1986.

51. Maisch, B., Lotze, U., Kochsiek, K., and Schneider, J. Myocarditis and rheumatic fever. predispose to cardiac conduction disturbances. An immunologic study. In: Cardiac Pacing and Electrophysiology. Belhassen, B., Feldman, S., and Copperman, Y. (eds.), Proceedings of the VIII World Symposium on Cardiac Pacing and Electrophysiology, R & L Creative Communications Ltd., Tel Aviv, 1987, pp. 241–252.

52. Maisch, B., Lotze, U., Schneider, J., and Kochsiek, K. Antibodies to human AV node and conducting tissue in atrioventricular block (submitted).

53. Maisch, B., Berg, P.A., and Kochsiek, K. Clinical significance of immunopathological

findings in patients with postpericardiotomy syndrome. I. Relevance of antibody pattern. *Clin. Exp. Immunol.* **38**: 189–197, 1979.

54. Maisch, B., Berg, P.A., and Kochsiek, K. Autoantibodies and serum inhibition factors (SIF) in patients with myocarditis. *Klin. Wochenschr.* **58**: 219–225, 1980.

55. Maisch, B., Maisch, S., and Kochsiek, K. Immune reactions in tuberculous and chronic constrictive pericarditis. Clinical data and diagnostic significance of antimyocardial antibodies. *Am. J. Cardiol.* **50**: 1007–1013, 1982.

56. Maisch, B., Trostel-Soeder, R., Stechemesser, E., Berg, P.A., and Kochsiek, K. Diagnostic relevance of humoral and cell mediated immune reactions in patients with acute viral myocarditis. *Clin. Exp. Immunol.* **48**: 533–545, 1982.

57. Hawkins, B.R., McDonald, M., and Dawkins, R.C. Characterization of immunofluorescent heterophil antibodies which may be confused with autoantibodies. *J. Clin. Pathol.* **30**: 299–301, 1977.

58. Maisch, B. Immunologic regulator and effector functions in perimyocarditis, postmyocarditic heart muscle disease and dilated cardiomyopathy. *Basic. Res. Cardiol.* **81** (Suppl. 1): 217–242, 1986.

59. Maisch, B. The sarcolemma as antigen in the secondary immunopathogenesis of myopericarditis. *Eur. Heart J.* **8** (Suppl. J): 155–166, 1987.

60. Maisch, B., Schwab, D., Bauer, E., Sandhage, K., Schmaltz, A.A., and Wimmer, M. Antimyolemmal antibodies in myocarditis in children. *Eur. Heart J.* **8** (Suppl. J): 167–174, 1987.

The Possible Role of Autoantibodies in the Development of Electrical Disorders in Postinfectious Heart Muscle Disease

H.-P. Schultheiss* and U. Kühl**

* Department of Internal Medicine, University of Düsseldorf, Düsseldorf, FRG
** Department of Internal Medicine, University of Munich, Munich, FRG

ABSTRACT

We recently described autoantibodies (AB) to the ADP/ATP carrier of the inner-mitochondrial membrane as an organ-specific autoantigen in myocarditis and dilated cardiomyopathy. These AB crossreact with components of the cardiac myocyte surface. The crossreacting sarcolemmal epitopes could be identified as the calcium channel complex and the connexon, a cardiac gap junction protein. Using patch clamp technique we could show that the AB caused a potentiated calcium inward current and slowed calcium channel in activation leading to calcium overload and cell death.

Binding of AB to the gap junctions may interfere with channel gating and block spread of rapid impulse conductance in the heart. Both calcium channels and gap junctions play a central role in cardiac contractility. Disturbance of channel gating may be involved in the generation of complex cardiac arrhythmias often seen in association with myocarditis and dilated cardiomyopathy.

The relevance of the experimental data to the human situation is explored and the mechanisms for arrhythmias and conduction disturbances encountered in humans are discussed.

Dilated cardiomyopathy is characterized by dilation of one or generally both ventricles associated with impaired pump function, low cardiac output, increased filling pressures, and decreased ejection fraction. Although by definition dilated cardiomyopathy is a heart muscle disease of unknown cause, it is now believed that viral myocarditis, which has either become inactive or continues as a smoldering process, might be etiologic in a significant portion of genetically predetermined patients with dilated cardiomyopathy.[1-5] This assumption has been confirmed by the recent finding of Bowles and Kandolf and their coworkers[6-9] demonstrating the presence of enterovirus RNA in the human myocardium from patients with myocarditis and dilated cardiomyopathy. Thus the viral infection may act as a trigger initiating the autoimmunologic process by altering the host's immune system, by causing the release or expression of sequestered antigens, or through antigenic determinants shared by the virus and the host cell.[10,11] Although it is now believed that myocarditis more often follows a viral infection, confirmation of a definite viral etiology in clinical cases of myocarditis is often difficult if not impossible. Clinical presentations of myocarditis show wide variations ranging from a total absence of clinical manifestations to severe heart failure or sudden unexpected death.[3] Fatal arrhythmia, high degree AV block, or circulatory failure may be the cause of death in postmyocarditic cardiomyopathy.[12-14] Although the pathophysiology of viral myocarditis is only vaguely substantiated and understood, immunologic mechanisms are presumed to be important.[1,2,15–17] Humoral autoimmunity as a possible mechanism of myocardial injury in myocarditis and dilated cardiomyopathy is evidenced by autoantibodies in the serum and within the myocardium.[15–16] Although it is quite likely that most of the autoantibodies to membrane-related or intracellular antigens reflect a nonspecific process of myocardial injury, a subset of antibodies may yet prove to be immunopathogenetic.[15–18] Principally, autoantibodies to cell membrane receptors have been documented in a number of autoimmune diseases in humans. There is good evidence for a pathogenic role of autoantibodies to the nicotine acetylcholine receptor in myasthenia gravis, to the thyroglobulin receptor in certain types of diabetes, or to the β-adrenergic receptor in asthma.

Recently, we identified and characterized immunologically the ADP/ATP carrier, a protein localized within the inner mitochondrial membrane, as an organ- and conformation-specific autoantigen in myocarditis and dilated cardiomyopathy.[16,19]

The ADP/ATP carrier protein is one of the most abundant and active transport systems within biomembranes of eukaryotic cells enabling directed nucleotide transport between the intra- and extramitochondrial compartments.[20,21] It is responsible for maintenance of cellular energy metabolism, providing transport of ATP to energy-consuming cytosolic processes as well as transport of ADP back into the mitochondria for rephosphorylation.[22] Binding of autoantibodies at the cytosolic side of the carrier protein causes a drastic decrease in the nucleotide transport in vitro.[16,17] In experimental studies an action of the autoantibodies against the ADP/ATP carrier could be documented not only in vitro but also in vivo.[18,23] As a result of this antibody-mediated inhibition of the ADP/ATP carrier in vivo, the cytosolic concentration of ATP decreases while the mitochondrial ATP content increases dramatically. Based on these results, it has been suggested that autoantibodies against the ADP/ATP carrier play an important pathophysiologic role in dilated cardiomyopathy by causing an imbalance between energy delivery and demand.[18,46,47] Regardless of the mechanism of action of the antibodies in vivo, a specific binding of the antibodies to the cell surface is postulated as a prerequisite step.

In this paper, we describe data indicating that the antibodies against the ADP/ATP carrier specifically bind to 2 proteins at the cardiac myocyte plasma membrane—the connexon and the calcium channel—and discuss their possible role in the pathogenesis of myocarditis and dilated cardiomyopathy.

IMMUNOCHEMICAL CHARACTERIZATION OF THE ANTIBODIES AGAINST THE ADP/ATP CARRIER

To characterize the targets of the antibodies specific for the carboxyatractylate protein complex, different methods such as radioimmunoassay, immunoprecipitation, and Western blotting were used. To test the possible effect of the antibodies on nucleotide transport in vitro, the exchange rate of mitochondria was determined by the inhibitor-stop method combined with back exchange.[19] Such studies have shown that the antibodies against the ADP/ATP carrier are organ- and conformation-specific.[18,19] Functionally they inhibit nucleotide transport in vitro by binding specifically to the substrate/ligand binding site of the carrier protein.[18] The remarkable organ specificity of the ADP/ATP carrier was previously interpreted as reflecting isoenzyme distribution of the carrier in various organs. Although the concept of isoenzymes seemed at first bold and premature, it has been extended to several other instances. The organ specificity of the ADP/ATP carrier, which was confirmed by peptide maps,[25] and studies of the cDNA sequence[26] may reflect tissue-specific regulation of nucleotide transport. This regulation may be adapted to specific requirements in different tissues by the expression of specific isoenzymes.

SPECIFIC BINDING OF THE ANTIBODIES AGAINST THE ADP/ATP CARRIER TO THE CELL SURFACE OF CARDIAC MYOCYTES

Evidence for cross-reactivity between the ADP/ATP carrier and cell surface proteins was first obtained by indirect immunofluorescence. Incubation of frozen sections of heart tissue with the above characterized anti-ADP/ATP carrier antibodies showed, in addition to intracellular staining, antibody binding to the plasma membrane (Fig. 1). This was confirmed by positive staining of isolated cardiac myocytes showing a sarcolemmal immunofluorescence (Fig. 1). After neutralization of anti-ADP/ATP carrier antibodies by preadsorption with the isolated ADP/ATP carrier, intracellular staining and staining of the cell surface disappeared (Fig. 1). Preimmune sera did not react with the cell surface.

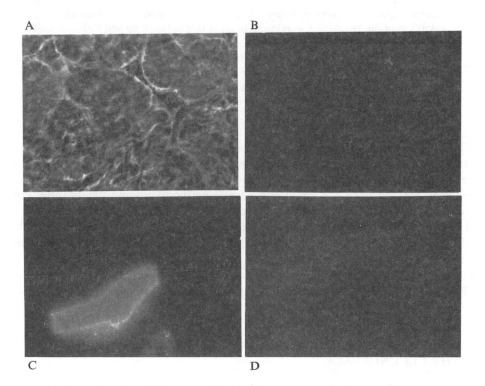

Fig. 1.   A and B: Immunofluorescence localization of antibodies to the ADP/ATP carrier: rabbit antibodies to the ADP/ATP carrier show intracellular staining of mitochondria and a reaction to the cell surface in cross-sections of cardiac tissue (A); disappearance of cell surface and intracellular reaction after neutralization of antibodies with purified ADP/ATP carrier (B). C and D: Binding of anti-ADP/ATP carrier antibodies to cardiac myocyte cell surface (C) and inhibition of antibody binding to cardiac myocytes by preincubation with the ADP/ATP carrier (D).

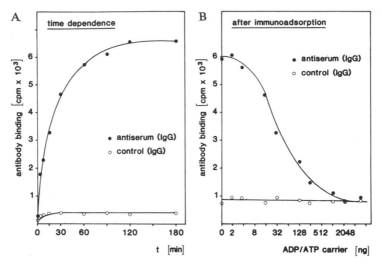

Fig. 2. The binding of antibodies against the ADP/ATP carrier on living cardiac myocytes is time-dependent. Cells were incubated with antibodies in a 1:3500 dilution, reaching a maximum binding rate between 60 and 120 min. Cell surface-bound antibodies were detected using ^{125}I-labeled protein A (A). After preincubation of antibodies with increasing amounts of purified ADP/ATP carrier, the binding of antibodies to the cell surface was decreased in a concentration-dependent manner (B). Incubation of cells with the antibodies was carried out for 90 min at 10°C. Control binding was done using preimmune IgG.

This cross-reactivity between antibodies and the cell surface was also demonstrated by radioimmunobinding assay. Figure 2 shows a time-dependent binding of antibodies to myocytes. After 60 min most of the antibodies were bound to the cell. Prolonged incubation for up to 180 min could not increase antibody binding significantly. Preimmune serum IgG (control) did not bind to myocytes. Antibody dilution from 1:1000 to 1:6000 resulted in a reduction of antibody binding until 1:5000, where no significant binding could be detected. The specificity of the antigen-antibody reaction was demonstrated by suppression of the binding to myocytes by immunoadsorption. Figure 2 shows that preincubation of the antibody with increasing amounts of the isolated ADP/ATP carrier (1 to 2,048 ng) resulted in a concentration-dependent decrease in antibody binding.

IDENTIFICATION OF THE CONNEXON AS A CROSSREACTING EPITOPE ON THE CELL SURFACE

Two protein hexamers consisting of 6 identical polypeptide subunits, termed the connexon (47,000 Dalton), compose the architectural picture of the gap junction channel.[27,28] Gap junctions are specialized membrane structures that enable the intercytoplasmic exchange of small molecules and ions between contracting cells.[29,30] The functional sequence of the expression of such transcellular pathways has long been postulated for excitable tissues like the heart, where gap junctions conduct electrical impulses and are involved in the synchronization of electrical activity. Immunofluores-

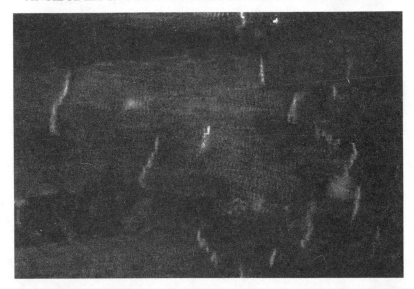

Fig. 3. Immunofluorescence localization of the binding of antibodies against the ADP/ATP carrier at the cardiac myocyte plasma membrane. After high antibody dilutions longitudinal sections of heart tissue revealed prominent staining of intercalated discs.

cence staining of cardiac myocytes resulted in a typical dotted pattern on the cardiac myocyte cell surface with a concentration of the labeled antibodies at both ends of the cells. These more intensively stained areas are the sites of close cell contacts forming the intercalated discs in heart tissue. In sections of heart tissue, in addition to cell surface staining, antimitochondrial-bound antibodies are found. At higher antibody dilutions staining of the total cell surface decreases, leaving remaining antibodies mainly bound at the intercalated discs (Fig. 3). Quantification of immunofluorescence staining intensity is not possible, because one cannot exclude different accessibilities of the antigens for the antibodies. Nevertheless, these observations suggest that the crossreacting epitope, at least in part, is concentrated within this specialized membrane region of intensive cell contact. These data are in good agreement with our electron microscopic data. If animals are immunized with the purified ADP/ATP carrier protein, cell surface and intracellular IgG deposits are found. While intracellular antibodies are bound to the mitochondrial membrane, cell surface-bound IgG can be detected on the whole plasma membrane and coinciding with the immunofluorescence staining within the intercalated discs. Antibody binding structures of these cell-cell contact sites were identified as gap junctions (Fig. 4). To identify cell surface components recognized by the anti-ADP/ATP carrier antibodies, cardiac myocyte membranes were purified on discontinuous sucrose gradients according to Cates and Holland[31] with some modifications. The resulting fraction yielding a product enriched in plasma membranes was tested by immunoblot analysis after SDS polyacrylamide electrophoresis. Antibody binding is specific for 3 proteins of molecular weights of 47,000, 32,000, and 29,000 Daltons, respectively (data not shown). The 32,000 Dalton protein has the electrophoretic mobility of the purified ADP/ATP carrier protein. It is the only protein recognized by the antibodies when purified mitochondrial membranes are tested in immunoblot analysis (not shown),

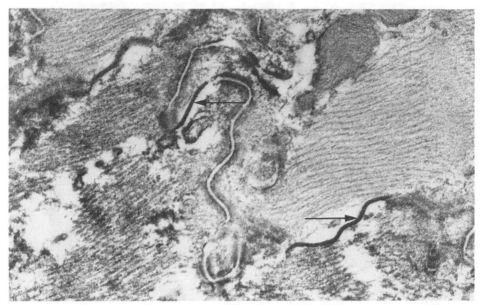

Fig. 4. Binding of antibodies against the ADP/ATP carrier at the cardiac myocyte plasma membrane: for immune electronmicroscopy, heart tissue of rabbits immunized with the purified ADP/ATP carrier was stained with protein A-peroxidase. Deposition of IgG molecules was seen at the plasma membrane and at gap junctions, localized within the intercalated discs. × 30,000.

indicating that part of the intracellular ADP/ATP carrier copurifies with the plasma membrane fraction. To discriminate between intracellular and cell surface membrane proteins, living adult cardiac myocytes were iodinated by lactoperoxidase-glucose oxydase. By this method, only plasma membrane components are labeled. Immunoprecipitation of the detergent solubilized membrane proteins by anti-ADP/ATP carrier antibodies is shown in Fig. 5c. The 47,000 and 29,000 Dalton proteins but not the 32,000 Dalton mitochondrial membrane protein were labeled with iodine, demonstrating their cell surface origin. Electrophoretic mobility of the 47,000 and 29,000 Dalton proteins is identical with that of isolated gap junction proteins (Fig. 5d). The ratio between the 47,000 and the 29,000 Dalton components obtained in different plasma membrane preparations was found to be dependent on different isolation conditions and on the amount of the added protease inhibitors, especially PMSF. These observations indicate that the 47,000 and the 29,000 Dalton components are related to each other and that the 29,000 Dalton component might be a degradation product of a 47,000 Dalton membrane protein. This fact was also demonstrated by Manjunath and Page.[24] Our results provide strong experimental arguments in support of the idea that antibodies against the ADP/ATP carrier of the inner mitochondrial membrane crossreact with a cell surface protein. This crossreacting cell surface binding site recognized by the anti-ADP/ATP carrier antibodies is the 47,000 Dalton subunit of the gap junctions—the connexon. Immunofluorescent staining of intercalated discs which contain concentrated sheets of the gap junctions in cardiac tissue, biochemical data obtained from immunoblot analysis and immunoprecipitation, and localization of antibodies seen in electron microscopy are compatible with this suggestion.

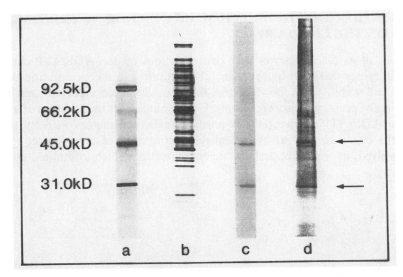

Fig. 5. Crossreaction of ADP/ATP carrier antibodies with cardiac gap junction proteins: In immunoprecipitations of rat cardiac myocyte membranes selectively labeled with ^{125}iodine only 2 proteins, with molecular weights of 47,000 and 29,000 Daltons, were detected after radiography (c). Electrophoretic mobility of the precipitated proteins is identical with that of isolated gap junction proteins (d). Samples were run on a linear 5–18% SDS polyacrylamide gradient gel. (a) Molecular weight marker proteins, (b) rat cardiac myocyte membranes, stained by silver nitrate.

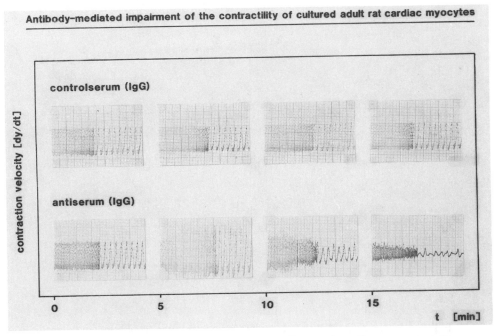

Fig. 6. Contraction characteristics of externally paced cardiac myocytes after addition of preimmune serum (control serum) and antibodies against the ADP/ATP carrier (antiserum).

IDENTIFICATION OF THE CALCIUM CHANNEL AS A CROSSREACTING EPITOPE ON THE CELL SURFACE

Incubation of cardiac myocytes with concentrations of anti-ADP/ATP carrier antibodies (affinity-purified IgG) higher than 1:1000 resulted in a concentration-dependent decrease in cell viability. As shown in Fig. 6, externally paced myocytes beat regularly after addition of preimmune sera (control). Five minutes after the addition of antibodies against the ADP/ATP carrier (affinity-purified IgG), contraction velocity increased, and the cells began to beat arrhythmically. Deterioration of myocytes as monitored visually involved, in sequence: arrhythmic concentrations, bleb formation, contracture

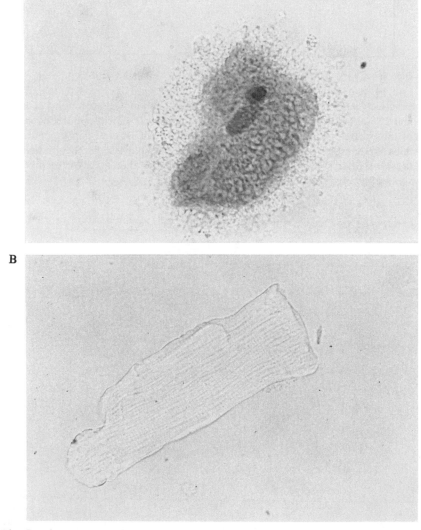

Fig. 7.   Appearance of isolated cardiac myocytes after incubation with antibodies to the ADP/ATP carrier (A) or control serum (B). After incubation with the anti-ADP/ATP carrier antibody the cells lost their membrane integrity and took up trypan blue, a marker of cell death.

to an almost cuboid shape, cell rounding, and finally cell death. These cells took up trypan blue very rapidly (Fig. 7). This antibody-mediated cytotoxic effect was strictly calcium-dependent. Using an antibody concentration of 1:100 and a calcium concentration of 1 mM, 20% of myocytes died after 30 min, 40% after 1 hr, and about 80% after 3 hr. In contrast, only 10% of myocytes incubated with preimmune serum IgG (control) did not survive 3 hr (Fig. 8). With decreasing amounts of calcium the effect of antibody-mediated cytotoxicity is gradually diminished. With an antibody-concentration of 1:100 and nominally no calcium only 10% of cells died in 3 hr. The corresponding control shows a mortality of 5% in 3 hr.

The use of calcium channel antagonist together with anti-ADP/ATP carrier antibodies (IgG 1:100) in myocyte suspension (1 mM Ca^{2+}) reduced dramatically the cytotoxic effect of antibodies. Nifedipine and nitrendipine (both 10^{-6} M) seemed to be more potent in protecting the cells than did verapamil (10^{-6} M). Without antibodies none of the calcium channel antagonists had a significant influence on cell viability. The use of the β-receptor antagonist propranolol (10^{-7} M) together with anti-ADP/ATP carrier antibodies had no protective effect on the cells.

The results thus far suggest that the antibody binds specifically to the cell surface of cardiac myocytes and enhances their calcium permeability, leading to cell damage. To gain further evidence for a direct interaction of the anti-ADP/ATP carrier antibodies with the calcium channel, we isolated the calcium channel protein complex according to the method of Campbell.[32] After SDS gel electrophoresis and transfer of the proteins

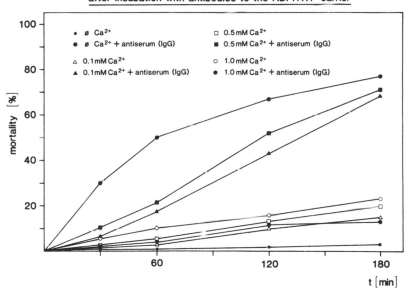

Fig. 8. Calcium concentration-dependent mortality of cardiac myocytes incubated with antibodies against the ADP/ATP carrier: Ca^{2+} concentration 1.0 mM + antiserum (solid circles); open circles, control. Ca^{2+} concentration 0.5 mM + antiserum (solid squares); open squares, control. Ca^{2+} concentration 0.1 mM + antiserum (solid triangles); open triangles, control. Ca^{2+} concentration 0 + antiserum (circled asterisks); asterisks, control. Antibody (IgG) dilution: 1:100.

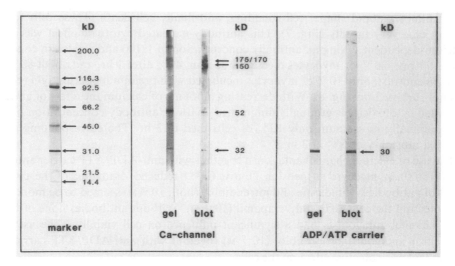

Fig. 9. SDS gel electrophoresis of the calcium channel and the ADP/ATP carrier and subsequent immunblot analysis with affinity-purified antibodies against the ADP/ATP carrier.

to nitrocellulose paper, immunoblot analysis showed that the affinity-purified antibodies against the ADP/ATP carrier protein bind to the calcium channel subunits (Fig. 9). These data clearly indicate a crossreactivity between the ADP/ATP carrier of the inner mitochondrial membrane and the calcium channel located within the cell surface membrane. Therefore, in another series of experiments we examined the possible effects of the antibody on the calcium current in isolated myocytes. Myocytes were patch-clamped in control tyrodes (1–5 mM Ca^{2+}), and the magnitude of I_{Ca} and its kinetics

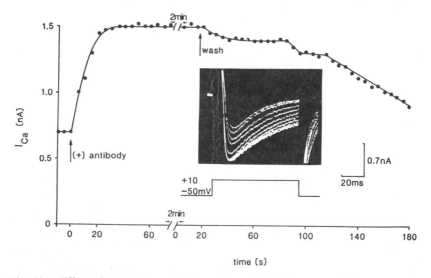

Fig. 10. Effect of antibody on calcium current (I_{Ca}) of rat ventricular myocytes: time course of effect of antibodies and its reversal on removel of antibodies. Inset, original superimposed traces of I_{Ca}, activated at +10 mV from holding potential (HP) of −50 mV, on addition of antibodies (IgG).

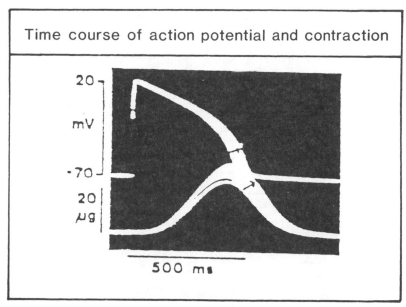

Fig. 11. Effect of the antibodies to the ADP/ATP carrier on action potential contraction, I_{Ca} of frog heart, and time course of action potential and contraction in frog ventricular strip subjected to 1:100 concentration of antibody (IgG). Action potential was prolonged, and contraction was potentiated.

were examined. Cells were dialyzed with high concentrations of Cs^+ and TEA^+ in order to block the K^+ current. Intracellular calcium concentration was buffered at $\approx 10^{-8}$ M, using 11 mM EGTA and 1 mM Ca^{2+}. I_{Na} was inactivated and blocked using a combination of TTX (10^{-5} M) and holding potentials of -40 to -50 mV. I_{Ca} was then activated by step depolarization to different potentials from -50 mV.[33] The addition of antibodies markedly enhanced I_{Ca} and slowed its inactivation. The effect of the antisera (isolated affinity purified IgG) on the inactivation time course was often more marked in rat than in frog myocytes. Figure 10 shows the time course of potentiation of I_{Ca} (induced by pulsing from -50 to $+10$ mV) in a rat ventricular myocyte, which was dialyzed with a solution containing high concentrations of CsCl and TEA-Cl to block outward currents. The onset of enhancement of I_{Ca} was rapid, and generally 20–30 s were sufficient for the full effect of antibodies to take place. The enhancement of I_{Ca} was only slowly reversible. In frog ventricular strips, addition of antibodies prolonged the action potential twitch tension (Fig. 11). The tension-potentiating effect of antibodies was complete within 2 min of the solution exchange and was reversible, although reversal required a much longer time. The enhancing effect of antibody on I_{Ca} could be blocked by addition of nifedipine (10^{-6} M-10^{-5} M). β-blockers (propranolol or atenolol, 10^{-6} M) did not alter the enhancement of I_{Ca} by the antibody. Figure 12 illustrates the effect of antibodies on an isolated ventricular cell in which I_{Ca} and contraction velocity were measured simultaneously. Contraction was monitored by measuring cell shortening using a 256-photodiode array. This cell was dialyzed against only 100 μM EGTA in order to allow it to contract (generally about 1.0 mM EGTA was necessary to completely suppress contraction). Note that both I_{Ca} and contraction are strongly enhanced in the presence of antibody. The enhancement of calcium current is reflected in a marked potentiation of tension. Since this effect is not mediated through the β-adrenergic recep-

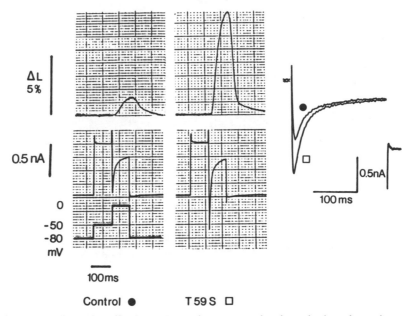

Fig. 12.   Effect of antibody on I_{Ca} and concentration in a single guinea pig ventricular myocyte. Simultaneous recording of I_{Ca} (lower panels) and cell shortening (upper panels) in control and antibody (T 59)-containing solutions. In this example immunized serum rabbit was used. Contraction and I_{Ca} were markedly enhanced. The calcium current in the presence and absence of antibody is shown superimposed in traces on the far right. The experimental double-pulse procedure is shown below.

tor and the effect was blocked by nifedipine, we conclude that the antibody against the ADP/ATP carrier may crossreact with the calcium channel, possibly the DHP receptor. This finding is consistent with the observation that exposure of isolated rat myocytes for 2–3 hrs to high concentrations of antibody leads to cell deterioration and death, which can be prevented with pretreatment of organic calcium antagonists.

Since the antibodies against the ADP/ATP carrier are also found in patients with myocarditis and dilated cardiomyopathies,[16-18] we examined possible effects of sera from such patients on the calcium current in isolated mammalian myocytes. Exposure of whole cell-clamped guinea pig and rat cardiac myocytes to sera of such patients (1 : 100 dilution) cause a marked potentiation of I_{Ca} in 2 of 5 cases. The onset of the antibody effect was about 10 times faster than its washout. Calcium current was potentiated by about 40%, and its inactivation was markedly slowed. We also tested the effect of normal human and rabbit sera and found little, or often an inhibitory, effect on calcium current of the isolated rat ventricular myocytes. Thus, we concluded that antibodies in human sera may crossreact with the sarcolemmal calcium channel, causing an enhancement of the current which may eventually lead to calcium overload and cell toxicity.[34]

DISCUSSION

The experiments described here provide evidence for a crossreactivity of antibodies against the ADP/ATP carrier of the inner mitochondrial membrane with 2 cell surface

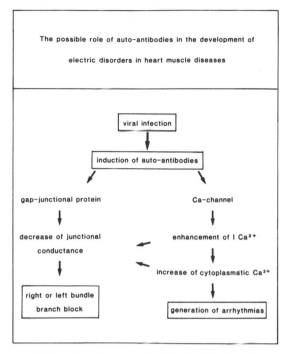

Fig. 13. The possible role of autoantibodies in the development of electric disorders in heart muscle diseases.

proteins—the calcium channel and the connexon. Cell surface proteins of cardiac myocytes were obtained from several experiments.

Let us extrapolate these findings to the human situation. Although sudden death is a major clinical problem in patients with dilated cardiomyopathy, data on the causes are limited.[12] It has been suspected that many cases of unexplained dilated cardiomyopathy result from myocarditis.[1,2,5,36] On the other hand, patients with myocarditis often have significant arrhythmias, conduction disturbances, and sudden death.[3,14] The association of ventricular arrhythmias with acute viral myocarditis is well documented, although cases of myocarditis are often subclinical. Whether the inflammatory cells are primarily responsible for the observed arrhythmias is not yet known. Conduction abnormalities may be an electrocardiographic marker of increasing interstitial myocardial fibrosis or due to increasing left ventricular hypertrophy.[37]

Based on the data presented in this paper it seems possible that autoantibodies reacting with cell surface proteins—the calcium channel and the connexon—may play a role in the development of electric disorders in heart muscle diseases (Fig. 13). Thus, the antibody binding to cell surface gap junctions might be responsible for clinical observations such as branch block, arrhythmias, or excitation spreading disorder. Although made up of discrete cells, electrophysiologically the heart muscle is a functional syncytium, synchronized by ion-permeable junctions that are important for providing efficient current spread or promoting rapid impulse conductance.[38] Gap junctional conductance is regulated by the number of channels between coupled cells (the balance between the formation and loss of these channels) and by the channel fraction that is open. Disorder in gating of these channels, which might lead to partial or complete decoupling is influenced by changes in intracellular calcium or pH[27,38] as well as by antibodies raised to the gap junctional protein.[39,40]

Cytotoxicity was delayed or completely suppressed when organic calcium channel blockers (verapamil, nitrendipine, and nifedipine) were used in addition to the antibody. Abnormalities in calcium metabolism of the myocardium are thought to be involved in the pathogenesis of cardiomyopathies.[44,45] So far the mechanism underlying disturbed calcium metabolism is not clear. Limas[44] suspected a lower calcium uptake rate by the sarcoplasmic reticulum; Gwathmey,[45] an increased calcium entry through a voltage-dependent sarcolemmal channels and a diminished capacity to restore resting calcium levels during diastole. As we can show that antibodies against the ADP/ATP carrier, also found in myocarditis and dilated cardiomyopathy, crossreact with the calcium channel, these antibodies could be responsible for the disturbance of calcium homeostasis by enhancing calcium current. This may lead to an antibody-mediated calcium overload with the consequences discussed above (see Fig. 13). Thus, the data presented here could be of clinical relevance in the understanding of the pathogenesis of postinfectious cardiomyopathies.

REFERENCES

1. Gravanis, M.B. and Ansari, A.A. Idiopathic cardiomyopathies. *Arch. Pathol. Lab. Med.* **111**: 915–929, 1987.

2. Kereiakes, D.J. and Parmley, W.W. Myocarditis and cardiomyopathy. *Am. Heart J.* **108**: 1318–1326, 1984.

3. Kawai, C., Matsumori, A., and Fujiwara, H. Myocarditis and dilated cardiomyopathy. *Ann. Rev. Med.* **38**: 221–239, 1987.

4. Dec, G.W., Palacios, I.F., Fallon, J.T., Aretz, T., Mills, J., Lee, D.C.S., and Johnson, R.A. Active myocarditis in the spectrum of acute dilated cardiomyopathy. *N. Engl. J. Med.* **312**: 885–890, 1985.

5. Fallon, J.T. Myocarditis and dilated cardiomyopathy: Different stages of the same disease? In: Contemporary Issues in Cardiovascular Clinics, Waller, B. (ed.), **18**: 1987, pp. 155–162.

6. Bowles, N.E., Richardson, P.J., Olsen, E.G.J., and Archard, L.C. Detection of Coxsackie B virus specific RNA sequences in myocardial biopsy samples from patients with myocarditis and dilated cardiomyopathy. *Lancet* **1**: 1120–1122, 1986.

7. Archard, L.C., Freeke, C.A., Richardson, P.J., *et al.* Persistence of enterovirus RNA in dilated cardiomyopathy: A progression from myocarditis. In: New Concepts in Viral Heart Disease. Schultheiss, H.P. (ed.), Springer-Verlag, Berlin, Heidelberg, New York, London, Tokyo, 1988, pp. 349–362.

8. Kandolf, R., Ameis, D., Kirschner, P., Canu, A., and Hofschneider, P.H. *In situ* detection of enteroviral genomes in myocardial cells by nucleic acid hybridization: An approach to the diagnosis of viral heart disease. *Proc. Natl. Acad. Sci.* USA **84**: 6272–6276, 1987.

9. Kandolf, R., Kirschner, P., Ameis, D., Canu, A., Erdmann, E., Schultheiss, H.P., Kemkes, B., and Hofschneider, P.H. Enteroviral heart disease: Diagnosis by *in situ* hybridization. In: New Concepts in Viral Heart Disease. Schultheiss, H.P. (ed.), Springer-Verlag, Berlin, Heidelberg, New York, London, Paris, Tokyo, 1988, pp. 337–348.

10. Southern, P. and Oldstone, M.B.A. Medical consequences of persistent viral infection. *N. Engl. J. Med.* **314**: 359–366, 1986.

11. Shoenfeld, Y. and Schwartz, R.S. Immunologic and genetic factors in autoimmune diseases. *N. Engl. J. Med.* **311**: 1019–1029, 1984.

12. Brandenburg, R.O. Cardiomyopathies and their role in sudden death. *J. Am. Coll. Cardiol.* **5**: 185B-189B, 1985.

13. Strain, J.E., Grose, R.M., Factor, S.M., and Fisher, J.D. Results of endomyocardial biopsy

in patients with spontaneous ventricular tachycardia but without apparent structural heart disease. *Circulation* **68**: 1171–1181, 1983.

14. Sekiguchi, M., Hiroe, M., Hiramitsu, S., and Izumi, T. Natural history of acute viral or idiopathic myocarditis: A clinical and endomyocardial biopsy follow-up. In: New Concepts in Viral Heart Disease. Schultheiss, H.P. (ed.), Springer-Verlag, Berlin, Heidelberg, New York, London, Paris, Tokyo, 1988, pp. 33–50.

15. Maisch, B., Deeg, P., Liebau, G., and Kochsiek, K. Diagnostic relevance of humoral and cytotoxic immune reactions in primary and secondary dilated cardiomyopathy. *Am. J. Cardiol.* **52**: 1072–1078, 1983.

16. Schultheiss, H.P. The mitochondrium as antigen in inflammatory heart disease. *Eur. Heart J.* 8, Suppl. J: 203, 1987.

17. Schultheiss, H.P. and Bolte, H.D. The immunochemical analysis of autoantibodies against the adenine nucleotide translocator in dilated cardiomyopathy. *J. Mol. Cell. Cardiol.* **17**: 603–617, 1985.

18. Schultheiss, H.P. The significance of autoantibodies against the ADP/ATP carrier for the pathogenesis of myocarditis and dilated cardiomyopathy—clinical and experimental data. *Springer Semin. Immunopathol.* **11**: 15–30, 1989.

19. Schultheiss, H.P. and Klingenberg, M. Immunochemical characterization of the adenine nucleotide translocator: Organ- and conformation specificity. *Eur. J. Biochem.* **143**: 599–605, 1984.

20. Klingenberg, M. The ADP/ATP carrier in mitochondrial membranes. In: The Enzymes of Biological Membranes. Martonosi, A.N. (ed.), Plenum Publishing, 1985, vol. 4, pp. 511–553.

21. Vignais, P.V. and Lauguin, G.J.M. Mitochondrial adenine nucleotide transport and its role in the economy of the cell. *TIBS* **4**: 90–92, 1979.

22. Klingenberg, M. and Heldt, H.W. The ADP/ATP translocation in mitochondria and its role in intracellular compartmentation. In: Metabolic Compartmentation. Sies, H. (ed.), Academic Press, London, 1982, pp. 101–122.

23. Schulze, K., Becker, B., and Schultheiss, H.P. Autoimmunity to an intracellular protein: Antibodies to the ADP/ATP carrier penetrate into myocardial cells and disturb energy metabolism *in vivo*. *Circ. Res.* **64**: 179–192, 1989.

24. Merle, P. and Kadenbach, B. Kinetic and structural differences between cytochrome C oxidase from liver and heart. *Eur. J. Biochem.* **125**: 239–244, 1982.

25. Rasmussen, U.B. and Wohlrab, H. Conserved structural domains among species and tissues-specific differences in the mitochondrial phosphate-transport protein and the ADP/ATP carrier. *Biochim. Biophys. Acta* **852**: 306–314, 1986.

26. Neckelmann, N., Li, K., Wade, R.P., Shuster, R., and Wallace, D.C. cDNA sequence of a human skeletal muscle ADP/ATP translocator: Lack of a leader peptide, divergence from a fibroblast translocator cDNA and coevolution with mitochondrial DNA genes. *Proc. Natl. Acad. Sci. USA* **84**: 7580–7584, 1987.

27. Manjunath, C.K. and Page, E. Cell biology and protein composition of cardiac gap junctions. *Am. J. Physiol.* **248** (Heart Circ. Physiol. 17): H783–H791, 1985.

28. Manjunath, C.K., Goings, G.E., and Page, E. Human cardiac gap junctions: Isolation, ultrastructure, and protein composition. *J. Mol. Cell. Cardiol.* **19**: 131–134, 1987.

29. Unwin, P.N.T. and Ennis, P.D. Two configurations of a channel-forming membrane protein. *Nature* **307**: 609–613, 1984.

30. Hertzberg, E.L., Lawrence, T.S., and Gilula, N.B. Gap junctional communication. *Ann. Rev. Physiol.* **43**: 479–491, 1981.

31. Cates, G.A. and Holland, P.C. Biosynthesis of plasma membrane proteins during myogenesis of skeletal muscle *in vitro*. *Biochem. J.* **174**: 873–881, 1978.

32. Leung, A.T., Imagawa, T., Block, B., Franzini-Armstrong, C., and Campbell, K.P. Biochemical and ultrastructural characterization of the 1,4-dihydropyridine receptor from rabbit skeletal muscle. *J. Biol. Chem.* **263**: 994–1001, 1988.

33. Morad, M., Davies, N., Ulrich, G., and Schultheiss, H.P. Antibodies against ADP/ATP carrier enhance the calcium current in isolated cardiac myocytes. *Am. J. Physiol.* **24**: H960–H964, 1988.

34. Schultheiss, H.P., Ulrich, G., Janda, I., Kühl, U., and Morad, M. Antibody-mediated enhancement of calcium permeability in cardiac myocytes. *J. Exp. Med.* **168**: 2105–2119, 1988.

35. Unwin, N. Is there a common design for cell membrane channels? *Nature* **323**: 12–13, 1986.

36. Zee-Cheng, C.S., Tsai, C.C., Palmer, D.C., Codd, J.E., and Pennington, D.G. High incidence of myocarditis by endomyocardial biopsy in patients with idiopathic congestive cardiomyopathy. *J. Am. Coll. Cardiol.* **3**: 63–70, 1984.

37. Wilensky, R.L., Yudelman, P., Cohen, A.I., Fletcher, R.D., Atkinson, J., Virmani, R., and Roberts, W.C. Serial electrocardiographic changes in idiopathic dilated cardiomyopathy confirmed at necropsy. *Am. J. Cardiol.* **62**: 276–283, 1988.

38. Spray, D.C., White, R.L., Mazet, F., and Bennett, M.V.L. Regulation of gap junctional conductance. *Am. J. Physiol.* **248** (Heart Circ. Physiol. 17): H753–H764, 1985.

39. Hertzberg, E.L., Spray, D.C., and Bennett, M.V.L. Reduction of gap junctional conductance by microinjection of antibodies against the 27-kDA liver gap junction polypeptide. *Proc. Natl. Acad. Sci.* USA **82**: 2412–2416, 1985.

40. Warner, A.E., Guthrie, S.C., and Gilula, N.B. Antibodies to the gap junctional protein selectively disrupt junctional communication in the early amphibian embryo. *Nature* **311**: 127–131, 1984.

41. Vaughan-Jones, R.D. Excitation and contraction in heart: The role of calcium. *Br. Med. Bull.* **42**: 413–420, 1986.

42. Kass, R.S., Lederer, W.J., Tsien, R.W., and Weingart, R. Role of calcium ions in transient inward currents and after contractions induced by strophanthidin in cardiac Purkinje fibres. *J. Physiol.* **281**: 187–208, 1978.

43. Cranefield, P.F. Action potentials, after potentials and arrhythmias. *Circ. Res.* **41**: 415–423, 1977.

44. Limas, C.J., Olivari, M.T., Goldenberg, I.F., Levine, T.B., Benditt, D.G., and Simon, A. Calcium uptake by cardiac sarcoplasmatic reticulum in human dilated cardiomyopathy. *Cardiovasc. Res.* **21**: 601–605, 1987.

45. Gwathmey, J.K., Copelas, L., MacKinnon, R., Schoen, F.J., Feldman, M.D., Grossman, W., and Morgan, J.P. Abnormal intracellular calcium handling in myocardium from patients with end-stage heart failure. *Circ. Res.* **61**: 70–76, 1987.

46. Schulze, K., Becker, B.F., Schaner, R., and Schultheiss, H.P. Antibodies to ADP-ATP carrier an autoantigen in myocarditis and dilated cardiomyopaty-impair cardiac function. *Circulation* **81**: 959–969, 1990.

47. Schulze, K., Kuhl, U., Chaner, R., Schulze, K., Kemkes, B., and Becher, B.F. Antibodies against the ADP-ATP carrier alter myocardial function by disturbing cellular energy metabolism. In: New Concepts in Viral Heart Disease. Schultheiss, H.P. (ed.), Springer Verlag, 1988, pp. 243–258.

Left Ventricular Involvement in Right Ventricular Cardiomyopathy

Fulvio Camerini, Bruno Pinamonti, Gianfranco Sinagra, Andrea Di Lenarda, Alessandro Salvi, Tullio Morgera, Furio Silvestri, and Rossana Bussani

Department of Cardiology and Morbid Anatomy, Ospedale Maggiore and University, Trieste, Italy

INTRODUCTION

A disease (or a group of diseases) of unknown etiology characterized by right ventricular involvement, usually with preservation of the left ventricle, has been described in the last decades by many authors. The first detailed observation was probably that of Uhl,[1] who published in 1952 a report on an 8-month-old infant with "almost total absence of the myocardium of the right ventricle," normal valves, normal coronary arteries, and severe heart failure. In the following decade sporadic observations were reported, but the first systematic approach to the disease was that by the group of Fontaine.[2-4] In 1982 Marcus et al.[4] reported on a group of 24 patients with localized and in some instances also with diffuse right ventricular involvement and, in the great majority of cases, recurrent ventricular tachycardia with a peculiar left bundle branch block configuration.

From a pathoanatomic point of view, the right ventricular abnormalities were characterized by a marked decrease in cardiac myocytes, usually replaced by fatty tissue with varying amounts of fibrosis. Marcus et al. called this entity "arrhythmogenic right ventricular dysplasia."[4] However, analyzing the cases previously reported in the literature, they noted that ventricular tachycardia may not be the most important clinical manifestation; in fact the majority of patients (21 of 34) reported in the literature had "presenting signs or symptoms other than ventricular tachycardia, including cardiomegaly or right ventricular failure of unknown etiology." This discrepancy might be explained by the interest of those authors in cardiac electrophysiology and surgical treatment of ventricular tachycardia.

Another contribution to the knowledge of this disease was that of Fitchett et al.,[5] who reported on 14 patients with "right ventricular dilated cardiomyopathy." In those patients the right ventricle was severely involved, with left ventricular function usually preserved. However, the authors' opinion was that the right ventricular involvement was a manifestation of a more diffuse myocardial disease, which could involve also the left ventricle.

In the past 3 years a series of important contributions has come from a group[6-12] working in Padua, Italy, who described the polymorphous clinical and echocardiographic aspects of the disease, the characteristics of hereditary transmission (autosomic dominant with variable penetrance), and the frequency of sudden death. The disease is considered rare,[13] although Nava et al.[11] in a systematic study observed a total of 126 patients.

The disease has been called by many names, the majority of them stressing the characteristic of being the cause of frequent and sometimes severe arrhythmias: right ventricular dysplasia, arrhythmogenic right ventricular dysplasia, right ventricular dilated cardiomyopathy, arrhythmogenic right ventricle, arrhythmogenic right ventricular cardiomyopathy, primary arrhythmogenic disease of the right ventricle, right ventricular lipomatosis, isolated dilatation of the right ventricle, Uhl's anomaly, parchment heart, etc.[11,13] However, the most comprehensive is probably "right ventricular cardiomyopathy," which indicates a myocardial disease of unknown origin involving mainly the right ventricle.[13]

The clinical expression of right ventricular cardiomyopathy is likely to vary according to patient age and the extent and severity of pathologic changes. According to Bharati *et al*.[14] the pathologic changes depend on the patient age. In infancy or early childhood the myocardium of the right ventricle is usually absent; the walls are very thin, parchment-like, and usually free of fat or inflammatory reaction. In infants or children the dominant symptomatology is congestive heart failure, usually with rapid deterioration. When seen later in life, the disease may be more localized and may frequently not involve the right ventricle massively. Pump function may be good or slightly impaired and longer survival is possible.

Symptomatology may be characterized by a high incidence of ventricular arrhythmias and sudden death is relatively frequent. However, in a subset of adult patients (Refs. 4, 5, and personal observations) the right ventricle may be very large, and Bharati *et al*.[14] suggested that the absent myocardium, replaced by fat and/or fibrous tissue, is the cause of progressive distension of the right ventricle. Also other authors[12] considered right ventricular cardiomyopathy a form of "progressive right ventricular atrophy, bringing about fibro-fatty infiltration and replacement of the right ventricular free wall."

However, at the present time it is not certain whether Uhl's anomaly, arrhythmogenic right ventricular dysplasia, and right ventricular (dilated) cardiomyopathy are different expressions of the same disease. Nevertheless, pathologic, clinical, and laboratory observations suggest that it is probable that there is a continuum in the degree and timing of right ventricular involvement.[15] Right ventricular cardiomyopathy is not always strictly localized in one ventricle, but sometimes also involves the left ventricle.[16–18]

The aims of the present study were: 1) to summarize present knowledge about right ventricular cardiomyopathy; and 2) to analyze the frequency, extent, and characteristics of left ventricular involvement in right ventricular cardiomyopathy.

RIGHT VENTRICULAR CARDIOMYOPATHY: CLINICAL OUTLINE

The age of onset of symptoms usually ranges from 20 to 40 years, according to the largest published series.[4,5,11,19] Sometimes, however, isolated right ventricular involvement may be discovered in infants presenting with severe right-sided heart failure,[1,20–22] or in children with ventricular arrhythmias.[23,24] Cases of right ventricular cardiomyopathy may be recognized also in very old persons, as in the 84-year-old man described by Sugiura *et al*.[25]

The disease seems more frequent in males.[4,19] The presenting symptoms in adult patients are generally related to arrhythmias, and are characterized by palpitations and syncope; less frequent are attacks of dyspnea and chest pain.[5,19] Some patients are asymptomatic but they may die suddenly and the pathologic changes are discovered at postmortem examination.[10,26,27] Symptoms due to right heart failure may occur.[5] They are very frequent in infants,[1,20–22] but they may also appear later in the course of the disease.[4,19,28] In some instances the diagnosis is occasionally made in asymptomatic patients who show abnormalities during routine clinical examination,[4] or by studying families of affected patients.[11] Familial occurrence is frequently reported.[8,12,27,29–34]

Physical examination may be completely normal in presence of an enlarged heart.[4] Cyanosis may be present, especially in children, usually due to a right-to-left shunt across a patent foramen ovale,[22,35,36] or an atrial septal defect,[37–40] but sometimes without an obvious intracardiac shunt.[1,21,41,42]

Asymmetry of the precordium, with prominence of the left anterior hemithorax, has been reported in rare instances.[4] A splitting of the first heart sound, third and fourth heart sounds, and systolic murmurs over the lower left sternal border may be heard upon auscultation.[4,19] A widely split second heart sound, sometimes not varying with respiration, is sometimes reported, and it is believed to depend on the slow contraction of the right ventricle.[4,19,43] In some patients abnormally prominent "a" waves are seen upon jugular inspection, while in other cases predominant "v" waves suggest tricuspid regurgitation.[4] Right ventricular failure, with high venous pressure, hepatomegaly, and peripheral edema may be present, characteristically in the absence of signs of left ventricular failure or of pulmonary hypertension.[5,19]

In chest X-ray the configuration of the heart is usually globular, sometimes showing a convexity of the left lateral border due to an enlarged right ventricular outflow tract.[4,19] The largest hearts are seen in patients with right heart failure.[19] In all cases, pulmonary congestion is characteristically absent.

Electrocardiographic recording during sinus rhythm may be helpful in the diagnosis. The most characteristic findings include right precordial (V1-V4) T wave inversion, incomplete or complete right bundle branch block, and ventricular postexcitation waves (epsilon potentials).[4,19] Ventricular postexcitation waves were suspected at admission in 6 of the 15 patients studied by Blomstrom-Lundqvist et al.[19] and in 7 of the 24 patients of Marcus et al.[4] In the last series the epsilon potentials were evident in almost all patients when high-amplitude and signal-averaging techniques were employed.[4] Epsilon potentials are rapid single or multiple small deflections, which may be seen in right precordial leads at the end of the QRS complex or in the first part of the ST segment (Fig. 1). They correspond to a late activation of small zones of the right ven-

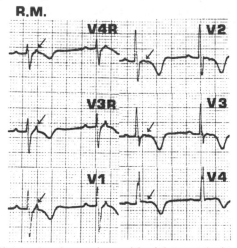

Fig. 1. Precordial leads of a patient with right ventricular cardiomyopathy, showing: a) negative T waves from V4R to V4; and b) postpotentials (arrows) in the first part of the ST segment.

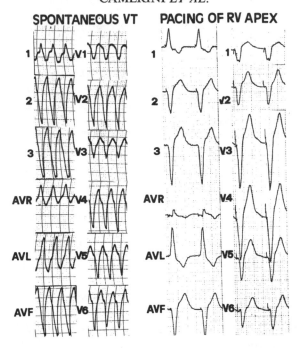

Fig. 2. Left: Electrocardiogram during sustained ventricular tachycardia in a patient with right ventricular cardiomyopathy. The ventricular complexes show a left bundle branch block morphology: QS in V1, V2; R in aVL. The mean QRS axis in the frontal plane is markedly deviated upward and to the left (about −90°). Right (pacing of the RV apex): the ventricular complexes during pacing of right ventricular apex are very similar to the complexes of spontaneous ventricular tachycardia, suggesting that the arrhythmia originated from that site.

tricle. It is believed that if delayed activations occur beyond the refractory period of the surrounding myocardium, they may be able to reactivate the ventricles, generating reentrant arrhythmias.[4]

Right atrial enlargement, first-degree to complete AV block, and low-voltage QRS, the last in cases of severe right ventricular dilatation, have also been reported.[1,4,19] Ventricular arrhythmias, in the form of ventricular ectopic beats, and repetitive nonsustained or sporadic sustained ventricular tachycardia of left bundle branch block configuration are important findings of the disease.[4,19] Ectopic QRS axis in the frontal plane ranges from −75 to +105 degrees; QRS axes between −30 and +60 degrees, however, are uncommon (Fig. 2).[19]

The evolution of ventricular arrhythmias associated with right ventricular cardiomyopathy is unpredictable. Remission of sustained ventricular tachycardia for up to several years, with or without therapy, has been reported.[19] In rare instances, the ventricular ectopic beats are polymorphous, or show a right bundle branch block pattern (Refs. 11, 18, 19, 28, and personal data). This finding suggests the possibility of left ventricular involvement (Refs. 11, 18, 19, 28, and personal data). Supraventricular arrhythmias have also been reported.[4,5]

Sudden death occurs in a substantial percentage of patients,[4,5,19] but it is not necessarily observed in the most severe forms of right ventricular involvement.[19] Thiene *et al.*[10] recently reported that 12 of the 60 persons who died suddenly under the age of 35 had pathologic changes typical of right ventricular cardiomyopathy. In 5 of them, sudden death was the first sign of disease; the remaining 7 had a history of palpitations and/or syncopal episodes, and in 5 of those 7 ventricular arrhythmias had previously been recorded on electrocardiographic examination. In no patient was the diagnosis of right ventricular cardiomyopathy made before death.

A number of noninvasive and invasive techniques have been employed to characterize the right ventricular morphology and function in right ventricular cardiomyopathy. M-mode echocardiography frequently shows an increased right ventricular diameter,[4,5,16,17,28,40,43-47] sometimes associated with paradoxical septal motion, simulating right ventricular volume overload.[5,17,28,44-48] In some instances a premature opening of the pulmonic valve was reported.[40,44] This technique, however, is neither very sensitive nor specific for the diagnosis of the disease.

Cross-sectional echocardiography, in contrast, gives a good appreciation of the morphology, dimensions, and function of the right ventricle. In some reported cases the right ventricle appears globally dilated and diffusely hypokinetic,[43-45,47,49,50] while in other instances localized wall motion abnormalities are seen, characterized by hypokinetic areas or akinetic-dyskinetic bulges at various locations.[4,45,47,49-51] Nonstandard oblique sections may be required for their recognition.[51] Manyari *et al.*[45] reported in their study that 2-dimensional echocardiography had a sensitivity of 80% and a specificity of 100% in recognizing the presence of right ventricular cardiomyopathy, compared with angiography as a reference method. Ribeiro *et al.*,[47] using 2-dimensional echocardiography, reported that it was possible to distinguish between right ventricular dilated cardiomyopathy, characterized by diffuse hypokinesis of the right ventricle with normal thickness of its walls, and Uhl's anomaly, where localized right ventricular wall thinning and paradoxical motion are present. Nevertheless, the distinguishing features are very subtle and difficult to apply in clinical practice.

Radionuclide ventriculography has been employed in the evaluation of right ventricular cardiomyopathy by several authors to quantify right ventricular volumes, ejection fraction, and regional wall motion at rest and during exercise.[16,28,43,45,50,51] In the group of patients studied by Manyari *et al.*[45] radionuclide ventriculography had a sensitivity of 100% and a specificity of 90% in the diagnosis of right ventricular "dysplasia." Yet this technique appears less accurate than 2-dimensional echocardiography and angiography in the identification and localization of wall motion abnormalities.[52]

Right ventricular ventriculography is considered the reference technique for diagnosis.[4,5,45,49,52-54] In some cases it demonstrates a dilated right ventricle with diffuse hypokinesis.[4,5,28,40,43,49,50,52-56] In other patients one or more asynergic areas are seen, with or without global dilatation and depressed ejection fraction.[4,17,24,46,52,54,57] In some of these patients the abnormal zones were described as "bulgings," "outpouchings," or "aneurysms," with diastolic deformation of the cavity contour and systolic akinesia or dyskinesia.[4,24,51,52,54] The most frequent localizations of abnormalities are the apex, the anterior wall of the infundibulum, and the inferior wall ("triangle of dysplasia").[4] In the most advanced forms the right ventricle can assume a bizarre, honeycombed, or cauliflower-like appearance.[43,50] Other, less specific signs are deep fissuring of the walls and stagnation of contrast medium near an abnormal wall.[4,52-54] In some patients, especially those with the most dilated and dysfunctioning ventricles, various degrees of tricuspid regurgitation and right atrial enlargement have been demonstrated.[5,43,46,52,53,55,56]

Cardiac output and index may be normal or depressed,[4,5] while intracavitary pressures are usually normal.[4,24,46,51,58] In some patients with severe right ventricular involvement, prominent "a" waves may be seen in right atrial pressure tracings. These "a" waves are sometimes transmitted to the right ventricle and to the pulmonary artery, with near equalization of the diastolic pressure.[4,5,17,20,40,44,46,56,59,60]

The systolic pressures in the right ventricle and in the pulmonary artery, although normal, are sometimes characterized by a slowly rising, broad curve.[44] These hemodynamic findings have been interpreted as due to the severe dysfunction of the right ventricle. A substantial contribution to the forward flow depends on forceful right atrial contraction,[20,40,44,59] and perhaps also on paradoxical septal motion.[44,59]

MORBID ANATOMY

The majority of papers in which the anatomopathologic changes of right ventricular cardiomyopathy have been considered reported only one or a small number of cases,[1,5,8,17,20,22,25-27,29,31,32,40,44,52,55,56,60,64] whereas more observations were presented in the studies of Marcus *et al.*[4] (13 cases: 12 at surgery and one at necropsy) and Thiene *et al.*[10] (12 cases of sudden death in young adults).

Although the disease has been called by several names, the anatomic abnormalities described seem to have many features in common.[65] In the few patients who died in severe heart failure during the first months or years of life (defined by the authors as Uhl's anomaly, or congenital aplasia of the myocardium of the right ventricle),[1,20-22,35] the right ventricular free walls were characteristically paper-thin, with an almost absent myocardium, and apposition of the endocardium to epicardium.[1] The endocardium was described as dense and gray, the epicardium as thickened and fibrous, sometimes with fat deposits.[1] In postmortem studies of adults who died suddenly, or after a period of chronic congestive right heart failure, pathologic changes are less homogeneous.

An almost constant feature is a marked decrease or absence of contractile elements in the right ventricular walls. This pattern is sometimes widespread, and similar to that observed in infants.[29,39,40,44,55,56,59,60-62,65] In these hearts the right ventricular walls are sometimes described as paper-thin or parchment-like.[39,44,59,61,62] Histologically, a few myocardial cells, usually located in the trabeculae and in the subendocardium, are interspersed in fatty and/or fibrous tissue. Various degrees of endocardial thickening and fibrosis, and of degenerative changes in the few remaining myocells are frequently noted. The epicardial fat is described as abundant in some cases.[4,29,44,52,55,63] Inflammatory infiltrates may be present.[4,5,10] Other patients may show in the right ventricle only one or a few abnormal zones with a similar histology while the remaining parts of the ventricular walls are relatively well preserved. These areas may appear as aneurysms[4,10,17,63] and generally correspond to a similar pattern at angiography.[4,17,52]

Thiene *et al.*[10] distinguished 2 histologic patterns of the disease: the lipomatous and the fibrous/fibrolipomatous pattern. In 6 patients with the lipomatous pattern there was a massive replacement of the myocytes with adipose tissue, mainly at the apex and infundibulum, without significant fibrosis. The wall thickness was normal. In 6 other patients with the fibrous/fibrolipomatous pattern, large areas of myocardial sclerosis were observed, with or without lipomatosis, which were more frequently located at the posteroinferior wall, and were macroscopically characterized by aneurysmal dilatations, scars, and wall thinning. Histologically, in these cases the fibrosis predominated in the subepicardium, and mononuclear infiltration surrounding degenerated or necrotic myocells was sometimes observed. A different pathogenesis was hypothesized for the 2 groups.[10]

In the 3 anatomic observations of "right ventricular dilated cardiomyopathy" reported by Fitchett et al.[5] several foci of fibrous replacement in both ventricles were described. Fatty infiltration was not mentioned, nor were histologic or anatomic specimens presented.

A few papers have reported data from endomyocardial biopsy in right ventricular cardiomyopathy.[11,27,46,58,66] The most systematic study was that of Hasumi et al.[58] who analyzed the histologic findings of right ventricular endomyocardial biopsy in 9 patients with "right ventricular dysplasia" and ventricular arrhythmias, and compared them with 2 control groups, one of patients with dilated cardiomyopathy, and one of patients with right ventricular overload. The histologic specimens of "right ventricular dysplasia" were characterized by advanced interstitial fibrosis and fatty infiltration. Hypertrophy and degeneration of the myocytes, disarrangement of muscle bundles, and endocardial thickening were also observed. After semiquantitative grading, the extent of fibrous and fatty infiltration was clearly more prominent in the 9 with right ventricular dysplasia than in the 2 control groups. It was concluded, therefore, that these findings were characteristic of the disease. The possibility of false negative endomyocardial biopsy was also considered by Hasumi's group, and in one case without typical biopsy findings massive fatty infiltration of the right ventricle was present at subsequent necropsy.

LEFT VENTRICULAR INVOLVEMENT IN RIGHT VENTRICULAR CARDIO-MYOPATHY

Data from the literature: Right ventricular cardiomyopathy has generally been considered a disease with isolated right ventricular involvement,[4] but in many reports concomitant abnormalities of the left ventricle have been described.[5,10,11,14,16-20,28,29,31,32,40, 46,51,52,54,59,64] The first observation of left ventricular involvement was perhaps in a patient studied in 1905 by Osler, who described necropsy findings of "parchment-like" thinning of the walls of all 4 cardiac chambers.[61]

More recently, Manyari et al.,[16] studying a group of patients with stress radionuclide angiography, suggested that right ventricular dysplasia might represent a "generalized cardiomyopathy." In this series 4 of the 6 tested patients demonstrated a latent left ventricular dysfunction, while the remaining 2 showed a depressed left ventricular ejection fraction at rest as well.

The problem of the left ventricular involvement in right ventricular cardiomyopathy was only marginally studied in several other reports, with few exceptions.[5,18] Fitchett et al.,[5] in their study on "right ventricular dilated cardiomyopathy," outlined that their patients had a diffuse myocardial disease and that for reasons as yet undetermined the right ventricle failed first.

Characteristics of Left Ventricular Involvement

The most common finding is the presence of wall motion abnormalities, characterized by hypo-a-dyskinetic areas, sometimes with diastolic bulging. The inferoposterior wall and the apex are more frequently involved.[4,17,18,46,51,52,54,57,64] In some cases the left ventricular ejection fraction is mildly or moderately depressed.[16,18,19,28,56,58] Severe left ventricular dysfunction is only rarely demonstrated.[18,58] The cavity was severely dilated in 2 reported cases only,[51,57] while more frequently the enlargement was mild or absent.[5,11,16,46,54]

At cardiac catheterization, some authors observed an increase in left ventricular end-diastolic pressure.[5,15,20,40,59,64] In the patients studied by Manyari *et al.*[16] and Webb *et al.*[18] with radionuclide angiography, the ejection fraction of the left ventricle did not increase adequately during exercise, and in some cases new asynergic areas appeared.

Left ventricular hypokinesia may develop in the context of a progressive disorder, in which the right ventricle only is initially involved.[5,19,28,56] In a patient described by Fitchett *et al.*[5] the left ventricle, initially normal at angiography, appeared after 8 years moderately dilated and showed histologic abnormalities at necropsy. Also Higuchi *et al.*[28] described a patient in whom during follow-up there was progressive dilatation and functional deterioration of the right ventricle, followed by progressive left ventricular dysfunction.

Reported observations on the pathologic changes found in the left ventricle are scarce. Marked fibrosis and/or fatty infiltration, usually associated with similar findings in the right ventricle, may be present.[5,10,14,17,55,56] In the case described by Letac *et al.*[55] the outer half of the walls of the left ventricle was constituted of fat; fatty infiltration with thinning of the myocardium was also present at the level of the apex. The left ventricular aneurysms documented by Waller *et al.*[17] in 2 patients were similar in appearance to those of the right ventricle, and were characterized by a thinned wall with very few myocardial cells and fibrous and fatty infiltration. The fatty tissue occupied the outer layers of the wall. In the exceptional case described by Yutani *et al.*[56] a typical right ventricular cardiomyopathy (characterized at necropsy by severe fibrosis, fatty infiltration, and a paper-thin appearance) was associated with a hypertrophic left ventricle, consistent with a diagnosis of hypertrophic cardiomyopathy. The left ventricular ejection fraction was depressed and the cavity dilated, with marked fibrosis and myocellular disarray at necropsy. The case was interpreted by the authors[56] as "an unusual type of idiopathic cardiomyopathy."

PERSONAL DATA

Patients and Methods

In order to evaluate the prevalence and the characteristics of left ventricular involvement in right ventricular cardiomyopathy and its possible evolution, 31 patients with right ventricular cardiomyopathy were studied. Right ventricular cardiomyopathy was diagnosed when morphologic and functional right ventricular abnormalities and localized (hypo-a-dyskinetic bulges of right ventricular walls) and/or diffuse (global dilatation and depressed systolic function) were detected by 2-dimensional echocardiography in the absence of major left ventricular dysfunction (LVEF $\geq 45\%$) and without any detectable cause.

All patients were studied by M-mode and 2-dimensional echocardiography. Left ventricular dimensions and systolic function were evaluated by standard M-mode diameters and shortening fraction, and by 2-dimensional volume calculations, using an area-length, single-plane method from the apical 4-chamber view.[67]

Right ventricular dimensions and systolic function were evaluated by measuring from the apical 4-chamber view the right ventricular end-diastolic and end-systolic areas, and the fractional contraction of areas.[68]

The data were normalized for body surface area and were compared with a group of normal subjects.

In the qualitative analysis, the study was focused on the possible presence of "bulges" of ventricular walls, and regional wall motion abnormalities.

Twenty-four patients, usually with the most severe disease, were also studied by cardiac catheterization and angiography, and in 20 of them endomyocardial biopsy was performed.

At first examination the patients were arbitrarily divided into 2 groups: group 1 with right ventricular cardiomyopathy and normal left ventricle; and group 2 with right ventricular cardiomyopathy and left ventricular involvement (presence of localized left ventricular wall motion abnormalities and/or mild left ventricular dysfunction [LVEF: 46–52%]. Patients in the 2 groups were followed up clinically and with serial 2-dimensional echo examinations.

Clinical Presentation

Of the 31 patients, 16 were males and 15 females; their ages ranged from 5 months to 59 years at first diagnosis. Twenty-three patients presented with complex ventricular arrhythmias without overt heart disease (ventricular tachycardia in 18: sustained in 10, nonsustained in 8; frequent ectopic beats in 5 cases). The extrasystoles were monomorphous with left bundle branch block pattern (Fig. 2) in 15, and polymorphous in the other 8. Four patients presented with congestive heart failure, predominantly right; 4 were asymptomatic but had electrocardiographic (Fig. 1) and/or chest X-ray abnormalities.

Echocardiographic Data

At first examination, 19 patients showed right ventricular abnormalities (localized, with normal dimensions and global function in 7 (Fig. 3); associated with dilatation and depressed systolic function in 12 (Fig. 4)) in absence of any left ventricular abnormalities, and were classified in group 1. In the other 12 patients (group 2) the right

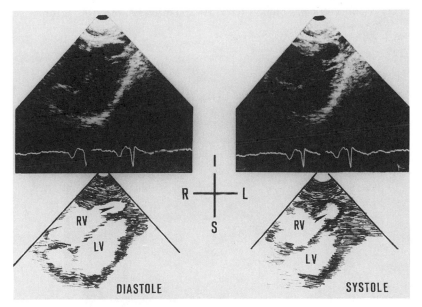

Fig. 3. Two-dimensional echocardiogram (modified subcostal 4-chamber view) in a patient with right ventricular cardiomyopathy and localized abnormalities. A dyskinetic bulge is present (arrow) at right ventricular apex. RV, right ventricle; LV, left ventricle.

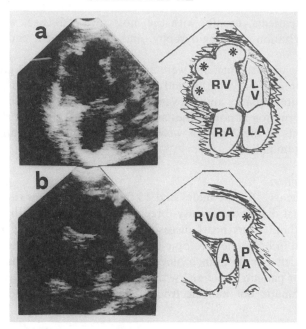

Fig. 4. Two-dimensional echocardiogram of a patient with right ventricular cardiomyopathy and diffuse abnormalities. a) Modified apical 4-chamber view; b) modified parasternal short-axis view at the level of pulmonary artery. Multiple akinetic bulges (*) are present at the level of right ventricular apex, lateral wall, and right ventricular outflow tract. The right ventricle is globally dilated and hypokinetic.

RV, right ventricle; LV, left ventricle; RA, right atrium; LA, left atrium; RVOT, right ventricular outflow tract; PA, pulmonary artery; A, aorta.

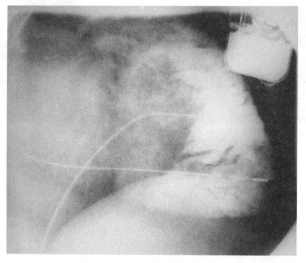

Fig. 5. Right ventricular angiography (right anterior oblique projection–end-systole) in a patient with right ventricular cardiomyopathy and diffuse abnormalities. The right ventricle is dilated and diffusely hypokinetic, with multiple akinetic areas. Tricuspid regurgitation is present.

ventricular abnormalities (localized in 4 patients, diffuse in 8) were associated with left ventricular involvement.

Left ventricular abnormalities were characterized by the presence of one or more asynergic areas (localized at the apex in 4, in the septum in 3, and in the inferoposterior wall in 5) or by mild diffuse hypokinesia (2 cases). The ejection fraction was mildly depressed in 5 patients. In no patient did the left ventricle appear severely dilated (maximal end-diastolic volume index 73 cc/m²).

Cardiac Catheterization

At catheterization, right ventricular abnormalities were confirmed in all patients (Fig. 5). Left ventricular function was normal in all group 1 patients studied. Left ventricular end-diastolic pressure was slightly increased in one of them (13 mmHg). On the contrary, the left ventricle was considered abnormal in 9 of 10 patients in group 2 studied by catheterization: 6 patients showed an increased left ventricular end-diastolic pressure (14–20 mmHg), 7 showed areas of left ventricular asynergy (Fig. 6), and 4 showed mild depression of ejection fraction. In no patient was the left ventricle severely dilated (maximal end-diastolic volume index: 138 cc/m). In addition, one patient in group 1 and 2 patients in group 2 showed one or 2 small diverticula at level of the inferior wall of the left ventricle.

Right ventricular endomyocardial biopsy was performed in 20 patients. It revealed fatty infiltration frequently associated with fibrosis (10 patients) (Fig. 7). In the others nonspecific abnormalities were present, or the biopsy was completely normal. Two patients also underwent left ventricular biopsy that in both cases demonstrated nonspecific abnormalities.

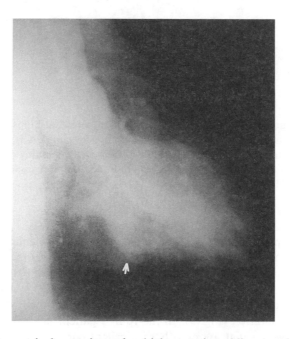

Fig. 6. Left ventricular angiography (right anterior oblique projection–end-systole) in a patient with right ventricular cardiomyopathy and left ventricular involvement. A dyskinetic bulge is present at the level of diaphragmatic wall (arrow).

A

B

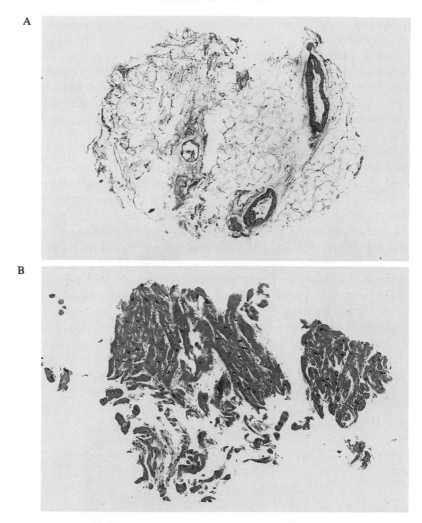

Fig. 7. A and B: Two right ventricular endomyocardial biopsy specimens in a patient with right ventricular cardiomyopathy. Specimen A is constituted exclusively of adipous tissue (H-H, ×20). Specimen B contains muscular tissue without any fatty infiltration, but with slight interstitial fibrosis and lymphocytic infiltration (H-H, ×20).

Follow-up

During follow-up (22 patients; 13–65 months) right ventricular function worsened in 4 patients in group 1 and in 2 in group 2 (Fig. 8). The left ventricle became abnormal in 4 patients in group 1 (in one associated with a worsening of right ventricular function). In 3 of them paradoxical septal motion with decreased systolic thickening and diffuse hypokinesis of the left ventricular free wall developed slowly during the follow-up, without chamber dilatation (Fig. 9). In the fourth patient, a small dyskinetic area appeared at the left ventricular apex, with an excellent contraction of the remaining segments of the ventricular walls.

Left ventricular function deteriorated in one patient in group 2, with depression of

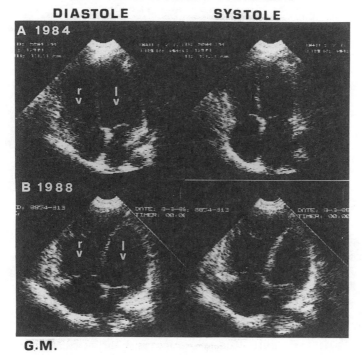

Fig. 8. Two-dimensional echocardiograms (apical 4-chamber views) in a patient in group 1. At first examination (upper panels, –A–), the right ventricle was only slightly dilated and showed apical hypokinesia. The left ventricle was normal. Four years later (lower panels, –B–) the right ventricle was massively enlarged, with multiple bulges, and severe diffuse hypokinesia. The left ventricle is also hypokinetic, but not dilated. RV, right ventricle; LV, left ventricle.

ejection fraction (48→40%), and a thrombus formation at the apex, but without cavity dilatation.

Four patients (3 in group 1 and 1 in group 2) died in congestive heart failure. One of them was a 5-month-old child, who died in shock a few days after the diagnosis. The other 3 patients showed a deterioration of left ventricular function, and died in chronic congestive heart failure, several years after the appearance of the first symptoms.

Postmortem Study

Postmortem data were available in one patient in group 1, and in 2 additional patients not included in the clinical series (a 58-year-old woman with a clinical picture of dilated cardiomyopathy and her 21-year-old son, who died suddenly). In all 3 the right ventricular free walls appeared parchment-like and showed massive fatty infiltration and fibrosis, with very few myocardial cells at histology (Fig. 10).

Massive fibrosis of the the right side of the interventricular septum and a fatty infiltration and fibrosis of the left ventricular apex were observed in one and 2 patients, respectively. The left ventricular free walls in all 3 of these patients revealed degenerative changes of the myocytes with moderate fibrosis (Fig. 11). This pattern may not be distinguishable from that commonly observed in dilated cardiomyopathy.

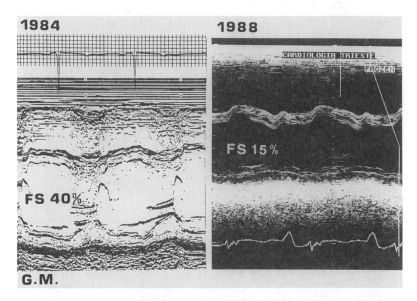

Fig. 9. M-mode echocardiographic tracings at ventricular level in the same patient as in Fig. 7. The first tracing (1984) was normal, whereas 4 years later (1988) the right ventricular diameter was increased, the interventricular septum showed a paradoxical motion, and left ventricular fractional shortening (FS) was decreased (from 40% to 15%).

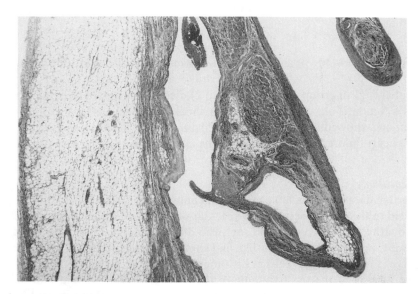

Fig. 10. Postmortem section of the right ventricular free wall (at the level of the outflow) in the same patient as in Fig. 7. The ventricular wall is almost completely constituted of fatty tissue. Subendocardial fibrosis and irregular endocardial thickening are present. Small residual muscular bundles are present only within a trabecula, surrounded by fatty and fibrous infiltration (H-H, ×4.5).

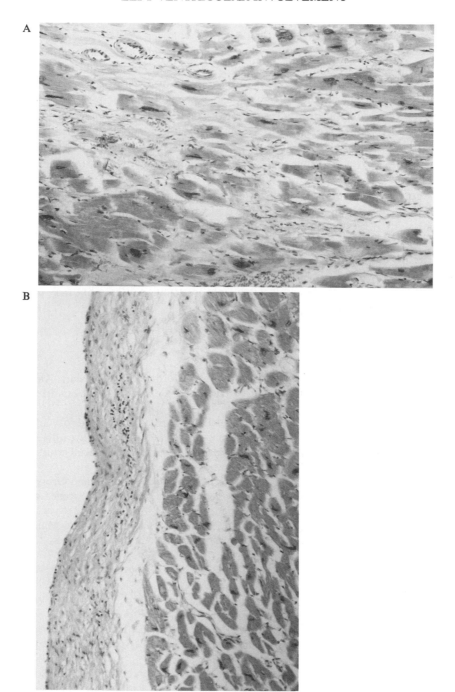

Fig. 11. A and B: Postmortem sections of the left ventricular free wall in another patient with right ventricular cardiomyopathy. In A, hypertrophy and attenuation of the myocelles, associated with marked diffuse interstitial fibrosis, are present (H-H, ×40). In B, evident endocardial fibrosis is seen (H-H, ×40). The clinical and hemodynamic pattern of this patient was compatible with dilated cardiomyopathy. The right ventricular free wall was massively infiltrated by fat, with very few myocardial cells, similarly to the pattern in Fig. 10.

CONCLUSIONS

A disease of unknown etiology involving mainly the right ventricle (right ventricular cardiomyopathy) has been described in the past by many authors. In this article, a comprehensive literature review and result of analysis of 31 cases of this disease at the author's department are presented. The disease is probably characterized by a spectrum of abnormalities, ranging from a severe form presenting in infancy with severe intractable heart failure, to a form seen later in life which is more localized and frequently characterized by ventricular arrhythmias of left bundle branch block configuration. However, in some of these patients cardiomegaly and right heart failure may be present.

Right ventricular cardiomyopathy is often accompanied by abnormalities of the left ventricle also, with the presence of localized wall motion (hypo-a-dyskinetic areas), sometimes with diastolic bulgings, and/or diffuse hypokinesis with a depression, usually moderate, of left ventricular ejection fraction. Sometimes it is also possible to observe the development of left ventricular abnormalities in the context of a progressive disorder, in which the right ventricle is initially involved. Right ventricular cardiomyopathy is thus not always an isolated right ventricular disease but may be a more generalized cardiomyopathy.

REFERENCES

1. Uhl, H.S.M. A previously undescribed congenital malformation of the heart: Almost total absence of the myocardium of the right ventricle. *Bull. Johns Hopkins Hosp.* **91**: 197–205, 1952.
2. Fontaine, G., Guiraudon, G., Frank, R., Vedel, J., Grosgogeat, Y., Cabrol, C., and Falquet, J. Stimulation studies and epicardial mapping in ventricular tachycardia: Study of mechanisms and selection for surgery. In: Reentrant Arrhythmias. Kulbertus, H. (ed.), Lancaster, MTP Publishing, 1977, p. 334.
3. Frank, R., Fontaine, G., Vedel, J., Mialet, G., Sol, C., Guiraudon, G., and Grosgogeat, Y. Electrocardiologie de quatre cas de dysplasie ventriculaire droite arythmogene. *Arch. Mal. Coeur* **71**: 963–972, 1978.
4. Marcus, F.I., Fontaine, G.H., Guiraudon, G., Frank, R., Laurenceau, J.L., Malergue, C., and Grosgogeat, Y. Right ventricular dysplasia: A report of 24 adult cases. *Circulation* **65**: 384–398, 1982.
5. Fitchett, D.H., Sugrue, D.D., MacArthur, C.G., and Oakley, C.M. Right ventricular dilated cardiomyopathy. *Br. Heart J.* **51**: 25–29, 1984.
6. Nava, A., Bottero, M., Fasoli, G., Scognamiglio, R., and Thiene, G. Arrhythmogenic right ventricular dysplasia: A familiar form. *Pace* **8**: 32, 1985.
7. Nava, A., Canciani, B., and Scognamiglio, R. La tachicardia e la fibrillazione ventricolare nel ventricolo destro aritmogeno (displasia aritmogena del ventricolo destro). Spettro clinico ed elettrocardiografico. *G. Ital. Cardiol.* **16**: 741, 1986.
8. Nava, A., Scognamiglio, R., Thiene, G., Canciani, B., Daliento, L., Buja, G., Stritoni, P., Fasoli, G., and Dalla Volta, S. A polymorphic form of familial arrhythmogenic right ventricular dysplasia. *Am. J. Cardiol.* **59**: 1405–1409, 1987.
9. Scognamiglio, R., Fasoli, G., and Nava, A. Two-dimensional echocardiographic features in patients with spontaneous right ventricular tachycardia without apparent heart disease. *J. Cardiovasc. Ultrasound* **6**: 113–118, 1987.
10. Thiene, G., Nava, A., Corrado, D., Rossi, L., and Pennelli, N. Right ventricular cardiomyopathy and sudden death in young people. *N. Engl. J. Med.* **318**: 129–133, 1988.

11. Nava, A., Martini, B., Thiene, G., et al. La displasia aritmogena del ventricolo destro. Studio su una popolazione selezionata. G. Ital. Cardiol. 18: 2–9, 1988.

12. Nava, A., Canciani, B., Daliento, L., et al. Juvenile sudden death and effort ventricular tachycardias in a family with right ventricular cardiomyopathy. Int. J. Cardiol. 21: 111–123, 1988.

13. Maron, B.J. Right ventricular cardiomyopathy: Another cause of sudden death in the young. N. Engl. J. Med. 318: 178–180, 1988.

14. Bharati, S., Ciraulo, D.A., Bilitch, M., Rosen, K.M., and Lev, M. Inexcitable right ventricle and bilateral bundle branch block in Uhl's disease. Circulation 57: 636–644, 1978.

15. Bewick, D.J., Chandler, B.M., and Montague, T.J. Dilated right ventricular cardiomyopathy: Uhl's disease. Chest 90: 300–302, 1986.

16. Manyari, D.E., Klein, G.J., Gulamhusein, S., Boughner, D., Guiraudon, G.M., Wyse, G., Mitchell, L.B., and Kostuk, W.J. Arrhythmogenic right ventricular dysplasia: A generalized cardiomyopathy? Circulation 68: 251–257, 1983.

17. Waller, B.F., Smith E.R., Blackbourne, B.D., Arce, F.P., Sarkar, N.N., and Roberts, W.C. Congenital hypoplasia of portions of both right and left ventricular myocardial walls. Clinical and necropsy observations in two patients with parchment heart syndrome. Am. J. Cardiol. 46: 885–891, 1980.

18. Webb, J.G., Kerr, C.R., Huckell, V.F., Mizgala, H.F., and Ricci, D.R. Left ventricular abnormalities in arrhythmogenic right ventricular dysplasia. Am. J. Cardiol. 58: 568–570, 1986.

19. Blomstrom-Lundqvist, C., Sabel, C-G., and Olsson, S.B. A long-term follow-up of 15 patients with arrhythmogenic right ventricular dysplasia. Br. Heart J. 58: 477–488, 1987.

20. Arcilla, R.A. and Gasul, B.M. Congenital aplasia or marked hypoplasia of the myocardium of the right ventricle (Uhl's anomaly). J. Pediatr. 58: 381–388, 1961.

21. Perez Diaz, L., Quero Jimenez, M., Moreno Granados, F., Perez Martinez, V., and Merino Batres, G. Congenital absence of myocardium of right ventricle: Uhl's anomaly. Br. Heart J. 35: 570–572, 1973.

22. Cumming, G.R., Bowman, J.M., and Whytehead, L. Congenital aplasia of the myocardium of the right ventricle (Uhl's anomaly). Am. Heart J. 70: 671–676, 1965.

23. Tomisawa, M., Onouchi, Z., Masakutsu, G., Nakata, K., Mizukawa, K., and Kusunoki, T. Right ventricular aneurysm with ventricular premature beats. Br. Heart J. 36: 1182, 1974.

24. Dungan, W.T., Garson, A., Jr., and Gillette, P.C. Arrhythmogenic right ventricular dysplasia: A cause of ventricular tachycardia in children with apparently normal hearts. Am. Heart J. 102: 745–750, 1981.

25. Sugiura, M., Hayashi, T., and Ueno, K. Partial absence of the right ventricular muscle in an aged. Jpn. Heart J. 11: 582, 1970.

26. Voigt, J. and Agdal, N. Lipomatous infiltration of the heart. An uncommon cause of sudden, unexpected death in a young man. Arch. Pathol. Lab. Med. 106: 497–498, 1982.

27. Ruder, M.A., Winston, S.A., Davis, J.C., Abbott, J.A., Elder, M., and Scheinman, M.M. Arrhythmogenic right ventricular dysplasia in a family. Am. J. Cardiol. 56: 799–800, 1985.

28. Higuchi, S., Caglar, N.M., Shimada, R., Yamada, A., Takeshita, A., and Nakamura, M. 16-year follow-up of arrhythmogenic right ventricular dysplasia. Am. Heart J. 108: 1363–1365, 1984.

29. Hoback, J., Adicoff, A., From, A.H.L., Smith, McK., Shafer, R., and Chesler, E. A report of Uhl's disease in identical adult twins. Evaluation of right ventricular dysfunction with echocardiography and nuclear angiography. Chest 79: 306–310, 1981.

30. Diggelmann, U. and Baur, H.R. Familial Uhl's anomaly in the adult. Am. J. Cardiol. 53: 1402–1403, 1984.

31. Ibsen, H.H.W., Baandrup, U., and Simonsen, E.E. Familial right ventricular dilated cardiomyopathy. Br. Heart J. 54: 156–159, 1985.

32. Rakovec, P., Rossi, L., Fontaine, G., Sasel, B., Markez, J., and Voncina, D. Familial arrhythmogenic right ventricular disease. *Am. J. Cardiol.* **58**: 377–378, 1986.

33. Zanardi, F., Occari, G., Cavazzini, L., Grandi, E., and Tomasi, A.M. Displasia aritmogena del ventricolo destro ad incidenza familiare. *G. Ital. Cardiol.* **16**: 4–12, 1986.

34. Laurent, M., Descaves, C., Biron, Y., Deplace, C., Almange, C., and Daubert, J.C. Familial form of arrhythmogenic right ventricular dysplasia. *Am. Heart J.* **113**: 827–829, 1987.

35. Haworth, S.G., Shinebourne, E.A., and Miller, G.A.H. Right-to-left interatrial shunting with normal right ventricular pressure. *Br. Heart J.* **37**: 386–391, 1975.

36. Reeve, R. and McDonald, D. Partial absence of the right ventricular musculature-partial parchment heart. *Am. J. Cardiol.* **14**: 415–419, 1964.

37. Taussig, H. Congenital Malformation of the Heart: II. Specific Malformations. Commonwealth Fund, Harvard University Press, Cambridge, Massachusetts, 1960, pp. 138–145.

38. Neimann, N., Pernot, C., and Rauber, G. Aplasie du myocarde du ventricle droit (ventricule droit papyracé congenitale). *Arch. Mal. Coeur* **58**: 421–430, 1965.

39. Vecht, R.J., Carmichael, D.J.S., Gopal, R., and Philip, J. Uhl's anomaly. *Br. Heart J.* **41**: 676–682, 1979.

40. French, J.W., Baum, D., and Popp, R.L. Echocardiographic findings in Uhl's anomaly. *Am. J. Cardiol.* **36**: 349–353, 1975.

41. Perrin, E.V. and Mehrizi, A. Isolated free wall hypoplasia of the right ventricle. *Am. J. Dis Child.* **109**: 558–566, 1965.

42. Kinare, S.G., Panday, S.R., and Deshmukh, S.M. Congenital aplasia of the right ventricular myocardium (Uhl's anomaly). *Dis Chest* **55**: 429–431, 1969.

43. Rossi, P., Massumi, A., Gillette, P., and Hall, R.J. Arrhythmogenic right ventricular dysplasia: Clinical features, diagnostic techniques, and current management. *Am. Heart J.* **103**: 415–420, 1982.

44. Child, J.S., Perloff, J.K., Francoz, R., Yeatman, L.A., Henze, E., Schelbert, H.R., and Laks, H. Uhl's anomaly (parchment right ventricle): Clinical, echocardiographic, radionuclear, hemodynamic and angiocardiographic features in two patients. *Am. J. Cardiol.* **53**: 635–637, 1984.

45. Manyari, D.E., Duff, H.J., Kostuk, W.J., *et al.* Usefulness of noninvasive studies for diagnosis of right ventricular dysplasia. *Am. J. Cardiol.* **57**: 1147–1153, 1986.

46. Cherrier, F., Floquet, J., Cuilliere, M., and Neimann, J.L. Les dysplasies ventriculaires droites. A propos de 7 observations. *Arch. Mal. Coeur* **72**: 766–773, 1979.

47. Ribeiro, P.A., Shapiro, L.M., Foale, R.A., Crean, P., and Oakley, C.M. Echocardiographic features of right ventricular dilated cardiomyopathy and Uhl's anomaly. *Eur. Heart J.* **8**: 65–71, 1987.

48. Bahler, A.S., Meller, J., Brik, H., Herman, M.V., and Teichholz, L.E. Paradoxical motion of the interventricular septum with right ventricular dilatation in the absence of shunting. Report of two cases. *Am. J. Cardiol.* **38**: 654–657, 1976.

49. Robertson, J.H., Bardy, G.H., German, L.D., Gallagher, J.J., and Kisslo, J. Comparison of two-dimensional echocardiographic and angiographic findings in arrhythmogenic right ventricular dysplasia. *Am. J. Cardiol.* **55**: 1506–1508, 1985.

50. Foale, R.A., Nihoyannopoulos, P., Ribeiro, P., McKenna, W.J., Oakley, C.M., Krikler, D.M., and Rowland, E. Right ventricular abnormalities in ventricular tachycardia of right ventricular origin: Relation to electrophysiological abnormalities. *Br. Heart J.* **56**: 45–54, 1986.

51. Baran, A., Nanda, N.C., Falkoff, M., Barold, S.S., and Gallagher, J.J. Two-dimensional echocardiographic detection of arrhythmogenic right ventricular dysplasia. *Am. Heart J.* **103**: 1066–1967, 1982.

52. Daubert, C., Descaves, C., Foulgoc, J-L., Bourdonnec, C., Laurent, M., and Gouffault, J. Critical analysis of cineangiographic criteria for diagnosis of arrhythmogenic right ventricular dysplasia. *Am. Heart J.* **115**: 448–459, 1988.

53. Drobinski, G., Verdière, C., Fontaine, G.H., Frank, R., Fechner, J., and Grosgogeat, Y.

Diagnostic angiocardiographique des dysplasies ventriculaires droites. *Arch. Mal. Coeur* **78**: 544–551, 1985.

54. Blomstrom-Lundqvist, C., Selin, K., Jonsson, R., Johansson, S.R., Schlossman, D., and Olsson, S.B. Cardioangiographic findings in patients with arrhythmogenic right ventricular dysplasia. *Br. Heart J.* **59**: 556–563, 1988.

55. Letac, B., Tayot, J., and Barthes, P. Infiltration graisseuse du coeur et maladie de Uhl. A propos d'une observation de lipomatose cardiaque. *Arch. Mal. Coeur* **70**: 107–113, 1977.

56. Yutani, C., Imakita, M., Ishibashi-Ueda, H., Nagata, S., Sakakibara, H., and Nimura, Y. Uhl's anomaly as a result of progression to ventricular dilation from hypertrophic cardiopathy. *Acta Pathol. Jpn.* **37**: 1477–1488, 1987.

57. Halphen, C., Beaufils, P., Azancot, I., Baudouy, P., Manne, B., and Slama, R. Tachycardies ventriculaires récidivantes par dysplasie ventriculaire droite. Association a des anomalies du ventricule gauche. *Arch. Mal. Coeur* **74**: 1113–1118, 1981.

58. Hasumi, M., Sekiguchi, M., Hiroe, M., Kasanuki, H., and Hirosawa, K. Endomyocardial biopsy approach to patients with ventricular tachycardia with special reference to arrhythmogenic right ventricular dysplasia. *Jpn. Circ. J.* **51**: 242–249, 1987.

59. Viola, A.P., Adaro, F.V.M., and Roncoroni, A.J. Idiopathic myocardiopathy resulting in failure of contractility of the right ventricle. *Am. J. Med.* **48**: 235–238, 1970.

60. Froment, R., Perrin, A., Loire, R., and Dalloz, C. Ventricule droit papyracé du jeune adulte par dystrophie congénitale. A propos de 2 cas anatomo-cliniques et de 3 cas cliniques. *Arch. Mal. Coeur* **61**: 477–503, 1968.

61. Segall, H.N. Parchment heart (Osler). *Am. Heart J.* **40**: 948–950, 1950.

62. Castleman, B. and Sprague, H.B. Case records of the Massachussets General Hospital: Weekly clinicopathological exercises. *N. Engl. J. Med.* **246**: 785–790, 1952.

63. Gould, L., Guttman, A.B., Carrasco, J., and Lyon, A.F. Partial absence of the right ventricular musculature. A congenital lesion. *Am. J. Med.* **42**: 636–641, 1967.

64. Purcaro, A., Capestro, F., Ciampani, N., *et al.* La displasia ventricolare destra aritmogena. A proposito di 3 osservazioni. *G. Ital. Cardiol.* **14/II**: 1087–1096, 1984.

65. Fontaine, G., Guiraudon, G., Frank, R., *et al.* Dysplasie ventriculaire droite arythmogéne et maladie de Uhl. *Arch. Mal. Coeur* **75**: 361–372, 1982.

66. Morgera, T., Salvi, A., Alberti, E., Silvestri, F., and Camerini, F. Morphological findings in apparently idiopathic ventricular tachycardia. An echocardiographic, haemodynamic and histologic study. *Eur. Heart J.* **6**: 323–334, 1985.

67. Whar, D.W., Wang, Y.S., and Schiller, N.B. Left ventricular volumes determined by two-dimensional echocardiography in a normal adult population. *J. Am. Coll. Cardiol.* **1**: 863–868, 1983.

68. Kaul, S., Chuwa, T., Hopkins, J.M., and Sham, P.M. Assessment of right ventricular function using two-dimensional echocardiography. *Am. Heart J.* **107**: 526–531, 1984.

Spectrum of Restrictive Cardiomyopathy: A Report of a National Survey

Yuzo Hirota,* Gen Shimizu,* Yoshio Kita,* Yasushi Nakayama,* Michihiro Suwa,* Keishiro Kawamura,* Seiki Nagata,** Toshitami Sawayama,*** Toru Izumi,† Takeshi Nakano,† Hironori Toshima,§ and Morie Sekiguchi#

* The Third Division, Department of Internal Medicine, Osaka Medical College, Osaka, Japan
** Department of Internal Medicine, The National Cardiovascular Center, Osaka, Japan
*** Department of Cardiology, Kawasaki Medical College, Okayama, Japan
† The First Department of Internal Medicine, Niigata University Medical School, Niigata, Japan
† The First Department of Internal Medicine, Mie University Medical School, Mie, Japan
§ The Third Department of Internal Medicine, Kurume University School of Medicine Fukuoka Japan
# The Department of Internal Medicine, Japan Heart and Blood Pressure Institute, Tokyo Women's Medical College, Tokyo, Japan

ABSTRACT

This report describes clinical profiles, echocardiographic, hemodynamic, and histologic findings in 23 patients with restrictive cardiomyopathy (RCM) based on the diagnostic criteria of: 1) heart failure due to reduced left ventricular (LV) compliance; 2) normal LV size and systolic function; 3) absence of LV hypertrophy; and 4) etiology or association unknown.

Twelve were males. The patient ages ranged between 5 and 63 years. Eight patients died during a mean follow-up period of 145 months, 5 of whom died of congestive heart failure (CHF) after 10 years of illness. Three had a family history of hypertrophic cardiomyopathy (HCM). Thromboembolism was observed in 7 cases. Echocardiograms showed normal LV wall thickness and contraction, atrial enlargement, and pericardial effusion in patients with severe CHF. Hemodynamic characteristics included elevated right (RV) and LV filling pressures, LV filling pressure usually being higher than that of RV filling pressure. RV filling pressure was, however, elevated in patients with tricuspid regurgitation (TR), and equalization of biventricular filling pressures were seen in some patients with severe TR. The square root sign was seen in 48% in RV and 33% in LV diastolic pressures. Interstitial fibrosis (19 of 20) and endocardial thickening (11 of 18) were the most common histologic findings. Severe myocardial disarray consistent with HCM was seen in 2 patients.

Our observations indicate that the clinical course is long, RV and LV pressures could be equal when TR is severe, the square root sign is not diagnostic, and thromboembolism is common in RCM. Some of these may be atypical manifestations of HCM.

INTRODUCTION

Idiopathic cardiomyopathy is classified into 3 categories: hypertrophic, dilated, and restrictive. Restrictive cardiomyopathy (RCM) is the least common and not well understood. Even in the report of the WHO/ISFC Task Force, no definition or diagnostic criteria was proposed.[1] Restrictive physiology due to amyloid infiltration or hemosiderin deposition are well known as amyloid heart disease[2] or cardiac hemochromatosis.[2] Another category of heart disease which causes restrictive physiology is endomyocardial fibrosis as the sequelae of tropical or nontropical hypereosinophilia[2] or endocardial fibroelastosis in association with congenital heart disease.[2] These diseases, however, should be categorized into specific heart muscle diseases, as the associations or etiologies are known.

Idiopathic RCM can be defined as heart muscle disease of reduced myocardial compliance of unknown etiology. It has not been established yet whether such specific heart muscle disease could exist. This study was undertaken to clarify the incidence, clinical profile, natural history, and diagnostic criteria of RCM using a nationwide questionnaire survey in Japan.

METHODS

Letters were sent to 801 major hospitals in Japan, asking whether they had seen patients who fulfilled the following 4 criteria: 1) presence of heart failure due to stiff ventricle; 2) normal left ventricular (LV) cavity and normal or near normal systolic function; 3) absence of LV hypertrophy based on echocardiographic and/or angiographic observations; and 4) association or etiology unknown. Answers were obtained from 355 hospitals. Thirty-six patients were reported from 20 institutes, and clinical data on 31 were sent to us. We reviewed them, and eliminated 8 patients: 2 had constrictive pericarditis, 3 had severe LV hypertrophy by echocardiography, one had pheochromocytoma, and the existence of heart disease was doubtful in 2 patients. The names of the collaborating institutions are listed in Table 1.

Patient profiles are summarized in Table 2. Twelve were males, and the ages ranged from 5 to 63 years (36 ± 13). The duration of illness was defined as the time interval between the initial time of cardiac abnormality found by medical doctors and the last medical examination. One patient was lost to follow-up after 3 years, 8 patients died, and 14 others were alive as of the end of June 1988. Of the 8 who died, autopsy was

TABLE 1.   Collaborating Institutions

Osaka Medical College
National Cardiovascular Center
Kawasaki Medical School
Mie University School of Medicine
Niigata University School of Medicine
Kohchi Medical School
Kurume University School of Medicine
Tokyo Saiseikai Chuo Hospital
Nagasaki City Hospital
Tenri Yorozusoudansho Hospital
Tane Hospital
Faculty of Medicine, Kyoto University
Faculty of Medicine, Kyushu University
Yamagata University School of Medicine
Tachikawa Hospital
National Defense Medical College
Sapporo Medical College
Yamada Red Cross Hospital
Tokyo Municipal Toshima Hospital
Ohfune Hospital

TABLE 2. Profiles of 23 Patients with Restrictive Cardiomyopathy

Age	Sex	Duration of illness	Symptoms			Deaths	FH		TE
			RVF	LVF	Arrhythmias		RCM	HCM	
36	M = 12	145	17/23	16/23	19/23	8	3?	3	7
± 16	F = 13	± 121 (m)	(74%)	(70%)	(83%)	(CHF = 5)			(33%)

FH: family history, TE: thromboembolism, RVF: right ventricular failure, LVF: left ventricular failure, CHF: congestive heart failure, M: male, F: female; m, month.

performed in 6. Echocardiographic, hemodynamic, and angiographic findings were reported in the questionnaires by the primary physicians. The presence or absence of the square root sign of ventricular diastolic pressure was also judged by them. The degree of mitral and tricuspid regurgitation (TR) was judged on a scale of 4 as absent, mild, moderate, or severe based on the observations from angiography and echocardiography, or bedside assessment.

Data are presented as means ± one standard deviation of the mean (Mn ± SD). The unpaired Student's t-test was used for the statistical analysis.

RESULTS

Mean duration of illness was 145 ± 121 months. Symptoms of right ventricular (RV) and LV failure, and/or atrial fibrillation were commonly seen, and 7 patients had thromboembolic episodes. Eight patients died: 5 from congestive heart failure (CHF), one suddenly, one during tricuspid valve replacement, and one of gastric cancer. Only one died within one year; another died in the 5th year, and 5 others died after more than 10 years of illness. A pair of siblings were reported from different institutions, and another patient had a family history strongly suggestive of RCM in 2 brothers. Three patients had documented family history of hypertrophic cardiomyopathy (HCM).

Echocardiographic measurements of the LV are shown in Table 3. The LV wall was not thick, and indexes of contractility were normal. Very important findings were the presence of severely enlarged left atria and pericardial effusion (Fig. 1).

The hemodynamic and angiographic findings are summarized in Table 4. Biventricular filling pressures were elevated and LV volumes were in the normal range. The early diastolic dip and subsequent plateau pattern or the square root sign of ventricular diastolic pressure was seen in the RV in 54%, and in the LV in 33%. Figure 2A shows a typical square root sign in a patient with constrictive pericarditis, but this sign was absent in a patient with RCM (Fig. 2B). The fluid-filled system was used for the LV pressure recordings in all 7 patients who were reported to have this sign. Atrial pressures were compared between patients with and without the square root sign (Table 5). Right

TABLE 3. Echocardiographic Findings ($n = 23$)

IVS cm	LVPW cm	Dd cm	Ds cm	FS %	EF %
1.0	1.1	4.3	2.7	36	69
± 0.3	± 0.2	± 0.6	± 0.6	± 9	± 11

IVS: interventricular septum, LVPW: left ventricular posterior wall, Dd: end-diastolic dimension, Ds: end-systolic dimension, FS: fractional shortening, EF: ejection fraction.

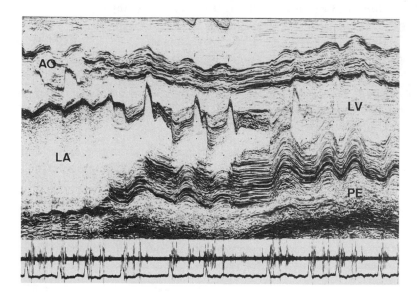

Fig. 1. M-mode echocardiographic scan in a patient with RCM. Marked left atrial (LA) enlargement and pericardial effusion are characteristic findings in association with normal left ventricular (LV) systolic function in patients with severe congestive failure in RCM. AO, aorta.

TABLE 4. Pressures (mmHg) and Left Ventricular Volumes (ml/m²)

RAm	PCWm	LVsp	LVedp	EDVI	ESVI
n = 21	20	22	22	16	16
10	16	111	19	82	29
± 6	± 8	± 13	± 7	± 24	± 12

RAm: mean right atrial pressure, PCWm: mean pulmonary capillary wedge pressure, LVsp: left ventricular systolic pressure, LVedp: left ventricular end-diastolic pressure, EDVI: end-diastolic volume index, ESVI: end-systolic volume index.

atrial pressure was significantly higher in patients with the square root sign, but no significant difference was observed in pulmonary wedge pressure.

Biventricular filling pressures were compared between patients with and without severe TR (Table 6). LV filling pressure was significantly higher than RV filling pressure in patients without TR. In the presence of severe TR, RV filling pressure was elevated and even equalization of biventricular filling pressure was seen in 5 patients.

Autopsy was performed in 6 patients, and endomyocardial biopsy in 17. Histologic examination was performed in 20 patients. There were no specific findings diagnostic for RCM. Biopsy or autopsy specimens showed some degree of myocardial fibrosis in almost all (19 of 20). Nonspecific endocardial thickening was present in 11 of 18 (less than 100 μm) (Fig. 3), and fine elastic fiber proliferation was seen in one autopsied heart (Fig. 4). Mild to moderate myocardial fiber disarray was seen in 10, and severe disarray consistent with HCM was seen in 2 patients. One was found to have a thick endocardium in the right ventricle at the time of pulmonary valvotomy for mild congenital pulmonary stenosis and severe CHF. This patient might be classified as endocardial fibroelastosis.

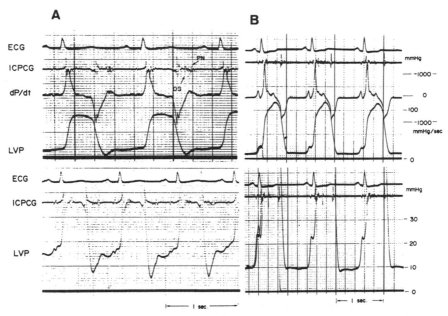

Fig. 2. Low gain (upper panel) and high gain (lower panel) pictures of LV pressure recordings in a patient with constrictive pericarditis (A) and RCM (B). While LV pressure of constrictive pericarditis showed a typical square root sign, this was not present in RCM. Markedly slow decay of LV pressure during isovolumic relaxation with a reduced peak negative dP/dt and prolonged time constant of the pressure decay are other characteristics of RCM.

TABLE 5. Differences of RV and LV Filling Pressures with and without Square Root Sign

	RAm		PCWm	
	SRS (+)	(−)	(+)	(−)
	n=10	n=9	n=7	n=14
	13 ± 6	6 ± 3	21 ± 9	14 ± 5
		$p < 0.005$		$0.05 < p < 0.1$

SRS: square root sign.

TABLE 6. Differences of RV and LV End-Diastolic Pressures (mmHg) with and without TR

RVedp		LVedp		LVedp − RVedp	
TR (+)	(−)	(+)	(−)	(+)	(−)
n=6	n=12	n=6	n=12	n=6	n=12
15 ± 5	7 ± 3	18 ± 7	18 ± 7	4 ± 2	11 ± 7
	$p < 0.005$		ns		$p < 0.01$

TR: tricuspid regurgitation.

DISCUSSION

Among the 3 types of idiopathic cardiomyopathies, RCM is the least common and least well understood. Even the diagnostic criteria have not been established yet. This disease can be defined as a heart muscle disease of unknown etiology with increased

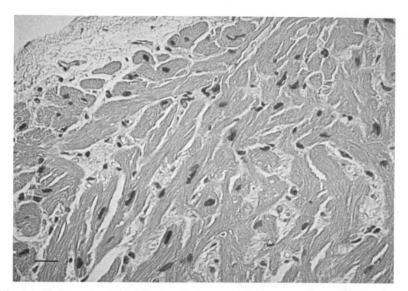

Fig. 3. Endomyocardial biopsy of the patient shown in Fig. 2B. Moderate myocardial fiber disarray, interstitial fibrosis, and mild thickening of the endocardium are shown in the picture taken from the right side of the interventricular septum. These findings are commonly seen in biopsy as well as autopsy specimens. Hematoxylin-eosin stain, × 375; scale indicates 20 μm.

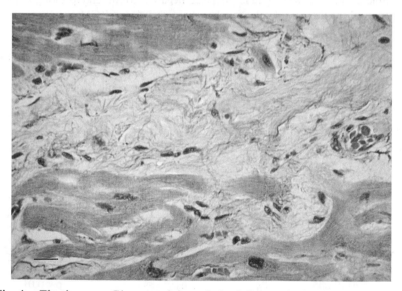

Fig. 4. Elastica van Gieson staining of the left ventricular free wall of the patient shown in Fig. 1. Fine elastic fiber proliferation was observed in the interstitial tissue of the autopsy specimen. × 375; scale indicates 20 μm.

muscle stiffness or reduced muscle compliance without definite LV hypertrophy. As hypertrophy per se causes a reduction in chamber compliance, hypertrophied hearts should be eliminated from RCM even when restrictive physiology is present. Two other

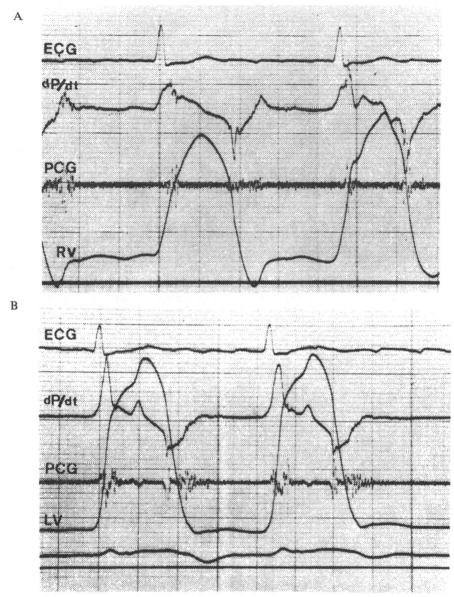

Fig. 5. RV (A) and LV pressures (B) recorded with the tip manometer system in a patient. While RV pressure showed a typical square root sign, it was not seen in the LV. The genesis of the square root sign in the RV is considered to be the results of rapid early diastolic filling due to elevated right atrial pressure and sudden cessation of the filling with the constriction of the RV due to elevated pericardial pressure or constraint by the other 3 chambers. The absence of this sign in the LV is probably related to slow relaxation and reduced compliance, both of which impede rapid filling.

conditions that are associated with restrictive physiology are infiltrative heart disease such as amyloidosis[2] or hemochromatosis,[2] and thickening of the endocardium, *i.e.*, endocardial fibroelastosis and endomyocardial fibrosis. Although infiltrative heart disease is recognized as a specific heart muscle disease, the question of whether endo-cardial disease should be included in RCM remains debatable.[1] In the discussion at the 2nd International Symposium on Cardiomyopathies held in Tokyo in 1988, there was general agreement[3] that endocardial disease should also be considered as a different disease entity (specific heart muscle diseases) as it is frequently seen as a sequela of hypereosinophilia or is associated with congenital anomalies.

Four major problems in the establishment of a diagnosis are: 1) whether the square root sign of the diastolic ventricular wave is necessary; 2) whether reduced systolic function in association with reduced muscle compliance should be included in this disease; 3) how high the ventricular filling pressure must be to qualify for RCM; and 4) what is the RV-LV filling pressure difference for the differential diagnosis from con-strictive pericarditis.

Although the square root sign was included in the diagnostic criteria in the report of Benotti *et al.*,[4] Tyberg *et al.*[5] found this sign in only 40% of their patients with amyloidosis, and one patient did not have this sign in the report of Siegel *et al.*[6] Hirota and associates[7] described the absence of this sign in 4 patients whose LV pressure was recorded with a tip manometer system in association with markedly prolonged relaxa-tion. As stiff ventricle with prolonged relaxation causes a slow decline in LV pressure during isovolumic relaxation and early diastolic filling periods, they postulated that this sign could be an artifact due to the resonance of the pressure recording system of the fluid-filled system. In our series of patients, the square root sign was seen in 11 patients in the RV and 7 in the LV. Both RV and LV pressures recorded with the tip manometer in one patient[8] are shown in Fig. 5. The square root sign was present only in the RV. From this evidence, the sign should be eliminated from the diagnostic criteria.

One of the diagnostic criteria of Benotti *et al.*[4] was normal or near normal systolic function, but patients with depressed ejection fraction were included in the report of the Stanford group.[9] We believe that patients with markedly reduced systolic function should not be included in this disease category, as RCM is a disease of the diastole.

No one knows how high the ventricular filling pressure must be for a diagnosis of RCM. As the filling pressure changes with numerous manipulations, no definite line can be drawn as a diagnostic criterion.

It is generally believed that LV filling pressure is higher than RV filling pressure since the LV is stiffer than the RV in RCM. Some authors have emphasized that a 5 mmHg difference is one important marker for the differential diagnosis from contrictive peri-carditis.[2] It is true in the absence of TR, but with the progression of the diasease, RV dilatation and the appearance of TR seems to be the natural course. In such advanced cases, it must be realized that even equalization of biventricular filling pressure could occur.

In our series of 23 patients, the possibility of amyloidosis was ruled out by endomyo-cardial biopsy, autopsy, or biopsies of other organs. Compared to amyloidosis, the natural history is very long, as has been reported by Benotti *et al.*[4] The importance of anticoagulation therapy must be emphasized, as 7 patients had thromboembolic epi-sodes.

Although the importance of differential diagnosis between RCM and constrictive pericarditis has been emphasized, it seems to be relatively easy with invasive and non-invasive investigations. On the other hand, differential diagnosis from atypical HCM, idiopathic or solitary TR, and effusive contrictive pericarditis is more difficult. As 3 patients had a family history of HCM, 2 had severe myocardial disarray, and the majority of biopsy specimens showed mild to moderate disarray, some patients may have an

TABLE 7. Proposed Diagnostic Criteria for Restrictive Cardiomyopathy

1. Evidence for stiff ventricle without
   endocardial or pericardial constriction
2. Normal or near normal left ventricular
   cavity and systolic function
3. Absence of left ventricular hypertrophy by
   echocardiography or cineangiography
4. Consistent findings in endomyocardial
   biopsy of stiff ventricle
5. Unknown etiology or association

atypical presentation of HCM, that is, HCM without LV hypertrophy, which has recently been reported by McKenna et al.[10] The genesis of stiff myocardium cannot be explained by the degree of endocardial thickening or myocardial fibrosis, and we do not have any suggestion for the pathogenesis of this stiff heart syndrome.

It is concluded that:

1) RCM is a rare disease, but with its recognition the incidence reported will increase.
2) The square root sign is not necessary for the diagnostic criteria.
3) Equalization of RV and LV filling pressures is seen in patients with severe TR.

Based upon these observations, we propose the diagnostic criteria of RCM shown in Table 7.

REFERENCES

1. Brandenburg, R.O., Charzov, E., Cherian, G., *et al.* Report of the WHO/ISFC Task Force on definition and classification of cardiomyopathies. *Circulation* **64**: 437A-438A, 1981.
2. Wynne, J. and Braunwald, E. Restrictive and infiltrative cardiomyopathies. In: Heart Disease. A Textbook of Cardiovascular Medicine, 3rd edition. Braunwald, E. (ed.), Chapter 42, The cardiomyopathies and myocarditides. W.B. Saunders Company, Philadelphia, 1988, pp. 1430–1440.
3. Olsen, E.G.J. Morphological overview and pathogenetic mechanism in endomyocardial fibrosis associated with eosinophillia. In this volume. pp. 1–8.
4. Benotti, J.R., Grossman, W., and Cohn, P.F. Clinical profile of restrictive cardiomyopathy. *Circulation* **61**: 1206–1212, 1980.
5. Tyberg, T.I., Goodyer, A.V.N., Hurst, V.W., III, Alexander, J., and Langou, R.A. Left ventricular filling in differentiating restrictive amyloid cardiomyopathy and constrictive pericarditis. *Am. J. Cardiol.* **47**: 791–796, 1981.
6. Siegel, R.J., Shah, P.K., and Fishbein M.C. Idiopathic restrictive cardiomyopathy. *Circulation* **70**: 165–169, 1984.
7. Hirota, Y., Kohriyama, T., Hayashi, T., Kaku, K., Nishimura, H., Saito, T., Nakayama, Y., Suwa, M., Kino, M., and Kawamura, K. Idiopathic restrictive cardiomyopathy: differences of left ventricular relaxation and diastolic wave forms from constrictive pericarditis. *Am. J. Cardiol.* **52**: 421–423, 1983.
8. Kodaka, M., Kubo, S., Kitaura, Y., Hirota, Y., Kino, M., Nishioka, A., Kawamura, K., Nakata, K., Ejiri, N., and Nakajima K. An autopsy case report of restrictive cardiomyopathy with cerebral embolism and diabetes insipidus. *J. Jpn. Med. Assoc.* **73**: 358–367, 1984. (in Japanese)
9. Appleton, C.P., Hatle, L.K., and Popp R.L. Demonstration of restrictive ventricular physiology by Doppler echocardiography. *J. Am. Coll. Cardiol.* **11**: 757–768, 1988.
10. McKenna, W.J., Nihoyannopoulos, P., and Davies, M.J. Hypertrophic cardiomyopathy

without hypertrophy: A description of two families with premature cardiac death and myocardial disarray in the absence of increased muscle mass. *Circulation* **78**: Suppl. III-375, 1988 (abstr.).

Clinical Recognition of Restrictive Cardiomyopathy

Oakley C.M.

Department of Clinical Cardiology, Royal Postgraduate Medical School, London, U.K.

Restrictive cardiomyopathies are characterised by preservation of normal or near normal ventricular systolic function with normal or reduced end-diastolic cavity size but raised filling pressures caused by a diastolic fault with prolonged active relaxation and/or increased passive stiffness.[1,2]

Primary restrictive cardiomyopathy can be difficult to distinguish from constrictive pericarditis.[3] The hyper-eosinophilic syndrome and endomyocardial fibrosis are usually readily recognised because of cavity deformity and atrioventricular valve involvement.[4] Restrictive syndromes are seen in infiltrations exemplified by amyloid but also in some forms of haemochromatosis and in thalassaemia.[2] Sarcoid infiltration can cause restrictive haemodynamics but can usually be recognised because it is focal rather than generalized.[5,6] Advanced hypertrophic cardiomyopathy (HOCM) can closely mimic amyloid heart disease.[2] Extracardiac tumors such as pericardial mesothelioma or primary cardiac tumors such as rhabdomyosarcoma or fibroma may produce a restrictive syndrome but are usually easily distinguished as is carcinoid heart disease.[7]

Diagnosis depends on echocardiographic differences and an endomyocardial biopsy. The diagnosis of primary rather than secondary restriction of filling of the heart is by exclusion.

Primary restrictive cardiomyopathy is characterized by a normal appearance of the ventricles on echo and angiographic examination. Apart from atrial dilatation the heart may appear grossly normal. Even the histology at both light microscopic and at ultrastructural level may show little detectably amiss. In some cases there is a very fine reticular interstitial fibrosis. Other cases show disarray sometimes with little or no increase in wall thickness and particularly in childhood distinction from hypertrophic cardiomyopathy may be blurred. The valves are structurally normal but considerable tricuspid regurgitation may develop and this can cause gross enlargement of the right atrium associated with atrial fibrillation.

The condition is rare accounting for only about 5% of cardiomyopathies and characterisation has been slow. A familial form exists but the condition is usually sporadic. It appears most commonly in children and young people but is seen at all ages. One form has been described as an "atrial cardiomyopathy" because of gross atrial dilatation culminating in atrial standstill sometimes preceded by clinical manifestations of sinoatrial disorder or advancing to atrioventricular conduction failure needing pacemaker implantation.

CLINICAL RECOGNITION OF PRIMARY RESTRICTIVE CARDIOMYOPATHY

As in constrictive pericarditis the presentation is usually with right sided congestive features of insidious onset.[1,3,8] Women may first complain of swelling of the ankles or varicose veins at a time when the chest X-ray and ECG are still normal. Presentation may even be with ascites and hepatomegaly simulating malignancy or cirrhosis but the jugular venous pressure is of course greatly raised and should not be missed. While sinus rhythm persists the venous pressure may show an M shape and small excursion as in constrictive pericarditis. With the onset of atrial fibrillation or in cases of atrial standstill, tricuspid regurgitation dominates and the venous wave form will reflect this with large V-waves which are not seen in pericardial constriction. Third heart sounds are usual, occasionally asynchronous right and left ventricular filling sounds reflect inequality of left and right ventricular diastolic pressures. Sometimes third heart sounds are so early that they are inaudible or not easily separated from the second heart sound which may be widely split. Regurgitant murmurs are usually absent or unimpressive even when tricuspid regurgitation is marked unless the right ventricular pressure is raised because of pulmonary hypertension.

Pulmonary congestion may give rise to pulmonary hypertension, uncommon in constrictive pericarditis but when patients have been over-treated with diuretics before referral the lungs may be radiographically clear. In some cases the chest X-ray may be normal. In others atrial dilatation may be responsible for seemingly gross cardiomegaly so the radiological spectrum is wide.

The electrocardiogram in sinus rhythm usually shows high voltage P-waves with prolongation indicating biatrial hypertrophy. Atrial arrhythmias or absent P-waves and a slow regular "sino-ventricular" rhythm may be seen. The QRS may be normal but the axis may be leftward with higher left ventricular voltage than is usual in constrictive pericarditis. Fascicular blocks sometimes occur as well and complete atrioventricular block is more common in restrictive than in any other form of cardiomyopathy.

The echocardiographic features are described by Dr. Nagata and suffice it to say that echocardiography, CT-scans and MRI are all able to display the normal structural anatomy of the heart, the atrial dilatation and the thickness of the ventricular walls and pericardium with echo and MRI able also to demonstrate flows and valvar regurgitation.

DIFFERENTIAL DIAGNOSIS

Constrictive Pericarditis

Constrictive pericarditis can be the most difficult differential diagnosis as well as the most important since it is a curable condition.[3] Primary restrictive cardiomyopathy also has to be distinguished from endomyocardial fibrosis, from myocardial infiltration and sometimes from hypertrophic cardiomyopathy.

In contrast to constrictive pericarditis atrial dilatation particularly of the right atrium, is usual in restrictive cardiomyopathy and may be gross. Tricuspid regurgitation when more than slight and associated with atrial fibrillation also suggests cardiomyopathy rather than constriction. A difference between the right and left ventricular filling pressures in restrictive cardiomyopathy may be shown by asynchronous third heart sounds from the right and left ventricles. Inspiratory decrease in the E-A ratio on inspiration on Doppler echo and recognition of a pericardial space on cross-sectional echo, usually best seen on inspiration and inferiorly help to exclude constriction by the pericardium. An impression of pericardial thickening often reported on CT and MRI scans should be viewed critically and carefully compared with the images from other

TABLE 1.   Key Features in the Differential Diagnosis of Restrictive Syndromes: A high jugular venous pressure is common to all

---

Primary Restrictive Cardiomyopathy

Sporadic
Familial with atrial standstill and atrioventricular block
Atriomegaly
Tricuspid regurgitation

Constrictive Pericarditis

Small atria
No or mild tricuspid regurgitation
No pulmonary congestion

Amyloid heart disease

Patient usually old and ill
Skin petechiae
Macroglossia
Hypotension and orthostatic hypotension
Quiet heart. No gallop sounds
Low voltage ECG

Sarcoid heart disease

Sarcoid elsewhere not invariable
Arrhythmias common
A-V block occasionally

Eosinophilic heart disease

Eosinophilic syndrome or Churg-Strauss variant of polyarteritis

Hypertrophic Cardiomyopathy (HOCM)

Previous typical HOCM not invariably known
ECG LV hypertrophy

Beta-thalassaemia major

---

patients known to have normal pericardium! Similarity in left and right ventricular filling pressures accounts for a sigmoid shape of the ventricular septum in constrictive pericarditis which is well seen on CT-scans, while higher left than right sided filling pressures will be recognised easily by echocardiographic short axis views of the ventricular septum and also by seeing which way the atrial septum bulges.

Resort to open pericardial biopsy should no longer be necessary in order to exclude constrictive pericarditis.

Amyloid Heart Disease

Differentiation from *amyloid heart disease* is usually readily made by echo. Clinically the patients with amyloid disease are usually (but not invariably) older and may have skin petechiae, macroglossia or enlarged peripheral nerves. The patient with amyloid commonly looks more ill, has a lower cardiac output, peripheral cyanosis, low pulse pressure and often orthostatic hypotension. Left ventricular third heart sounds are usually absent in amyloid but mitral or tricuspid regurgitant murmurs may be heard and there may be a filling sound at the left sternal edge when the systemic venous pressure is high. The ECG in amyloid nearly always shows strikingly low voltage and indeed this may provide the first clue to the diagnosis when the patient is initially seen. When fascicular blocks are present the voltage may be higher and the ECG less helpful in making the distinction. Sinoatrial disease may also be a feature both in restrictive cardiomyopathy and in amyloid pericardial effusions are not infrequently seen in amyloid heart disease due to amyloid infiltration of the pericardium.[2]

Haemochromatosis

Haemochromatosis may present with a restrictive picture particularly in younger men with a rapid onset of symptoms. The clinical features may not differ from those in primary restrictive cardiomyopathy but systolic function is impaired and the diagnosis is made quickly by the finding of raised serum iron, iron binding and serum transferrin and by myocardial biopsy. Myocardial iron may disappear and the haemodynamic fault improve after repeated venesection.[2]

Beta Thalassaemia Major

Beta thalassaemia major commonly leads to cardiac restriction. Both heart failure and arrhythmias are common in thalassaemia and blood pool (MUGA) scanning or echocardiography often reveal depressed systolic function before there is clinical, ECG or radiological abnormality. Doppler indices of diastolic function are abnormal and because of the major impairment to diastolic filling caused by myocardial iron overload, congestive failure or sudden death may occur at a stage when the ejection fraction is still relatively well maintained. Intensified desferrioxamine iron chelation therapy results in improvement in cardiac function which can be correlated with a fall in serum ferritin and an increase in urinary iron excretion.[2]

Sarcoid Heart Disease

Myocardial sarcoidosis classically presents with ventricular arrhythmias or atrioventricular block but numerous other clinical presentations are seen.[5,6] Very rarely this can be mitral regurgitation when the papillary muscles are infiltrated or mitral stenosis when the mitral leaflets are infiltrated. Heart failure with a restrictive picture results from massive though still focal infiltration which while not modifying the clinical picture is highly characteristic on echo. The site of election for sarcoid infiltration is typically in the proximal part of the left ventricle and ventricular septum sparing the apex. The contrast between a vigorously contracting apex and akinetic, often dilated, inflow portion of the left ventricle is very striking and contrasts with the much more usual finding of apical akinesia or dilatation in coronary heart failure with previous anteroapical infarction. In the active phase of sarcoidosis the akinetic segment may be of normal thickness or even thicker than normal. This progresses to a healed phase when the previous granuloma is replaced by thin fibrous bulging scar again well recognised on echo. Aneurysm formation is well recognized. Unlike in amyloid and haemochromatosis, endomyocardial biopsy in sarcoid may be negative because of its focal nature. The use of ultrasound to guide the bioptome can increase the chances of success.

CONCLUSION

The clinical features together with the ECG and chest X-ray usually permit the easy recognition of amyloid heart disease and sometimes also of hypertrophic cardiomyopathy in its restrictive form. Endomyocardial fibrosis is usually clinically silent until there is mitral or tricuspid regurgitation as cavity restriction and obliteration have to be advanced before clinical signs appear.

Constrictive pericarditis must always be considered lest it be missed but a positive clinical diagnosis can normally be made.

Primary restrictive cardiomyopathy is by contrast a diagnosis of exclusion and can only be made after echocardiography and endomyocardial biopsy have eliminated infiltrations, endomyocardial disease and hypertrophic cardiomyopathy in its restrictive form.

REFERENCES

1. Oakley, C.M. Specific heart muscle disorders. In: Oxford Textbook of Medicine. 2nd Ed. Weatherall, D., Ledingham, J. and Warrell, D. (eds.) Publ. oup 1987, p. 13 196–209.
2. Oakley, C.M. The cardiomyopathies. In: Oxford Textbook of Medicine. 2nd Ed. Weatherall, D., Ledingham, J. and Warrell, D. (eds.) Publ. oup 1987, p. 13 209–229.
3. Restrictive Cardiomyopathy or constrictive pericarditis? (Ed.). *Lancet* **ii**: 372–374, 1987.
4. Olsen, E.G.J. and Spry, C.J.F. The Pathogenesis of Loeffler's endomyocardial disease and its relationship to endomyocardial fibrosis. *Progress Cardiol.* **6**: 281–303, 1979.
5. Fleming, H.A. and Bailey, S.M. Sarcoid heart disease. *Brit. Heart J.* **36**: 54–68, 1974.
6. Oakley, C.M. Cardiac Sarcoidosis (ed.). *Thorax* **44**: 371–372, 1989.
7. Oates, J.A. The carcinoid syndrome. *N. Engl. J. Med.* **315**: 702–703, 1986.
8. Benotti, J.R., Grossman, W., and Cohn, E.F. Clinical profile of restrictive cardiomyopathy. *Circulation* **61**: 1206–1212, 1980.

Quantitative Analysis of Myofiber Disorganization and Fibrosis in Patients with Idiopathic Cardiomyopathy Characterized by Restrictive Physiology

Chikao Yutani,* Masami Imakita,* Hatsue Ishibashi-Ueda,* Seiki Nagata,** Yasuhara Nimura,*** and Shigeyuki Echigo[†]

* Division of Pathology, National Cardiovascular Center, Osaka, Japan
** Department of Internal Medicine, National Cardiovascular Center, Osaka, Japan
*** Research Institute, National Cardiovascular Center, Osaka, Japan
† Department of Pediatrics, National Cardiovascular Center, Osaka, Japan

ABSTRACT

The hearts of 4 patients with restrictive hemodynamic features were investigated morphologically. Three were females, one was male, and age ranged from 7 to 66 years (mean 45 years). All patients had symptoms of congestive heart failure, and 2 patients had received surgical valvular replacements because of tricuspid and mitral regurgitation. Two other patients had sudden cardiac death.

A dip and plateau pattern was present in the pressure tracings in 3 of 4 patients. Pathologic evaluation demonstrated biatrial dilatation, with mildly dilated left ventricles, and extensive myofiber disorganization ($47.4 \pm 23.4\%$, area percent), with small areas of fibrosis ($11.5 \pm 8.7\%$). Disproportionate hypertrophy was present in all patients but wall thickness was almost within 10 mm. There was no significant pericarditis, endocardial or valvular abnormalities, and no infiltrative myocardial disorders.

It is assumed that restrictive hemodynamic profile may be observed in the presence of myofiber disorganization and affected patients may exhibit years long clinical course. The findings in the present study suggest that the myofiber disorganization may limit diastolic relaxation and prevent ventricular dilatation, but does not always appear to be relevant to the myocardial hypertrophy.

INTRODUCTION

Cardiomyopathies have been divided into the dilated, hypertrophic, and restrictive types,[1,2] and a specific hemodynamic and clinical profile has been described for each class and correlated with specific etiologies.[3]

Restrictive cardiomyopathy (RCM) is characterized by normal or near normal ventricular size and systolic function but compromised ventricular relaxation leading to distinctive hemodynamic findings.[4] The pathologic basis for most cases of RCM includes infiltrative disorders such as amyloidosis, hemochromatosis, glycogen storage disease, mucopolysaccharidosis, endomyocardial fibrosis with or without eosinophilia, endocardial fibroelastosis, sarcoidosis, and collagen-vascular diseases like scleroderma.[5] Rarely has a primary or idiopathic form of the disease been reported in which histologic examination did not reveal specific changes.[6]

In this report, we describe the clinical, hemodynamic, and morphologic data from 4 patients who presented with RCM that was not associated with the usual pathologic entities responsible for this clinical-dynamic syndrome, but was associated with extensive myofiber disorganization and small areas of fibrosis.

CLINICAL PROFILES OF THE PATIENTS

Case Report No. 1: This 61-year-old woman was informed of cardiomegaly and arrhythmia at age 45. At age 51, she was easily fatigued, and developed edema of the lower legs and orthopnea. She was admitted to the National Cardiovascular Center in December 1979 for cardiac catheterization, which showed a dip and plateau pattern in the right ventricular pressure (Table 1). Chest X-ray showed cardiothoracic ratio (CTR) of 70%. Echocardiography revealed aortic dimension (AoD) 2.8 cm, left atrial dimension (LAD) 6.4 cm, LVDd 5.2 cm, LVDs 4.3 cm, IVS 0.9 cm, PWT 0.7 cm, EF 36%. In February 1982, a sudden attack of ventricular fibrillation occurred and she died.

Case Report No. 2: A 65-year-old woman was discovered to have cardiomegaly at age 39. She was first admitted to the National Cardiovascular Center in November 1984 with a diagnosis of arterial thromboembolism of the right lower leg followed by embolactomy, at which time she was found to have mitral regurgitation (MR). The data from her cardiac catheterization are listed in Table 1. Echocardiography revealed marked dilation of the left atrium and right ventricle, and MR (3/4), tricuspid regurgitation (TR) (4/4). ECG showed af. CTR was 80% on chest X-ray.

In May 1985, she was operated on with mitral valve replacement by Björk-Shiley valve, tricuspid annular plication, and left atrial appendage closure. Postoperatively, the EKG showed decreased p waves and increased ST in V2-V6. Echocardiography showed hematoma at the posterior wall of the left ventricle. In spite of intraaortic balloon pumping (IABP), the patient died of multiple organ failure.

Case Report No. 3: A 45-year-old woman was first admitted to the National Cardiovascular Center in 1981 with a 10-year history of dyspnea on effort. Cardiac catheterization showed PA 24/14/17 mmHg, AO 85/60/70 mmHg, RV 23/5 mmHg, RVEDP 16 mmHg, LA mean 13 mmHg, RA mean 15 mmHg, LV 91/6 mmHg, and LVEDP 12 mmHg, with a diastolic dip and plateau morphology in the right ventricular pressure curve (Table 1). Echocardiography revealed massive TR and moderate TR, which subsequently necessitated tricuspid valve replacement by Ionescu-Shiley valve. She complained, however, of fatigability and developed right pleural effusion and ascites. She died of congestive heart failure.

Case Report No. 4: A 7-year-old boy had an abnormal ECG at age 4, and cardiac catheterization showed a suspicion of RCM. Clinically, he occasionally had chest distress and dyspnea. In November 1986, he suddenly had severe chest pain and died.

AUTOPSY ANALYSIS

Autopsy of the 4 patients revealed no anatomic involvement of the heart valves, except for valvular replacement, or coronary artery stenosis. No structural defect such as congenital heart malformation was seen. Gross findings of the hearts are presented in Table 2. At autopsy, the hearts were weighed and the volume of the ventricles in 2 hearts was measured by placing water into the ventricles. After fixation, the hearts were cut transversely at a depth of 1 cm, and the cut surface of the upper third of the left ventricle was embedded in paraffin.

The whole cut surface was sectioned at approximately 5 μm thickness on a glass slide and stained with hematoxylin-eosin (HE) and trichrome, and used for histologic examination of fibrosis and myofiber disorganization.

The percentage area of fibrosis and myofiber disorganization was measured with a NIKON Cosmozone using an NEC PC9801 computer. Myofiber disorganization was

TABLE 1. Hemodynamic Valves

Patient no.	CO (l/min)/ CI (l/min/m²)	SAP (mmHg)	LVSP/ LVEDP (mmHg)	LVEDV/ LVESV (ml)	Mean PCWP or LAP (mmHg)	RVSP/ RVEDP (mmHg)	Mean RAP (mmHg)	EF	Dip and plateau	LV g	RV g
1	2.52/	142/94	108/18	61/27	19	41/1~5	7	0.53	(+)	MR(−)	TR(−)
2	3.98/2.82	120/72	115/~17	192/87	20	51/~11	11	0.55	(+)	MR2/4~3/4	TR 4/4
3	/2.77	110/60	91/6~12	110/49	13	23/5~16	17	0.55	(+)	MR2/4~3/4	TR 4/4
4	2.90/3.97	88/50	81/6(16)	41/9	11	34/0	3	0.78	(−)	MR(−)	TR(−)

CO: cardiac output, CI: cardiac index, SAP: systemic arterial pressure, LVSP: left ventricular systolic pressure, LVEDP: left ventricular end-diastolic pressure, LVEDV: left ventricular end-diastolic volume, LVESV: left ventricular end-systolic volume, PCWP: pulmonary capillary wedge pressure, RVSP: right ventricular systolic pressure, RVEDP: right ventricular end-diastolic pressure, RAP: right atrial pressure, EF: ejection fraction, LV gram left: ventriculogram.

TABLE 2.   Gross Findings in Hearts

Patient no.	Weight (g)	Volume (m*l*)		Wall thickness (mm)					Endocardial thickening	Dilatation	
		LV	RV	LV				RV		RA	LA
				Ant.	Lat.	Post.	Sept.				
1	450	N.D.		8	13	4	8	3	Lat. 1 mm	+	+
2	800*	N.D.		14	15	16	13	5	(−)	+	+
3	390	38	N.D.	7	9	10	8	4	(−)	+	+
4	210	20	20	10	8	7	9	3	(−)	+	+
Mean ± S.D.				9.8 ± 3.1	11.3 ± 3.3	9.3 ± 5.1	9.5 ± 2.4	3.8 ± 0.9			

* Including hematoma formed perioperatively.

evaluated according to the histologic criteria of Roberts and Ferrans[5] and Davies *et al.*[7]

CLINICOPATHOLOGICAL ASSESSMENT

Clinical Findings and Their Course (Table 1)

All patients had symptoms of congestive heart failure, and 2 patients had been operated on for valvular replacements because of TR and MR. Two other patients had sudden cardiac death.

Complete left and right heart catheterizations were performed in the 4 patients. Hemodynamic findings included elevated left ventricular filling pressures as well as elevated right ventricular end-diastolic pressure in 2 patients. A prominent early diastolic dip and middle-to-late diastolic plateau was noted in the ventricular pressure tracings of 3 patients.

Left ventriculography was performed in all patients and revealed 2+ to 3+ MR and 4+ TR in 2 patients. The left ventricular ejection fraction (determined by ventriculography) was 0.5 or greater in all 4 patients.

The analysis of regional left ventricular wall motion revealed normal contraction in all patients, and coronary arteries were normal.

Pathologic Findings (Table 2)

Right endomyocardial biopsy findings (Fig. 1). Two patients underwent right endomyocardial biopsy (case reports 1 and 4). Specimens taken from both patients showed moderate hypertrophy of the myocardium and myofiber disarrangement (unlike definite myofiber disorganization). Myocardial fibrosis was not found in these specimens; neither endocardial thickening or eosinophilic infiltration was seen. No evident proof of amyloidosis, hemochromatosis, or glycogen-storage disease was demonstrated.

Autopsy findings (Figs. 2–7). All patients were studied at autopsy. The heart weights were mildly to severely increased at 462.5 ± 247.0 g (range 210 to 800 g). The left ventricular volume of 2 patients was 38 ml and 20 ml, respectively. Marked biatrial dilatation was found in all patients and thrombi were present in the atrium in one patient. The atrioventricular and semilunar valves were structurally normal at autopsy. The anuli of the tricuspid valve and mitral valve were mildly dilated. Patient no. 2 had undergone mitral valve replacement 2 weeks and patient no. 3 tricuspid valve replace-

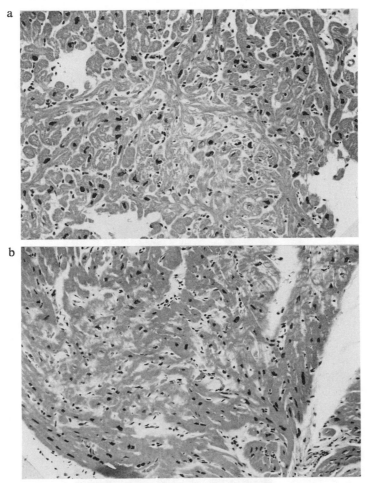

Fig. 1. Right endomyocardial biopsy findings. (a) Case 1 shows myocardial disarrangement and hyperchromatic nuclei with moderate hypertrophy. HE staining, ×100. (b) Case 2 shows moderate hypertrophy of the myocardium. HE staining, ×100.

ment 4 years before death. Right ventricular wall thickness was increased (>3 mm), measuring a mean 3.8 ± 0.9 mm, and increased left ventricular wall thickness (>15 mm) was present in one, showing that mean thickness in 4 segments of the left ventricles in these 4 patients was within normal limits. However, inappropriate wall thickness was present in all. No patients had asymmetric septal hypertrophy. The endocardium had patchy thickening in the lateral wall of the left ventricle in one patient, but was normal in the other 3 patients.

Gross and microscopic examination of the major epicardial coronary arteries demonstrated only minimal cross-sectional area luminal narrowing due to atherosclerosis in all patients.

Myocardial Fibrosis (Table 3)

The percentage area of the myocardial fibrosis in the anterior wall, lateral wall, posterior wall, septum, and right ventricular wall sections of the 4 hearts are given in

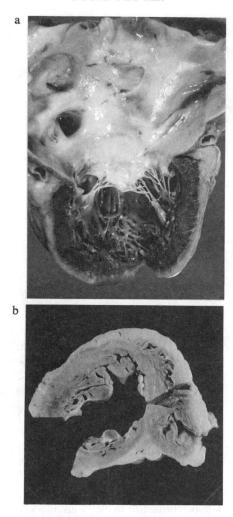

Fig. 2.   Gross photographs of case 1 showing (a) a marked dilatation of the left atrium and normal left ventricle cavity, and (b) disproportionate thickness of the left ventricle without fibrosis.

TABLE 3.   Fibrosis Percentage Areas

Patient no.	LV				RV	Mean ± S.D.
	Anterior	Lateral	Posterior	Septal		
1	18.6	2.6	42.5	10.8	5.6	16.0 ± 15.9
2	7.8	9.7	9.4	17.6	9.6	10.8 ± 3.9
3	6.7	9.8	12.1	13.9	9.5	10.4 ± 2.7
4	19.2	12.8	3.2	5.1	4.1	8.9 ± 6.9
Mean ± S.D.	13.1 ± 6.7	8.7 ± 4.3	16.8 ± 17.5	11.9 ± 5.3	7.2 ± 2.8	11.5 ± 8.7

Table 3. The mean percentage area of fibrosis was 11.5 ± 8.7 % (mean range 8.9 ± 6.9 % to 16.0 ± 15.9 %), and fibrotic areas were irregularly seen on the left ventricles. The largest area of fibrosis was noted in the posterior wall of the left ventricle.

Myofiber Disorganization (*Table 4*)

The percentage areas of myofiber disorganization in each segment of both ventricles are listed in Table 4. The mean percentage area of myofiber disorganization was 70.2 ± 9.5 % in the septum, which was the largest area, followed by the anterior, right ventricular, posterior, and lateral walls. The mean percentage area of myofiber disorganiza-

TABLE 4. Myofiber Disorganization Percentage Areas

Case	LV				RV	Mean ± S.D.
	Anterior	Lateral	Posterior	Septal		
1	49.0	34.1	46.6	59.8	37.0	45.3 ± 10.2
2	43.0	52.7	57.3	74.5	26.6	50.8 ± 17.7
3	44.6	6.7	0	65.2	15.0	26.3 ± 27.6
4	81.5	49.2	43.9	81.2	79.8	67.1 ± 18.8
Mean ± S.D.	54.5 ± 18.2	35.7 ± 20.9	36.9 ± 25.3	70.2 ± 9.5	39.6 ± 28.3	47.4 ± 23.4

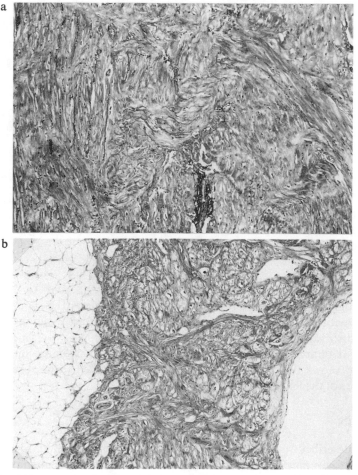

Fig. 3. Microscopic photographs showing (a) a type II myofiber disorganization in the septum, and (b) myofiber disorganization in the right ventricle. HE staining, ×100.

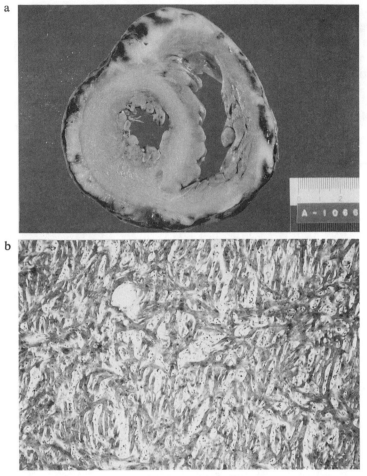

Fig. 4.   Patient no. 2: (a) gross photograph showing disproportionate thickness; (b) microscopic photograph taken from the septum showing typical myofiber disorganization. HE staining, ×100.

tion in the left ventricle was 47.4 ± 23.4 %, and in the right ventricle 39.6 ± 28.3 %.

The histologic pattern of myofiber disorganization was type II in Maron's classification[8] in all patients (Figs. 3 and 4); in particular, patient no. 3 showed a raft pattern of myofiber disorganization (Fig. 5).

Schematic diagrams of the localization of myofiber disorganization are drawn in Fig. 7, which shows that the area of disorganization tended to localize in the subendocardial zone of the left ventricles.

DISCUSSION

We have described 4 patients in whom clinical, hemodynamic, and morphologic features of hypertrophic cardiomyopathy (HCM) occurred in the absence of significant ventricular thickening, but in association with restrictive physiology as shown by cardiac catheterization.

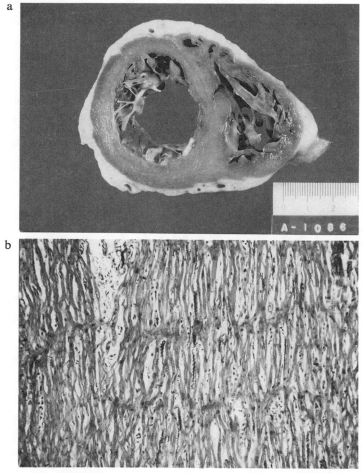

Fig. 5. Patient no. 3: (a) gross photograph showing moderately dilated left ventricle; (b) microscopic photograph taken from the septum showing raft-like appearance of myofiber disorganization. HE staining, × 100.

According to Maron et al.,[9] in order to make a diagnosis of HCM, disproportionate hypertrophy, septal disorganization, and systolic anterior motion of the anterior mitral leaflet (SAM) are essential. SAM, however, is not necessarily fundamental to recognize the morphologic hallmarks of HCM because of a clinical phenomenon under the left ventricular outflow tract obstruction (HOCM).[1] All patients in this study showed disproportionate thickening of the left ventricles and widespread myofiber disorganization, so that these 4 patients were morphologically considered to be consistent with classical HCM.

Regarding the absence of myocardial hypertrophy of more than 1.5 cm thick in the left ventricular wall, it has not been discussed yet whether HCM should be associated with a hypertrophic wall, where myofiber disorganization occurs, or not. We have previously published a report on HCM not associated with wall thickening.[10]

Normal left ventricular volume and the absence of left ventricular hypertrophy found in the present study are also essential for making a diagnosis of idiopathic RCM,[11]

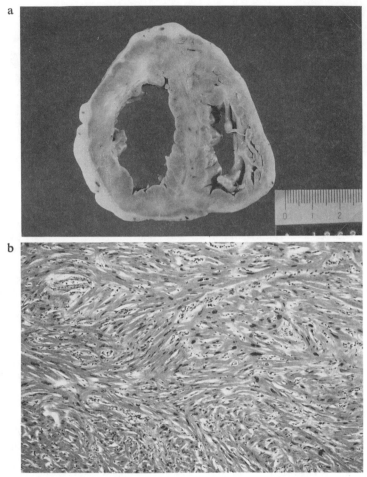

Fig. 6.   Patient no. 4: (a) gross photograph showing moderate dilation and focal fibrosis on anterior wall of left ventricle; (b) microscopic photograph taken from the left ventricular free wall showing type II myofiber disorganization. HE staining, ×100.

since the diagnostic criteria of idiopathic RCM are: 1) normal left ventricular volume and ejection fraction; 2) evidence of stiff ventricle; 3) absence of severe left ventricle hypertrophy; 4) absence of HCM; 5) histologic findings consistent with stiff ventricle; and 6) unidentifiable etiology of heart disease.[12] Therefore, it remains controversial whether idiopathic RCM may be associated with classical HCM.

On the other hand, the stiff ventricles found in our study might have resulted from myofiber disorganization, because widespread disorganization coexisting with plexiform fibrosis occurring in thin walls could be responsible for wall motion restriction, and moreover the raft pattern of myofiber disorganization seen in patient no. 3 compromised wall motion.

Waller *et al.*[14] mentioned HCM mimicking pericardial constriction or myocardial restriction. Although the patient they described had hemodynamic evidence of cardiac constriction or restriction, the mechanism by which HCM caused the hemodynamic

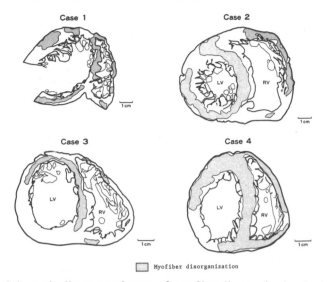

Fig. 7. Schematic diagrams of areas of myofiber disorganization in 4 patients.

alterations was uncertain, but probably was related to decreased left ventricular diastolic compliance.

In regard to the myofiber disorganization in patients with RCM, Arbustini et al.[15] reported that the irregular network of collagen fibrils and elastic fibers limits diastolic relaxation and prevents ventricular dilatation. More recently, Spirito et al.[16] wrote that the primary cardiomyopathic process in HCM may not be limited to areas of gross wall thickening, and nonhypertrophied regions of the left ventricle might contribute to impairment of diastolic function in patients with HCM.

The percentage area of fibrosis in the left ventricular wall in HCM, according to Tanaka et al.,[17] was $10.5 \pm 4.3 \%$, and therefore the 4 patients in our study showed smaller areas of fibrosis than in classical HCM. It is difficult to consider that diastolic restriction may be due to fibrosis of the left ventricle.

In 1987, Edwards[2] described RCM as encompassing 2 groups of idiopathic to ventricular filling, one associated with peripheral eosinophilia and the other not. Because of the absence of peripheral eosinophilia in our study, the 4 patients should have been included under the diagnosis of the noneosinophilic form of RCM.

REFERENCES

1. Gravanis, M.B. and Ansari, A.A. Idiopathic cardiomyopathies. A review of pathologic studies and mechanisms of pathogenesis. *Arch. Pathol. Lab. Med.* **111**: 915–929, 1987.
2. Edwards, W.D. Cardiomyopathies. *Hum. Pathol.* **18**: 625–635, 1987.
3. Wenger, N.K., Goodwin, J.F., and Roberts, W.C. Cardiomyopathy and myocardial involvement in systemic disease. In: The Heart, sixth edition. Hurt, J.W. (ed.), McGraw-Hill Book Company, 1986, pp. 1181–1248.
4. Benotti, J.R., Grossman, W., and Cohn, P.F. Clinical profile of restrictive cardiomyopathy. *Circulation* **61**: 1206–1212, 1980.
5. Roberts, W.C. and Ferrans, V.J. Pathologic anatomy of the cardiomyopathies. Idiopathic dilated and hypertrophic types, infiltrative types, and endomyocardial disease with and without eosinophilia. *Hum. Pathol.* **6**: 287–342, 1975.

6. Siegel, R.J., Shah, P.K., and Fishbein, M.C. Idiopathic restrictive cardiomyopathy. *Circulation* **70**: 165–169, 1984.

7. Davies, M.J., Pomerans, A., and Teare, R.D. Pathologic features of hypertrophic obstructive cardiomyopathy. *J. Clin. Pathol.* **27**: 529–535, 1974.

8. Maron, B.J. and Roberts, W.C. Quantitive analysis of cardiac muscle cell disorganization in the ventricular septum of patients with hypertrophic cardiomyopathy. *Circulation* **59**: 689–706, 1979.

9. Maron, B.J. and Epstein, S.E. Hypertrophic cardiomyopathy. Recent observations regarding the specificity of three hallmarks of the disease: Asymmetric septal hypertrophy, septal disorganization and systolic anterior mortion of the anterior mitral leaflet. *Am. J. Cardiol.* **45**: 141–155, 1980.

10. Yutani, C., Imakita, M., Ishibashi-Ueda, H., Nagata, S., Sakakibara, H., and Nimura, Y. Histopathological study of hypertrophic cardiomyopathy with progression to left ventricular dilation. *Acta. Pathol. Jpn.* **37**: 1041–1052, 1987.

11. Keren, A., Billingham, M.E., Weintrceub, D., Stinson, E.B., and Popp, R.L. Mildly dilated congestive cardiomyopathy. *Circulation* **72**: 302–309, 1985.

12. Hirota, Y., Kohriyama, T., Hayashi, T., Kaku, K., Nishimura, H., Saito, T., Nakayama, Y., Suwa, M., Saito, M., Kino, M., and Kawamura, K. Idiopathic restrictive cardiomyopathy: Differences of left ventricular relaxation and diastolic wave forms from constrictive pericarditis. *Am. J. Cardiol.* **52**: 421–423, 1983.

13. Anderson, K.R., St. J. Sutton, M.G., and Lie, J.T. Histopathological types of cardiac fibrosis in myocardial disease. *J. Pathol.* **128**: 79–85, 1979.

14. Waller, B.F., Maron, B.J., Morrow, A.G., and Roberts, W.C. Hypertrophic cardiomyopathy mimicking pericardial constriction or myocardial restriction. *Am. Heart J.* **102**: 790–792, 1981.

15. Arbustivi, E., Baonanno, C., Trevi, G., Pennelli, N., Ferrans, V.J., and Thiene, G. Cardiac ultrastructure in primary restrictive cardiomyopathy. *Chest* **84**: 236–238, 1983.

16. Spirito, P., Maron, B.J., Chiarella, F., Bellotti, P., Tramarin, R., Pozzoli, M., and Vecchio, C. Diastolic abnormalities in patients with hypertrophic cardiomyopathy: Relation to magnitude of left ventricular hypertrophy. *Circulation* **72**: 310–316, 1985.

17. Tanaka, M., Fujiwara, H., Onodera, T., Wu, D.J., Hamashima, Y., and Kawai, C. Quantitative analysis of myocardial fibrosis in normals, hypertensive hearts, and hypertrophic cardiomyopathy. *Br. Heart J.* **55**: 575–581, 1986.

Atrial and Ventricular Wall Properties Reflected in Filling Modes by Doppler Echocardiography in Myocardial Diseases with Restrictive Ventricular Physiology

Seiki Nagata, Shiro Izumi, Kunio Miyatake, and Yasuharu Nimura

Division of Cardiology, Hospital and Research Institute, National Cardiovascular Center, Osaka, Japan

ABSTRACT

We investigated the flow pattern in the superior caval vein and ventricular inflow by Doppler echocardiography in patients with restrictive ventricular physiology.

In the flow pattern in the superior caval vein in restrictive disease, peak velocity of the systolic wave (S wave) is smaller than that of the diastolic wave (D wave). The filling time of the S wave is shorter and that of the D wave is longer than in healthy subjects. These findings suggest that the reserve capacity of the right atrium is anatomically and functionally impaired, with a greater volume of blood flowing from the superior caval vein directly into the right ventricle, passing right through the right atrium.

Mitral inflow was characterized by a sharp peak followed by slurring in our patients with restrictive ventricular physiology. The sharpened peak of the rapid ventricular filling wave is assumed to be a specific feature of restrictive physiology.

INTRODUCTION

Restrictive cardiomyopathy is pathophysiologically characterized by impairment of distensibility of the heart wall and a dip and plateau pattern in the ventricular pressure curve.[1] Major underlying diseases in filling disturbances include restrictive cardiomyopathy, constrictive pericarditis, and some secondary myocardial diseases.[2,3]

The representative form of restrictive cardiomyopathy is endomyocardial fibrosis, as documented by Davies.[4] However, this disease is rarely observed in Japan, and therefore the present paper describes Doppler assessment of other myocardial diseases with a dip and plateau pattern of ventricular pressure curve presented in comparison with that of constrictive pericarditis. The underlying myocardial conditions were amyloidosis (three patients), hypertrophic cardiomyopathy with localized left ventricular hypertrophy, and nonspecific fibrosis documented by biopsy, surgery, or autopsy (three patients). Specific features of the patients are discussed concentrating on the flow pattern in the superior caval vein and of the ventricular inflow pattern.

DOPPLER FLOW VELOCITY IN THE SUPERIOR CAVAL VEIN

1) Specific Features of Superior Caval Vein Flow

The flow of the superior caval vein obtained by Doppler echocardiography usually consists of a systolic (S) wave and a diastolic (D) wave (Fig. 1). Here attention will focus on the peak velocity and filling time in each wave.

The flow shows a variety of patterns depending upon the underlying condition (Fig.

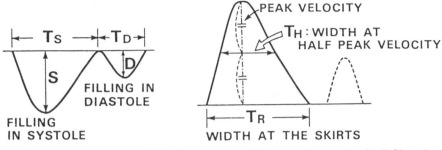

Fig. 1.   Measurements of the flow pattern of the superior caval vein (left) and of ventricular inflow wave (right).

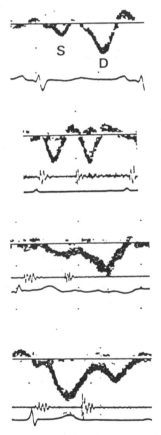

Fig. 2.   Doppler flow patterns in the superior caval vein in various conditions: from top, restrictive patients, constrictive pericarditis, lone atrial fibrillation and healthy subject.

2). In patients with restrictive physiology, the S wave is smaller than the D wave, while in healthy subjects the S wave is larger than the D wave. The flow patterns in patients with restrictive physiology are also similar to that in lone atrial fibrillation. The flow

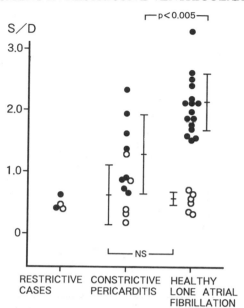

Fig. 3.   Doppler flow velocity in superior caval vein. Ratio of atrial filling in systole to that in diastole is shown. Closed circles represent the ratio in patients with sinus rhythm; open circles, that in patients with atrial fibrillation. The difference in the ratio of atrial filling in systole to that in diastole between constrictive pericarditis patients and healthy subjects with sinus rhythm was significant ($P < 0.005$); that between 2 groups with atrial fibrillation was not significant.

pattern in constrictive pericarditis is characterized by shortening of the filling time in both the S wave and the D wave.

The S-D ratio, the ratio of the peak velocity of the S wave to that of the D wave, is larger than 1.0 in healthy subjects (Fig. 3). It is smaller in constrictive pericarditis than in healthy subjects, including those with and without atrial fibrillation ($P < 0.005$). In those with atrial fibrillation, the ratio was small, regardless of the underlying condition.

2) Right Atrial Filling Time

The filling time of the S wave is shorter in constrictive pericarditis and restrictive disease patients than in healthy subjects (Fig. 4). The filling time of the D wave is longer in restrictive and lone atrial fibrillation patients than in healthy subjects, while it is shorter in constrictive pericarditis than in healthy subjects.

3) Mechanisms of Small S Wave and Tendency toward Prolonged D Wave

Possible mechanisms of small S waves are: 1) impairment of atrial contraction; 2) stiffness of the atrial wall; 3) maximal distension of the atrial wall; and 4) elevation of atrial pressure. The left atrium is usually enlarged in restrictive cases. In the present patients the echocardiographic left atrial dimensions were larger than 45 mm, and the reserve capacity of the atrium appeared to be anatomically and functionally impaired. The mechanisms of the tendency toward prolonged D waves are considered to be: 1) compensation for small S waves, *i.e.*, a greater volume of blood flows from the

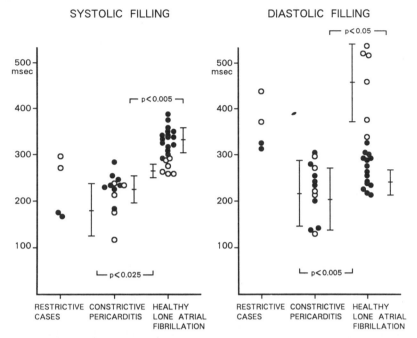

Fig. 4. Right atrial filling times in systole and diastole. Closed circles represent the filling times in patients with sinus rhythm. Open circles represent those in patients with atrial fibrillation. The differences in the systolic filling time and the diastolic filling time between constrictive pericarditis patients and healthy subjects with sinus rhythm and atrial fibrillation were significant.

superior caval vein directly into the right ventricle, passing right through the right atrium (Fig. 5); and 2) the ventricular wall retains potentiality of diastolic distension, although slow.

LEFT VENTRICULAR INFLOW PATTERN

1) Specific Pattern of Ventricular Inflow

Mitral inflow is characterized by a sharp peak in restrictive patients in comparison with that in healthy subjects.[5] However, in our patients, it was accompanied by a slurring of the descending limb. In constrictive pericarditis, the filling time measured at the "skirts" is usually shortened in both ventricles.

2) Width of Rapid Filling Wave

The width of the rapid filling wave of ventricular filling at half-peak velocity (TH) and that at the "skirts" (TR) as measured in our patients are shown in Figs. 1 and 6. In constrictive pericarditis, the width of the wave at the skirts in the right ventricle is shorter than in healthy subjects. In restrictive disease patients, the width at the half-peak velocity level in the left ventricle showed a tendency to shorten (Fig. 6). These characteristic features are more clearly demonstrated by the ratio of TH to TR (Fig. 7). The ratio in the left ventricle is significantly smaller in restrictive than in other conditions. This small ratio appears to correspond to the flow pattern of a sharp peak followed by a slurring (Fig. 5).

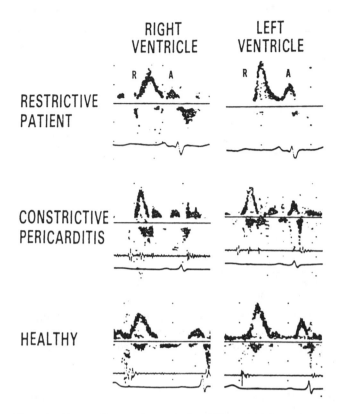

Fig. 5. Doppler flow patterns of ventricular filling wave in various conditions.

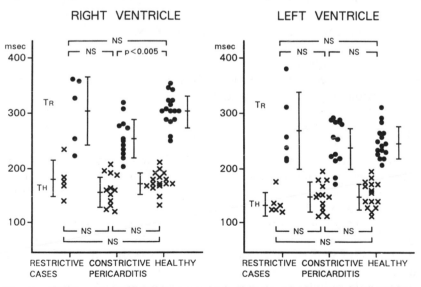

Fig. 6. Widths of rapid filling wave at half-peak velocity and at the skirts. Closed circles represent the width of rapid filling wave at the skirts (TR). Triangles represent those at the level of half peak velocity (TH). In constrictive pericarditis, the width of the wave at the skirts in the right ventricle is shorter than in that in healthy subjects.

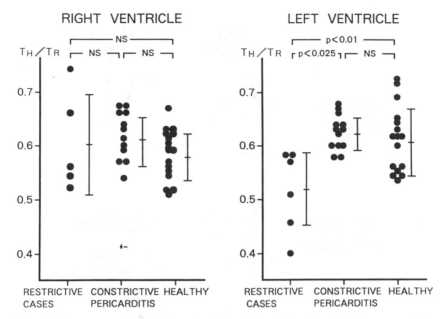

Fig. 7. Sharpness at the peak and width at the skirts of rapid filling wave. The ratio of TH to TR in the left ventricle in restrictive disease patients is significantly smaller than in constrictive pericarditis patients and healthy subjects.

The significance of the small ratio of TH to TR in restrictive patients is thought to be as follows: the sharp peak is assumed to result from high atrial pressure and impaired distensibility of the ventricular wall, although the slurring in the flow pattern shows that the ventricular wall still has the potential to distend. This is considered to correspond to the long D wave in the superior vena cava flow.

In constrictive pericarditis, the rapid filling time is shortened because of the difficulty of distension of the ventricular wall.[6] The flow pattern in restrictive patients exhibits features like those in constrictive pericarditis during the first half and like those in hypertrophic cardiomyopathy in the latter half.

DISCUSSION

A specific feature of patients with restrictive physiology appears to be that the S wave of the superior caval vein flow, *i.e.*, the atrial filling in the ventricular systole, is reduced in flow velocity and duration, and that the rapid ventricular filling wave is sharpened followed by a slurring (Fig. 8). However, Acquatella reported that the width of the rapid filling wave was shortened in patients with endomyocardial fibrosis.[7]

Appleton and coworkers reported similar results.[5] In our patients, the atrial filling wave and the rapid ventricular filling wave were generally shortened, suggesting impaired distensibility of the cardiac wall. In reference to these results, the sharpened peak of the rapid ventricular filling wave is assumed to be a specific feature of restrictive physiology. The underlying diseases were amyloidosis and hypertrophic cardiomyopathy, with hemodynamically with restrictive signs in the patients studied, who had some degree of ventricular wall hypertrophy. The slurring on the descending limb of the rapid filling wave probably resulted from this hypertrophy. If the restriction had become so intense

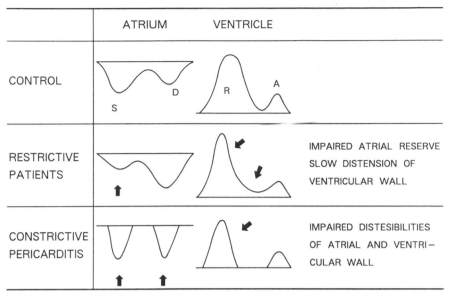

Fig. 8. Scheme of Doppler flow pattern of atrial filling wave and left ventricular inflow wave in healthy subjects, restrictive patients, and constrictive pericarditis patients.

that its effect would have overcome that of hypertrophy, the rapid filling wave might have been shortened. A few of the present patients showed a tendency toward a shortened rapid filling wave. Thus, the flow pattern of the rapid filling wave in patients with restrictive physiology might depend on the degree of restriction and wall hypertrophy.

Shortening of the atrial filling wave is assumed to result from the impaired distensibility of the atrial wall. Although the width of the atrial filling wave was observed in both our restrictive patients and those with constrictive pericarditis, the height of the wave was different in the 2 conditions. The reason for this difference is not known. It is speculated that it is related to central venous pressures in both conditions. This should be studied further in future.

REFERENCES

1. Siegel, R.J., Shah, P.K., and Fishbein, M.C. Idiopathic restrictive cardiomyopathy. *Circulation* **70**: 165–169, 1984.
2. Benotti, J.R., Grossman, W., and Cohn, P.F. Clinical profile of restrictive cardiomyopathy. *Circulation* **61**: 1206–1212, 1980.
3. Waller, B.F., Maron, B.J., Morrow, A.G., and Roberts, W.C. Hypertrophic cardiomyopathy mimicking pericardial constriction or myocardial restriction. *Am. Heart J.* **102**: 790–792, 1981.
4. Davies, J.N.P. Endocardial Fibrosis in Africans. *East African Medical Journal* **125**: 10–14, 1948.
5. Appleton, C.P., Hattle, L.K., and Popp, R.L. Demonstration of restrictive ventricular physiology by Doppler echocardiography. *JACC* **11**: 757–768, 1988.
6. Friedman, B.J., Drinkovic, N., Miles, H., Shih, W., Mazzoleni, A., and DeMaria, A.N. Assessment of left ventricular diastolic function: Comparison of Doppler echocardiography and gated blood pool scintigraphy. *JACC* **8**: 1348–1354, 1986.
7. Acquatella, H. *et al.* Echocardiographic recognition and Doppler abnormalities in eosinophilic endomyocardial disease and endomyocardial fibrosis. In this volume, pp. 35–48.

Ventricular Diastolic Function and the Pericardium

Eldon R. Smith and John V. Tyberg

Departments of Medicine and Medical Physiology, The University of Calgary, and the Cardiovascular Laboratories, Foothills Hospital, Calgary, Alberta, Canada

ABSTRACT

Ventricular end-diastolic pressure has generally been accepted as a reflection of preload. This is based on the belief that pericardial pressure is at or near zero. Recent studies have challenged this concept. Utilizing a balloon transducer (demonstrated experimentally to reflect accurately the constraining effect of the pericardium), both animal and clinical studies suggest that pericardial pressure is much greater than previously thought and not appreciably different from mean right atrial pressure. Thus, left ventricular end-diastolic pressure is not a reliable index of preload; moreover, a change in end-diastolic pressure may not be reflected by a change in preload. Whether or not pericardial pressure is increased in patients with restrictive cardiomyopathy and elevated end-diastolic pressure remains to be determined.

INTRODUCTION

Raised intracavitary end-diastolic pressure is a nonspecific but prominent feature of restrictive cardiomyopathy. Since the myocardium in restrictive cardiomyopathy is usually characterized by increased thickness (secondary to infiltration and/or fibrosis) the raised end-diastolic pressure is assumed to reflect loss of ventricular compliance. It is also accepted that the elevated filling pressure reflects the preload of the abnormal muscle. Whereas this may be so, it assumes that the external constraint on the heart (pericardial pressure) is negligible; that is, the intracavitary pressure equals the transmural pressure (preload) and increases in intracavitary pressure reflect an increase in preload.

In this paper, we will explore the validity of this concept in the light of recent observations concerning the role of the pericardium in both normal and certain disease states.

THE MEASUREMENT OF PERICARDIAL PRESSURE

Traditionally, pericardial pressure has been believed to be at or near zero and to vary little in response to alterations in cardiac volume. This concept is based primarily on the experimental observations of Kenner and Wood[1] who measured pericardial pressure with a fluid-filled catheter system and varied intracardiac pressures (and presumably volume) by alternate constriction of the pulmonary artery and aorta. Despite major changes in right atrial pressure, there was no significant change in pericardial pressure. Whereas these findings have been widely accepted, the possibility exists that the fluid-filled, open-ended catheter is not the appropriate means by which to measure pericardial pressure. Others,[2,3] in addressing the issue of pleural pressure, have been careful to distinguish between "liquid pressure," such as is measured with a fluid-filled catheter system, and "surface pressure." It is this latter pressure—actually a compressive contact stress—that is of importance when considering the function of the pericardium.

A transducer (liquid-containing flat silastic balloon) capable of measuring compressive contact stress had been previously used by Holt and coworkers[4] to measure pericardial pressure. With this device, those investigators noted a substantial increase in pericardial pressure in response to intravascular volume expansion. This finding, however, did not gain wide acceptance. Later, Smiseth et al.[5] used a similar transducer and demonstrated significant variation in pericardial pressure secondary to changes in preload and afterload in a model of left ventricular failure. Thus, 2 methods of measuring pericardial pressure (i.e., the open catheter and the balloon transducer) yielded very different results.

To develop a "gold standard" for pericardial pressure to which these 2 measurement techniques might be compared, we used a simple, static equilibrium concept. At the instant of end-diastole when all movement in the left ventricle has stopped, the blood in the cavity exerts a pressure against the endocardium which must be exactly opposed by the sum of the transmural pressure and the pericardial pressure. Thus, pericardial pressure must equal intracavitary pressure minus the transmural pressure. Moreover, with the pericardium removed (and the lungs retracted so that external constraint to the left ventricle is atmospheric pressure) transmural pressure must equal intracavitary pressure. The implication of this formulation is illustrated in Fig. 1. The upper curve depicts the diastolic portion of the pressure-volume relationship of the left ventricle with the pericardium intact. The pressure at end-diastole reflects the sum of transmural pressure and pericardial pressure. The bottom curve reflects the diastolic portion of the pressure-volume relationship after the pericardium has been removed and the volume of the ventricle adjusted to be equal at end-diastole to that in the upper curve. Thus, the end-diastolic pressure in this curve represents the transmural pressure for that ventricular volume. The end-diastolic pressure from the upper curve minus that from the lower curve (transmural pressure) represents the "theoretic" pericardial pressure.

This reasoning allowed us to conduct studies in a series of dogs[6] in which "theoretic" pressure over a range of left ventricular end-diastolic volumes was compared to measured pericardial pressure using both a fluid-filled catheter system and a liquid-containing

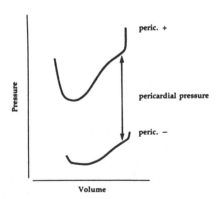

Fig. 1.   Scheme to illustrate how the theoretical value for pericardial pressure can be calculated. See text for description. Modified and reproduced with the permission of the American Heart Association.[6]

balloon. The results demonstrated that the balloon transducer measured a pressure equal to the theoretic pressure (gold standard) regardless of the presence or absence of fluid in the pericardial space. Conversely, the fluid-filled catheter system grossly underestimated pericardial pressure when the pericardium was emptied; only when there was at least 30–40 ml of fluid in the pericardium did the catheter record a pressure equal to that recorded with the balloon transducer, which was equal to the theoretic pressure. Even when we cut a number of slits in the pericardium, allowing all the fluid to drain, the balloon transducer accurately reflected pericardial pressure, whereas liquid pressure, as measured by the fluid-filled catheter, fell to zero.

On the basis of these experiments, we concluded that pericardial pressure can be accurately measured using a balloon transducer, whereas the traditional catheter system for measuring intravascular pressures seriously underestimates pericardial constraint—at least in the absence of a considerable amount of fluid within the pericardium.

PERICARDIAL PRESSURE AND RIGHT HEART FILLING PRESSURES

Although a balloon transducer can accurately measure pericardial constraint, this is not an easy device to use and is impractical for routine clinical use. An empirical observation in our laboratory has been that pericardial pressure, as measured with a balloon transducer, is not substantially different from mean right atrial or right ventricular diastolic pressure.[7] This observation implies that right ventricular end-diastolic transmural pressure is negligible in magnitude over the physiologic range of end-diastolic volumes.[8] Moreover, changes in pericardial pressure are mirrored by changes in right-sided filling pressure.[7] These observations suggested the presence of a means to estimate pericardial pressure clinically (right atrial pressure) and to calculate left ventricular end-diastolic transmural pressure (pulmonary capillary wedge minus right atrial pressure) by use of the flotation catheter.

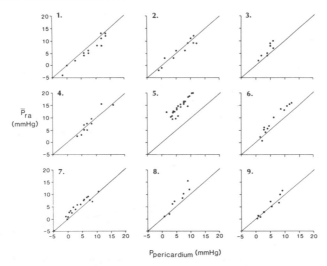

Fig. 2. Individual patient plots of mean right atrial pressure (Pra) on the ordinate versus pericardial pressure on the abscissa. The lines represent the lines of identity. In patient 5, the correlation coefficient was 0.94, although the data are shifted upward from the line of identity; this probably reflects an undetected error in baseline. Reproduced with permission of the American Heart Association.[9]

PERICARDIAL PRESSURE IN HUMANS

To determine the magnitude of pericardial pressure in humans and the correlation with right atrial pressure, 9 patients undergoing cardiac surgery were instrumented with a balloon transducer positioned in the pericardial space over the lateral left ventricle and a catheter in the right atrium.[9] Vascular volume was then expanded by infusion of crystalloid. The results are shown in Fig. 2. In each patient, there was a close linear relationship (mean $r = 0.94 \pm 0.03$) with slopes not different from unity between mean right atrial and pericardial pressure. Thus, pericardial pressure in humans is much greater than previously suspected and varies in response to changes in cardiac volume. Similar findings have also been reported by Boltwood and coworkers.[10]

THE PERICARDIUM AND LOAD-MEDIATED SHIFTS IN THE LEFT VENTRICULAR PRESSURE-VOLUME RELATION

The diastolic pressure-volume relation of the left ventricle is generally assumed to change significantly only in response to chronic processes, with the exception of interventions such as pacing in the presence of ischemia.[11] Alterations in ventricular loading conditions (e.g., vasodilator therapy) would therefore be expected to merely move the left ventricle along its diastolic pressure-volume curve. Several investigators,[12,13] however, using angiographic determination of left ventricular volume, have demonstrated that dilators, such as sodium nitroprusside and nitroglycerin, cause a parallel downward shift in the diastolic pressure-volume relation, whereas pressor agents, such as angiotensin, cause a parallel upward shift. Figure 3 illustrates this phenomenon in a patient before and after the administration of nitroglycerin. Since there is no experimental evidence that nitrates can alter the elastic properties of the myocardium, the mechanism for such an apparent improvement in left ventricular compliance has been controversial.

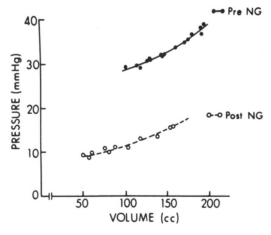

Fig. 3. The effect of nitroglycerin on the pressure-volume relationship in a patient undergoing cardiac catheterization. Pre-nitroglycerin (solid symbols), the end-diastolic pressure was approximately 40 mmHg and the ventricular volume (angiographically determined) was 190 m*l*. After nitroglycerin (open symbols) the end-diastolic pressure decreased to 15 mmHg although the volume decreased to only 160 m*l*. Modified and reproduced with permission from the American Heart Association.[12]

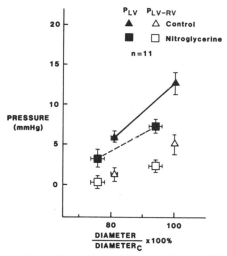

Fig. 4. Mean data from 11 patients who received sublingual nitroglycerin during cardiac catheterization. Left ventricular diameter (index of volume) was measured by echocardiography and has been normalized as a percent of control diameter at end-diastole. After administration of nitroglycerin (closed squares) the pressure-diameter relationship was shifted downward. The transmural curve (open symbols), calculated by using right ventricular diastolic pressure (Prv) as an estimate of pericardial pressure, was not shifted by nitroglycerin. Reproduced with permission of the Technical Publishing Company.[14]

One possible mechanism for such shifts could be an undetected change in pericardial pressure. We tested this hypothesis in a group of patients undergoing left and right heart catheterization.[14] Most of the patients had normal or near-normal hemodynamics at rest, with the group mean left ventricular end-diastolic pressure being 13 mmHg. Pressures were measured with catheter-tip manometers in both the right and left ventricles, with an estimate of left ventricular volume being derived from echocardiography. Recordings were obtained before and 3–5 min after the sublingual administration of nitroglycerin. Figure 4 shows the summary data from this study. The solid symbols show the mean normalized intracavitary diastolic pressure-diameter relation at the onset of diastole and at end-diastole and demonstrates a parallel downward shift after nitroglycerin, qualitatively similar to that seen in Fig. 3. The open symbols show the transmural diastolic pressure-diameter relation; left ventricular transmural pressure was estimated by subtracting right ventricular end-diastolic pressure from the instantaneous pressure in the left ventricle. Here, all data points, both before and after nitroglycerin, describe a single pressure-volume relation. Thus, nitroglycerin did not alter the elastic properties of the myocardium. Rather, the apparent improvement in left ventricular diastolic compliance resulted from an (undetected) reduction in pericardial pressure. In this way, nitroglycerin causes a major reduction in intracavitary pressure with only minor change in ventricular volume—this explains in part why nitroglycerin administration does not result in a major decrease in stroke volume, despite the often impressive decrease in filling pressure.

THE PERICARDIUM AND ACUTE LEFT VENTRICULAR FAILURE

Acute elevation of left ventricular end-diastolic pressure by volume loading in animals is largely explained by increases in pericardial pressure; transmural pressure actually changes very little. Acute myocardial infarction in humans is frequently associated with a marked increase in left ventricular end-diastolic pressure, often without depressed cardiac output. Although this has traditionally been attributed to an acute reduction in left ventricular compliance secondary to the infarcted segment, data to support this interpretation are minimal. In experimental studies,[15] the pressure-dimension relationship of acutely infarcted myocardium is shifted to the right (segment length is greater at any pressure); the relationship shifts leftward past the control values over several days, presumably secondary to developing fibrosis. Thus, it seems likely that the infarct-associated increase in left ventricular diastolic pressure reflects, at least in part, increased pericardial constraint. In support of this hypothesis is the observation that vasodilators, and particularly nitroglycerin, are very effective in reducing left ventricular filling pressure without a significant decrease in stroke volume. This would not be expected if the elevated left ventricular end-diastolic pressure reflected a true change in compliance.

THE PERICARDIUM AND CHRONIC HEART FAILURE

Whereas it has been generally accepted that the pericardium has a role in preventing acute cardiac dilation, it is obvious that in chronic heart failure the pericardium dilates progressively to accommodate larger cardiac chambers. Thus, the pericardium has not been considered important to diastolic function in chronic heart failure states. Recent data, however, suggest that this may not be true. Carroll and coworkers[16] studied a group of patients with dilated cardiomyopathy, all of whom exhibited abnormal diastolic properties. The administration of nitroprusside resulted in a significant reduction in left ventricular end-diastolic pressure; in 7 of 12 patients, this represented a parallel downward shift of the diastolic pressure-volume relation, whereas in the remainder, there was also an associated decrease in left ventricular volume. In the patients with the parallel downward shift, right atrial pressure was initially elevated and decreased by the same amount as left ventricular end-diastolic pressure, suggesting a nitroprusside-induced reduction in pericardial pressure. Herrmann and colleagues[17] obtained similar results when they studied the hemodynamic effect of a phosphodiesterase inhibitor and sodium nitroprusside. These results are in keeping with our recent observation (in an acute animal preparation) that nitroprusside decreases pericardial pressure, whereas angiotensin causes it to increase—both effects probably mediated through alteration in mesenteric venous capacitance.[18]

END-DIASTOLIC PRESSURE AND CHANGES IN PRELOAD

On the basis of both experimental and clinical studies, it seems clear that left ventricular end-diastolic (intracavitary) pressure is not an accurate indicator of preload. Moreover, as predicted by Katz,[19] changes in left ventricular end-diastolic pressure may not reflect a change in preload. In a recent study from our laboratory,[20] we assessed the effect of repeated pulmonary embolism on left ventricular performance. The embolism caused increased left ventricular end-diastolic pressure and reduced stroke work, although the dilatation of the right ventricle (secondary to increased pulmonary resistance) caused a greater increase in pericardial pressure and thereby a decrease in left ventricular transmural pressure. Thus, an increase in intracavitary end-diastolic pressure was associated with a decrease in transmural pressure; the decrease in stroke work occurred via the Frank-Starling mechanism.

THE PERICARDIUM AND RESTRICTIVE CARDIOMYOPATHY

We are unaware of any data that directly address this issue. The abnormal myocardial structure in this group of conditions would be expected to be less compliant than normal muscle; that is, ventricular intracavitary end-diastolic pressure should more closely reflect transmural pressure. However, since the atria are frequently dilated with markedly elevated pressures, pericardial pressure may also be substantially increased. Should this prove to be so, left ventricular intracavitary diastolic pressure would not provide an accurate reflection of the compliance characteristic of the myocardium. Moreover, changes in end-diastolic pressure would not necessarily reflect alterations in preload.

REFERENCES

1. Kenner, H.M. and Wood, E.H. Intrapericardial, intrapleural and intracardiac pressures during acute heart failure in dogs studied without thoracotomy. *Circ. Res.* **19**: 1071–1079, 1966.
2. Agostoni, E. Mechanics of the pleural space. *Physiol. Ref.* **52**: 57–128, 1972.
3. Permutt, S., Caldini, P., Bane, H.N., Howard, P., and Riley, R.L. Liquid pressure versus surface pressure of the esophagus. *J. Appl. Physiol.* **23**: 927–933, 1967.
4. Holt, J.P., Rhode, E.A., and Kines, H. Pericardial and ventricular pressure. *Circ. Res.* **8**: 1171–1180, 1960.
5. Smiseth, O.A., Refsum, H., Junemann, M., Sievers, R.E., Lipton, M.J., Carlsson, E., and Tyberg, J.V. Ventricular diastolic pressure-volume shifts during acute ischemic left ventricular failure in dogs. *J. Am. Coll. Cardiol.* **3**: 966–977, 1984.
6. Smiseth, O.A., Frais, M.A., Kingma, I., Smith, E.R., and Tyberg, J.V. Assessment of pericardial constraint in dogs. *Circulation* **71**: 158–164, 1985.
7. Smiseth, O.A., Refsum, H., and Tyberg, J.V. Pericardial pressure assessed by right atrial pressure: A basis for calculation of left ventricular transmural pressure. *Am. Heart J.* **108**: 603–608, 1984.
8. Traboulsi, M., Scott-Douglas, N.W., Smith, E.R., and Tyberg, J.V. Measurement of right ventricular transmural pressure. *Clin. Invest. Med.* **10**(5): C33, 1987.
9. Tyberg, J.V., Taichman, G.C., Smith, E.R., Douglas, N.W.S., Smiseth, O.A., and Keon, W.J. The relationship between pericardial pressure and right atrial pressure: An intraoperative study. *Circulation* **73**: 428–432, 1986.
10. Boltwood, C.M., Skulsky, A., Drinkwater, D.C., Lang, S., Mulder, D.G., and Shah, P.M. Intraoperative measurement of pericardial constraint: Role in ventricular diastolic mechanics. *J. Am. Coll. Cardiol.* **8**: 1289–1297, 1986.
11. Serizawa, T., Carabello, B.A., and Grossman, W. Effect of pacing-induced ischemia on left ventricular diastolic pressure-volume relations in dogs with coronary stenoses. *Circ. Res.* **46**: 430–439, 1980.
12. Ludbrook, P.A., Byrne, J.D., and McKnight, R.D. Influence of right ventricular hemodynamics on left ventricular diastolic pressure-volume relationships in man. *Circulation* **59**: 21–31, 1979.
13. Alderman, E.L. and Glantz, S.A. Acute hemodynamic interventions shift the diastolic pressure-volume curve in man. *Circulation* **54**: 662–671, 1976.
14. Kingma, I., Smiseth, O.A., Belenkie, I., Knudtson, M.L., MacDonald, R.P.R., Tyberg, J.V., and Smith, E.R. A mechanism for the nitroglycerin-induced downward shift of the left ventricular diastolic pressure-diameter relation. *Am. J. Cardiol.* **57**: 673–677, 1986.
15. Theroux, P., Ross, J., Jr., Franklin, D., Covell, J.W., Bloor, C.M., and Sasayama, S. Regional myocardial function and dimensions early and late after myocardial infarction in the unanesthetized dog. *Circ. Res.* **40**: 158–165, 1977.
16. Carroll, J.D., Lang, R.M., Neumann, A.L., Borow, K.M., and Rajfer, S.I. The differential

effects of positive inotropic and vasodilator therapy on diastolic properties in patients with congestive cardiomyopathy. *Circulation* **74**: 815–825, 1986.

17. Herrmann, H.C., Ruddy, T.D., Dec, G.W., Strauss, H.W., Boucher, C.A., and Fifer, M.A. Diastolic function in patients with severe heart failure: Comparison of the effect of enoximone and nitroprusside. *Circulation* **75**: 1214–1221, 1987.

18. Smiseth, O.A., Manyari, D.E., Lima, J.A., Scott-Douglas, N.W., Kingma, I., Smith, E.R., and Tyberg, J.V. Modulation of vascular capacitance by angiotensin and nitroprusside: A mechanism of changes in pericardial pressure. *Circulation* **76**: 875–883, 1987.

19. Katz, L.N. Analysis of the several factors regulating the performance of the heart. *Physiol. Rev.* **35**: 91–106, 1955.

20. Belenkie, I., Dani, R., Smith, E.R., and Tyberg, J.V. Ventricular interaction during experimental acute pulmonary embolism. *Circulation* **80**: 178–188, 1989.

Incidence of Each Clinical Type of Specific Heart Muscle Disease Studied by Endomyocardial Biopsy

Morie Sekiguchi,* Michiaki Hiroe,** Kiyomi Yamane,*** Shin-ichi Nunoda,**** and Minoru Hongo****

* The Heart Institute of Japan, Tokyo Women's Medical College, Tokyo, Japan
** Department of Radiology, Tokyo Women's Medical College, Tokyo, Japan
*** Department of Neurology, Tokyo Women's Medical College, Tokyo, Japan
**** The First Department of Internal Medicine, Shinshu University School of Medicine, Matsumoto, Japan

INTRODUCTION

In the recognition of heart muscle diseases, classification into hypertrophic (thickened) ventricular wall or dilated ventricular cavity is unproblematic.[1] However, difficulties arise when restrictive or electric (arrhythmias and/or conduction disturbances) disorders are seen and the clinician wants to know what type of heart muscle disease is present.[1-3] Endomyocardial biopsy[4-21] has solved this problem in many cases. For instance, a patient with complete right bundle branch block with left axis deviation was proven to have myocardial sarcoidosis.[9,10]

In this article, results of our trial in classifying the main clinical features of the 85 cases with specific heart muscle diseases are given in order to clarify the incidence of each clinical type and to stress the importance of the existence of the electric disturbance type of heart muscle disease.[11-15]

MATERIALS AND METHODS

In our series of studies in heart muscle diseases, patients who had obvious heart disease with or without symptoms underwent endomyocardial biopsy.[4-6] The purpose of the study was to establish the diagnosis or to investigate the pathomorphological background of heart muscle disease for a more precise understanding of possible treatment. The clinical features which we have taken into consideration for the study are cardiomegaly by roentgenogram, advanced arrhythmias or conduction disturbances, and obviously abnormal electrocardiograms and/or echocardiograms. When such abnormalities were found in patients with specific heart muscle diseases,[1,2] they underwent cardiac catheterization and right and/or left ventricular biopsy. Thereafter, routine histopathologic and, when needed, ultrastructural investigations were performed.

RESULTS

The biopsy findings were useful in establishing the diagnosis of specific heart muscle diseases because of the definitive pathomorphological and/or ultrastructural changes in 28 of 59 cases analyzed (Figs. 1–3). In many of the cases, the findings were not specific. However, significant pathology was seen by the biopsy in 22 out of the 31 cases where some pathological changes were observed (Fig. 4). Incorporating the diagnostic criteria for hypertrophic, dilated, restrictive and electric disturbance type of cardiomyopathy,[1]

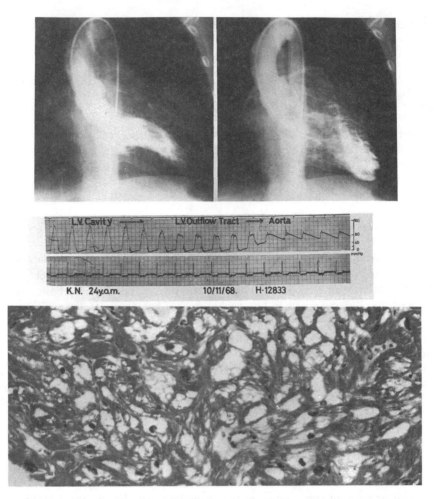

Fig. 1. An example case of hypertrophic type specific heart muscle disease. Note a marked left ventricular wall thickening in an anteroposterior view of a ventriculogram. A withdrawal precessure tracing from the left ventricle to the aorta revealed idiopathic hypertrophic subaortic stenosis. This 24-year-old male patient was finally diagnosed as having glycogenosis type III. A right ventricular biopsy reveals a lacework structure due to glycogen deposition.

the cases we studied could be classified into the four types (Table 1).[13] There were some overlapping in classifying the cases; however, they were categorized into the four types according to the main clinical features.

DISCUSSION

We were able to classify the cases with specific heart muscle disease into the hypertrophic, dilated, restrictive, and electric disturbance types. It was especially evident in cases with cardiac sarcoidosis[9,10] or in postmyocarditic disease where intraventricular conduction disturbance such as right branch block plus left axis deviation were common. As described by Puigbo *et al.*,[22] sick sinus syndrome (SSS), atrio-ventricular or

TABLE 1.   The Incidence of Each of the Clinical Type in Specific Heart Muscle Diseases

Disease	n	Hypertro.	Dilated	Restr.	Electric	Others
Sarcoidosis	20	0	3	0	14	3
Amyloidosis	27	16	1	6	7	4
Neuro-muscular disease	6	0	2	0	2	2
Eosinophilic heart disease	15	0	4	3	3	5
Myocarditis						
convalescent	10	0	1	0	7	2
Collagen disease	7	0	1	0	2	4

Hypertro.: hypertrophic, Restr.: restrictive

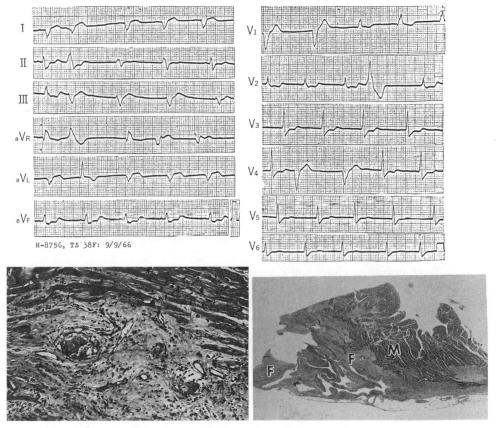

Fig. 2.   A case of cardiac sarcoidosis proven by right ventricular endomyocardial biopsy. An electrocardiogram reveals sinus arrest, complete right bundle
branch block with right axis deviation and premature ventricular contractions.
The biopsy revealed sarcoid granuloma in the myocardium (left lower). This
patient died suddenly at a later time, and the autopsy revealed a marked myocardial fibrosis (F) in the right side of the interventricular septum as well as in
the right ventricular free wall.

intraventricular conduction abnormalities, ventricular arrhythmias may be seen decades
after initial Chagasic myocarditis. Our analysis of cases with SSS showed that about
24% of the patients (18 out of 74) had a history of diphtheria in childhood, although
they had no concomitant heart disease at the time of infection.[23]

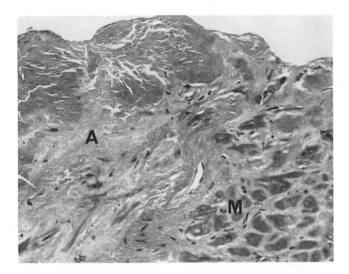

Fig. 3.   An example of a biopsy-proven case of cardiac amyloidosis (57-year-old male) with marked amyloid deposition (A) in the endomyocardium is seen in the left half of this micrograph. Only a small number of myocytes (M) are observable.

Patients who suffer from grave conditions such as congestive heart failure and ventricular arrhythmias presumably die at the acute stage, and therefore only the patients who suffer from atrial disease survive. The SSS may develop decades after the initial infection with diphtheria.

These facts regarding childhood disease with diphtheria may be applicable to viral myocarditis. In view of our experience, arrhythmias or conduction disturbances can be seen at the time of the postmyocarditic stage.[16-21] In our observation in performing serial biopsy in cases with viral or idiopathic myocarditis, we found that in 10 out of the 16 cases, recovery of the electrocardiographic changes was striking, and it returned to normal configuration in 3 cases. Another 6 cases showed either persistent A-V conduction disturbance or complete right bundle branch block plus left axis deviation. The patients were doing fairly well with or without pacemakers. A radionuclide follow-up study revealed that in all of the 10 cases, there was either depression or no rise of the ejection fraction after the ergometer exercise testing, and also there were defects in thallium scintigraphy in 7 cases. This indicates that subclinical heart disease is present.

In a nation-wide Japanese survey on cardiac sarcoidosis in 72 cases which consisted of 52 with fatal myocardial sarcoidosis and 20 cases of clinically diagnosed cardiac sarcoidosis, there were many cases where conduction disturbances such as complete A-V block, right bundle branch block, and ventricular arrhythmias were present.[9] We consider that many of the cases were not classifiable to any of the hypertrophic, dilated, and restrictive forms of heart muscle diseases, but were easily put into the group of electric disturbance (Fig. 5).

Literature reviews from other investigators[24] as well as our own may indicate that there exists an electric disturbance type of heart muscle disease.

It is well known that in amyloid heart disease, restrictive hemodynamics[2,3,25] are observed (Figs. 6, 7), and this gives us important concepts in the understanding of restric-

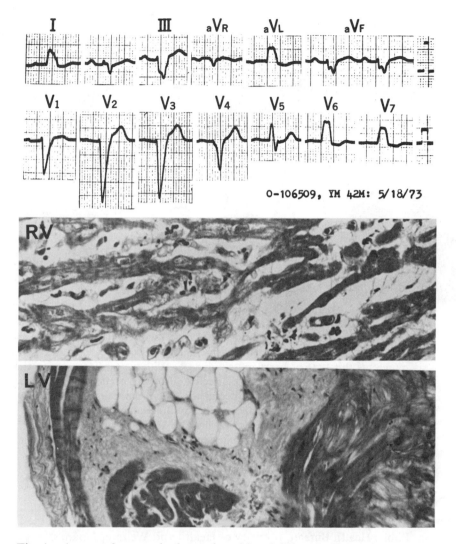

Fig. 4. A case of myotonic dystrophy with a left bundle branch block electrocardiogram underwent right (RV) and left (LV) endomyocardial biopsy. Interstitial fibrosis as well as fatty tissue infiltration and atrophic myocytes were observed the RV, and fibrosis and fatty tissue in the subendocardial myocardium in the LV biopsy.

tive cardiomyopathy.[3] We are postulating the importance of observing the clinical course of the disease as it progresses (Fig. 6).[30]

Recognition of restrictive heart muscle disease defines a problem. We found restrictive ventricular physiology in 6/27 (22.2%) of amyloid heart disease and 3/14 (21.4 %) in eosinophilic heart disease.

CARDIAC MANIFESTATIONS IN SARCOIDOSIS

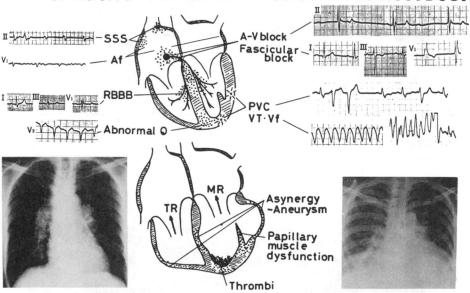

Fig. 5. A diagramatic representation of electric (arrhythmia and/or conduction disturbance) disorders in specific heart muscle diseases. Cardiac sarcoidosis represents this type of heart muscle disease. Without cardiomegaly in the chest X-ray picture, various forms of electric disorders occur because of the infiltration of the sarcoidosis (see dotted area). With a more diffuse infiltration, ventricles may develop dilatation and cardiac dysfunction may result.
SSS: sick sinus syndrome. Af: atrial fibrillation. RBBB: right bundle branch block. PVC: premature ventricular contraction. VT: ventricular tachycardia. Vf: ventricular fibrillation, TR and MR: tricuspid and mitral regurgitation.

ACKNOWLEDGEMENT

This work was supported in part by a Research Grant from the Intractable Diseases Division, Public Health Bureau, Ministry of Health and Welfare, Japan.

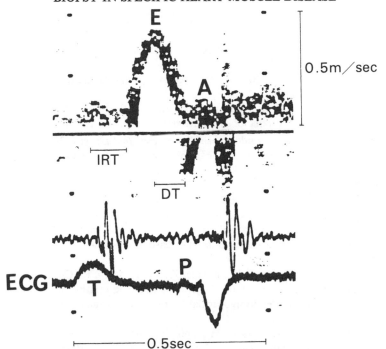

Fig. 6. A typical picture of restrictive ventricular physiology shown by a pulsed wave Doppler echocardiographic recording of the left ventricular inflow.

Note the restrictive flow pattern with increased E/A and short IRT and DT. (E: peak velocity of left ventricular rapid filling, A: peak velocity during atrial contraction, IRT: isovolunic relaxation time, DT: deceleration time)

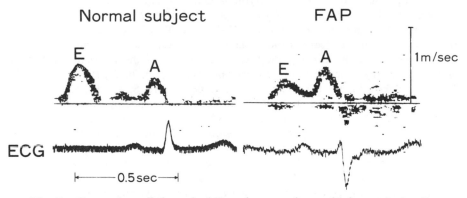

Fig. 7. Comparison of the pulsed Doppler wave form of left ventricular diastolic flow velocity in a healthy control (41 years old) and in a 38-year-old patient with familial amyloid polyneuropathy (FAP) who showed no evidence of overt heart disease or restrictive ventricular physiology in routine cardiological studies.

Note that the peak flow velocity during atrial contraction (A) is higher than the peak velocity of left ventricular rapid filling (E) in the FAP patient. This suggests that in patients with cardiac amyloidosis without restrictive heart muscle disease, abnormal left ventricular diastolic filling manifested by a reduction in the rate and volume of rapid diastolic filling with enhanced atrial contraction can be seen in the early stage of the disease. (From Kinoshita et al.,[28] reproduced with permission.)

REFERENCES

1. Report of the WHO/ISFC task force on the definition and classification of cardiomyopathies. *Br. Heart J.* **44**: 672–673, 1980.
2. Symons, C., Evans, T., and Mitchell, A.G. (eds.). Specific Heart Muscle Disease, Wright. PSG, Bristol, London, Boston, 1983.
3. Hirota, Y., Shimizu, G., Kita, Y., Kawamura, K., and Sekiguchi, M. Spectrum of restrictive cardiomyopathy: A report of the national survey. In this volume, pp. 275–284.
4. Sakakibara, S. and Konno, S. Endomyocardial biopsy. *Jap. Heart J.* **3**: 537–543, 1962.
5. Konno, S. and Sakakibara, S. Endomyocardial biopsy. *Dis. Chest* **44**: 345–350, 1963.
6. Konno, S., Sekiguchi, M., and Sakakibara, S. Catheter biopsy of the heart. *Radiol. Clin. North Am.* **9**: 491–510, 1971.
7. Sekiguchi, M., Hiroe, M., Ogasawara, S., and Nishikawa, T. Practical aspects of endomyocardial biopsy. *Ann. Acad. Med. Singappore* **10** (suppl.): 115–128, 1981.
8. O'Connell, J.B., Robinson, J.A., Subramanlian, R., and Scanlon, P.J. Endomyocardial biopsy: Technique and applications in heart disease of unknown cause. *Heart Transplantation* **3**: 132–143, 1984.
9. Sekiguchi, M., Numao, Y., Imai, M., Furuie, T., and Mikami, R. Clinical and histopathological profile of sarcoidosis of the heart and acute idiopathic myocarditis. Concepts through a study employing endomyocardial biopsy. I. Sarcoidosis. *Jpn. Circul. J.* **44**: 249–263, 1980.
10. Sekiguchi, M., Kaneko M., Hiroe M., and Hirosawa, K. Recent trends in cardiac sarcoidosis research in Japan. *Heart and Vessels* Suppl. 1: 45–49, 1985.
11. Sekiguchi, M., Hasumi, M., Hiroe, M., Kasanuki, H., Ohnishi, S., and Hirosawa, K. On the existence of non-hypertrophic, non-dilated cardiomyopathy as assessed by endomyocardial biopsy and a proposal for the term "electric disturbance type of cardiomyopathy". *Circulation* **72**: suppl. III-156, 1985.
12. Take, M., Sekiguchi, M., Hiroe, M. and Hirosawa, K. A clinicopathologic study on a cause of idiopathic cardiomyopathy and arrythmia and conduction disturbance employing endomyocardial biopsy. *Heart and Vessels* Suppl. 1: 159–164, 1985.
13. Sekiguchi, M., Hiroe, M., Hasumi, M., Nishikawa, T., Ohnishi, S., Kasanuki, H., and Hirosawa, K. Endomyocardial biopsy approach to various arrhythmias and condition disturbances: In: Proceedings of the Free Paper Session of the International Symposium on Cardiac Arrhythmias, Iwa T. (ed.) Excerpta Medica, pp. 76–79, 1987.
14. Take, M., Sekiguchi, M., Hiroe, M., Suzuki, S., Ogasawara, S., Omori, M., Hirosawa, K., Shirai, T., Ishide, T., and Okubo, S. Clinical spectrum and endomyocardial biopsy findings in eosinophilic heart disease. *Heart and Vessels* Suppl. 1: 243–249, 1985.
15. Hasegawa, A., Sekiguchi, M., Take, M., Hasumi, M., Hosoda, S., and Hiroe, M. Incidence of clinically diagnosed ECM (electric disturbance type of cardiomyopathy) cases in our 20 year study of cardiomyopathies. *Heart and Vessels* Suppl. 3, 1990. (in press)
16. Sekiguchi, M., Hiroe, M., Take, M., and Hirosawa, K. Clinical and histopathological profile of sarcoidosis of the heart and acute idiopathic myocarditis. Concepts through a study employing endomyocardial biopsy. II. Myocarditis. *Jpn. Circul. J.* **44**: 264–273, 1980.
17. Sekiguchi, M., Yu, Z.-X., Hasumi, M., Hiroe, M., Morimoto, S., and Nishikawa, T. Histopathologic and ultrastructural observations of acute and convalescent myocarditis. A serial endomyocardial biopsy study. *Heart and Vessels* Suppl 1: 143–153, 1985.
18. Yu, Z.-X., Sekiguchi, M., Hiroe, M., Take, M., and Hirosawa, K. Histopathological findings of acute and convalescent myocarditis obtained by serial endomyocardial biopsy. *Jpn. Circ. J.* **48**: 1368–1374, 1984.
19. Sekiguchi, M., Hiroe, M., Hiramitsu, S., and Izumi, T. Natural history of acute viral or idiopathic myocarditis: A clinical and endomyocardial biopsy follow-up. In: New Concepts in Viral Heart Disease: Virology, Immunology and Clinical Management. Schultheiss, H.-P. (ed.) Springer, pp. 33–50, 1988.

20. Take, M., Sekiguchi, M., Hiroe, M., and Hirosawa, K. Long-term follow-up of electocardiographic findings in patients with acute myocarditis proven by endomyocardial biopsy. *Jpn. Circ. J.* **46**: 1127–1234, 1982.
21. Hiroe, M., Sekiguchi, M., Take, M., Kusakabe, K., Shigeta, A., and Hirosawa, K. Long follow-up study in patients with prior myocarditis by radionuclide methods. *Heart and Vessels* Suppl. 1: 199–203, 1985.
22. Puigbo, J.J. Chagas' disease: Overview and perspectives. In this volume, pp. 341–354.
23. Sekiguchi, M., Nishino, H., Nishikawa, T., Morimoto, S., and Hiroe, M. An age-associated myocardial changes in various heart diseases. A clinicopathologic analysis in biopsied and autopsied myocardium. *Jpn. Circul. J.* **50**: 1023–1032, 1986.
24. James, T.N. Structure and function of the AV junction. *Jpn. Circul. J.* **47**: 1–47, 1983.
25. Chew, C., Ziady, G.M., Raphael, M.J. and Oakley, C.M. The functional defect in amyloid heart disease: the "stiff heart" syndrome. *Am. J. Cardiol.* **36**, 438–414, 1975.
26. Hongo, M. and Ikeda, S. Echocardiographic assessment of the evolution of amyloid heart disease: a study with familial amyloid polyneuropathy. *Circulation* **73**: 249–256, 1986.
27. Hongo, M., Fujii, T., Hirayama, J., Kinoshita, O., Tanaka, M., and Okubo, S. Radionuclide angiographic assessment of left ventricular diastolic filling in amyloid heart disease: A study of patients with familial amyloid polyneuropathy. *J. Am. Coll. Cardiol.* **13**: 48–53, 1989.
28. Kinoshita, O., Hongo, M., Yamada, H., Misawa, T., Kono, J., Okubo, S., and Ikeda, S. Impaired left ventricular diastolic filling in patients with familial amyloid polyneuropathy: A pulsed Doppler echocaidiographic study. *Br. Heart J.* **61**: 198–203, 1989.
29. Hongo, M., Kono, J., Okubo, S., Yamada, H., Misawa, T., and Kinoshita, O. Left ventricular systolic and diastolic time intervals in familial amyloid polyneuropathy. *Jpn. Circ. J.* **53**: 291–297, 1989.
30. Hongo, M., Misawa, T., Kinoshita, O., Yamada, H., Kono, J., Okubo, S., and Sekiguchi, M. Computerized M-mode echocardiographic assessment of left ventricular diastolic function in patients with familial amyloid polyneuropathy. *Jpn. Circ. J.* **54**:32–42, 1990.

Pathologic Aspects of Specific Heart Muscle Diseases with Restrictive and/or Electric Disorders

Ulrik Baandrup, Svend Aage Mortensen,** and Søren Høyer****

* University Institute of Pathology, Aarhus Kommunehospital, Aarhus, Denmark
** Department of Medicine B, Rigshospitalet, Copenhagen, Denmark
*** Department of Pathology, Sahlgrenska Sjukhuset, Gothenburg, Sweden

ABSTRACT

The term "restrictive" is used clinically when there is normal or nearly normal contractile function but impaired diastolic relaxation of the cardiac ventricles. The hemodynamic changes may be fickle and transient. The pathology includes a wide range of myocardial disorders, which will be illustrated with emphasis on the role of endomyocardial biopsy. Some of the disorders are rare or extremely rare.

The main focus is on (inborn) errors of metabolism, amyloid heart disease, and toxic conditions (Adriamycin).

Electric disorders may be combined with all of the disorders depending on the extent and target of the lesions. Electrophysiologic examination is mandatory if functional and structural changes are to be assessed and compared.

INTRODUCTION

Specific heart muscle diseases are defined as being of known cause or associated with disorders of other systems.[1] The term "restrictive" is used clinically when there is normal or nearly normal contractile function but impaired diastolic relaxation of the cardiac ventricles (mainly the left). Despite careful clinical, noninvasive, hemodynamic assessment of patients with restrictive/constrictive physiology, the differentiation of restrictive/obliterative endomyocardial disease from constrictive pericarditis remains difficult.[2] Further, these hemodynamic characteristics may be transient or "muddled" with other patterns, *e.g.*, congestion.

The pathology includes a wide spectrum of myocardial disorders. Some are rare or extremely rare, but the introduction of the endomyocardial biopsy procedure has made it possible to diagnose these disorders more frequently and also facilitated differential diagnosis.

METABOLIC DISORDERS

In only few of the metabolic disorders is the restrictive/infiltrative element dominant; often, however, it may be part of the hemodynamic pattern. In most instances, congestive heart failure is the end-stage, frequently due to concomitant valvar and/or vessel involvement.

As a general rule it should be stated that biochemical analysis of blood, urine, and tissue is necessary to categorize these various disorders correctly. There may be a characteristic, suggestive pattern of clinical and/or morphologic changes, but several are extremely rare (Pompe's disease, infantile type, one well-known disorder, is found in

TABLE 1. (Inborn) Errors of Metabolism

Diseases of carbohydrate metabolism	
Glycogen storage diseases	type IIa*
	type III*
Mucopolysaccharidoses	
Mucolipidoses	
Hyperoxaluria	
Diseases of amino acid and protein metabolism	
Ochronosis	
Homocystinuria	
Hemoglobinopathies	
Gout	
Amyloidosis	
Diseases of lipid metabolism	
Hyperlipoproteinemias	
Familial lipoprotein deficiency	
Storage of cholesterol and phytanic acid	
Sphingolipidoses and gangliosideroses	Fabry's disease*
Ceroid lipofuscinoses*	
Carnitine deficiency*	

Diseases of iron, copper, and calcium* metabolism

* See text.

1 of 145,000–246,000 live-borns) and the literature often consists of casuistic reports. This makes scrupulous and careful examination desirable whenever these disorders are suspected, including electron microscopic examination, and whenever possible histochemical and immunopathologic techniques.

The following text is limited to a table in brief (Table 1), and only a few disorders will be commented on in some detail. More have already been described (*e.g.*, Ref. 3) than can be found in standard textbooks on the topic (*e.g.*, Ref. 4), and certainly many more will be uncovered as studies continue. Histologic examination per se will not suffice; the use of refined biochemical/genetic methods are essential.

Glycogen Storage Disease Type IIa (*Pompe's Disease*)

The patient was a 1.5-year-old girl who developed normally during the first 6 months after birth, but subsequently showed signs of gradually increasing muscular hypotonia and failure to thrive. Her mental development was considered normal. She had several infections. Chest X-ray showed severe cardiac enlargement, and hypertrophic cardiomyopathy was suggested. The diagnosis was established by the very low activity of α-glucosidasis and as much as 0.9 glycogen/g protein in skeletal muscle, compared to the normal value which is below 0.01 g/g protein. At the age of one year cardiac failure was evident. The girl was treated with digitalis and diuretics, but died from viral pneumonitis. There was no familial history of metabolic disease.

At autopsy the heart showed severe biventricular hypertrophy (130 g, body weight 9.0 kg). The left ventricular endocardium was diffusely thickened and the myocardium was grayish-white and very stiff in both chambers. Microscopically the endocardium

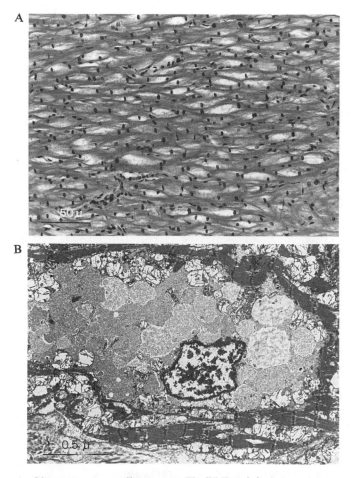

Fig. 1. A. Glycogen storage disease type IIa (H-E staining).
B. Glycogen storage disease type IIa, membrane-bound accumulation of glycogen (electron microscopy).

was thickened with lamellar elastic fibers, typical of elastofibrosis. Light microscopy
of the myocardium revealed severe myocyte vacuolization (Fig. 1a), which in cryostat
sections stained positively with PAS stain. Electronmicroscopically, the perinuclear
spaces were filled with membrane-limited structures containing a fine granular material
considered to be glycogen (Fig. 1b). Depositions of the same kind were found in the
liver, tubular epithelium of the kidneys, peripheral muscles, and neurons of the central
nervous system.

Glycogen Storage Disease Type III (Forbes' Disease)
    The disease is rarely symptomatic in the neonatal period. It is difficult to distinguish
clinically from type I (von Gierke's disease). The enzymatic deficiency is of amylo-1,
6-glucosidase, and amylo-1, 4→1, 4-glucan transferase. Involvement of the heart is seen
in about one-quarter of patients, but may even in those cases be asymptomatic.
    In our patient, a male 35 years old at the time of writing, glycogenosis, probably of

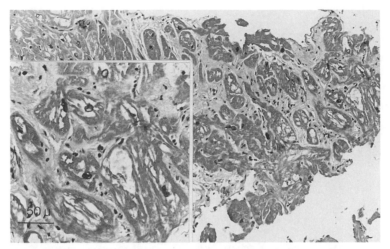

Fig. 2.   Glycogen storage disease type III (H-E staining).
Insert shows the vacuolated myocytes at larger magnification.

type I, had been diagnosed at the age of 11. At that time there was hepatomegaly and muscular weakness. The diagnosis was based on liver and skeletal muscle biopsies. In the following years he did well until a few years ago, when there was progression of the muscular weakness and at the same time signs of cardiac insufficiency. The patient had developed cardiomegaly. The coronary arteries were normal, but he had angina at effort. ECG showed left ventricular hypertrophy and strain. At exercise there was normal lactate production in the heart after 5 min, but later there was increased citrate release, indicating impaired glycogenolysis. These changes combined with the findings at light and electronmicroscopic investigation of endomyocardial biopsies (Fig. 2) (vacuoles; ultrastructurally normal-looking cytosolic glycogen deposits) pointed at type III, which was then confirmed by biochemical investigation.

A similar case was described by Olson *et al.*[5] in 1984.

Amyloidosis (Amyloid Deposits)—The β-Fibrilloses

An excellent review article on the topic of amyloid deposits and amyloidosis was published by Glenner.[6] Some of the mystery about the character of the "waxy, eosinophilic" tissue deposits, which Virchow believed in 1853 to be of polysaccharide composition and consequently designated as "amyloid" (starch-like or cellulose-like), has now been lit and has yielded to investigations employing a variety of chemical and physical techniques. Amyloid accumulation is not the consequence of a single disease process, and amyloidosis is not a single disease entity but a variety of different disease processes (Table 2). The unifying definition of amyloid deposits is that they are aggregates of proteinaceous, twisted β-pleated sheet fibrils of chemical diversity. This chemical diversity, however, is such that specific chemical types can be closely related to distinct clinicopathologic conditions.

Once the nature of the amyloid fibril protein is known, a simplified scheme recommended for the preliminary classification of amyloid syndromes can describe the disease in protein terms and further categorize it by one of three possible designations: associated with an underlying disease (*e.g.*, tuberculosis), familial, or idiopathic (*e.g.*, senile cardiomyopathy).

TABLE 2. Nosologic Classification of Amyloidosis

	Major fibril protein
Acquired systemic amyloidosis	
Immunologic dyscrasias with amyloidosis	AL
Reactive systemic amyloidosis	AA
Heredofamilial systemic amyloidosis	
(more subtypes)	
Organ limited amyloidosis	
e.g., cardiovascular (several subtypes)	
Localized deposition	
e.g., endocrine	
e.g., senile (cardiac, cerebral)	

AL, amyloid light chain; AA, amyloid associated (protein).

Incidence: The acquired β-fibrilloses disease complex (acquired amyloid deposits and acquired systemic amyloidosis) is directly associated with more morbid processes than is almost any other pathologic condition, and has greater clinical importance than previously appreciated. Amyloidosis is associated with rheumatoid arthritis in approximately 5% to 11% of patients. Although the incidence of systemic amyloidosis was reported to be 0.6% to 0.7% in one hospital population, the worldwide incidence of this disease complex is completely unknown.

The most common site of amyloid deposition outside the central nervous system in the elderly is the cardiovascular system, which is involved in so-called senile cardiac amyloidosis. The reported overall incidence is about 2.0%, with the frequency increasing to 50% after the age of 90 years. In this condition the amyloid distribution predominantly involves the heart: first the atrial myocardium, then the ventricles, and finally the aorticopulmonary trees.

Frederiksen et al.[7] in 1962 described a Danish family with a unique form of familial amyloid cardiac diasease which became clinically manifest between the ages of 30–40 years. Preliminary characterization of the amyloid protein[8] showed a partial amino acid sequence of a cyanogen bromide fragment, which corresponded to that in positions 14 to 19 in normal prealbumin. Nordlie et al.[9] have reported on the sequence of another fragment from the same patient which was shown to contain a single amino acid substitution of methionine for leucine in position 111.

Several families with occurrence of autosomal dominant amyloidosis like this Danish family have now been described. The fibril protein in the amyloid substance has been shown to be different variants of prealbumin. All amyloid proteins of this kind contain a single amino acid substitution derived from a single base change. If a DNA probe can be established it may be possible to carry out genetic mapping of live family members and thus by genetic counselling avoid continuation of the disorder.

Ceroid-Lipofuscinoses (Formerly Known as Amaurotic Idiocy)

Ceroid lipofuscinoses are rare disorders of autosomal recessive inheritance. The central nervous system is the target organ. Only very few reports refer to the accumulation of lipopigment in the heart of these patients. We described the morphology of the heart from all 13 patients in Denmark who died within a 7-year period[10] (Table 3). All compartments of the heart were involved, including the conduction system. Not only was very substantial deposition of lipopigment found in the myocytes (Fig. 3), but we also observed striking amounts of calcium and cholesterol compounds, indicating

TABLE 3.   Ceroid Lipofuscinosis Data

Patient no.	Sex	Age at diagnosis (years)	Age at death (years)	Last ECG recorded (age in years)	ECG diagnosis	Heart weight (g)	Body weight (kg)
1	F	7	16 4/12	10+	Right axis RAE	250	40
2	M	7	21 11/12	19	IRBBB	560	84
3	F	11	20 7/12	13+	LAE IRBBB ST-T changes	270	71
4	M	6	20 11/12	19	LAE IRBBB	350	52
5	M	6	26 6/12	25	Short P-Q RBBB Possible LVH	420	51
6	F	7	19 11/12	19 3/12	Sinusbradycardia LAE IRBBB	340	39.5
7	M	6	22 7/12	22 3/12	LVH	650	55
8	M	5	20 8/12	15 10/12	Normal	410	55.5
9*	F	6	21 11/12	21 9/12	IRBBB LAE	340	35
10*	F	12	19	18 9/12	ST-T changes	380	43
11	M	6	22 9/12	22 2/12	Possible LVH	260	41
12*	F	7	25 2/12	21 5/12	Normal	340	
13*	F	8	19 8/12	16 7/12	Normal	350	50

RAE: right atrial enlargement, IRBBB: incomplete right bundle branch block, RBBB: right bundle branch block, LVH: left ventricular hypertrophy, LAE: left atrial enlargement.
* patients in whom the entire heart was examined by the authors.
(Reproduced, by permission, from *Acta Pathol. Microbiol. Scand.*)

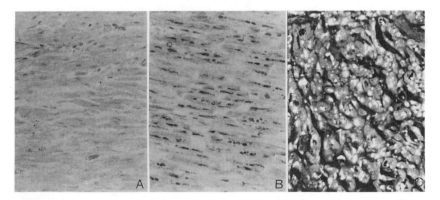

Fig. 3.   Ceroid lipofuscinosis. A) is a sex- and age-matched control to B), the patient. Heavy accumulation of lipopigment at the nuclear poles, the nuclei being almost unstained (Sudan B).

a restrictive type of heart muscle disorder. Because of the nature of the disease only rather poor information on the cardiac state is available. Eleven patients showed some cardiac enlargement. In 6 patients abnormal P-waves were recorded in the ECG, suggesting increased atrial and ventricular diastolic pressure. Two patients had bradycardia, probably due to sinus node involvement, and one patient developed complete right bundle branch block. However, in the 4 patients in whom the cardiac conduction system could be examined histologically no evidence of disturbance of cardiac impulse formation and conduction was seen in the few standard ECG strips available, in spite of extensive deposition of abnormal material throughout the conduction system. In our continued investigation of this disorder we have seen 2 cases of ceroid lipofuscinosis combined with changes mimicking hypertrophic cardiomyopathy.[11]

The association between Friedreich's ataxia and hypertrophic cardiomyopathy is well documented, as is the relation between lentiginosis and hypertrophic cardiomyopathy. What Fridreich's ataxia, lentiginosis, and ceroid lipofuscinoses have in common is not at all clear. They may all be metabolic disorders, or due to dysfunction of embryonic neural tube/neural crest elements, or both.

Fabry's Disease (Angiokeratoma Corporis Diffusum Universale)

The patient is a 67-year-old woman who developed mild cardiac failure in 1975. The decompensation was treated with digitalis and diuretics and she was stabilized in New York Heart Association functional class IIIa. Kidney function was reduced after renal

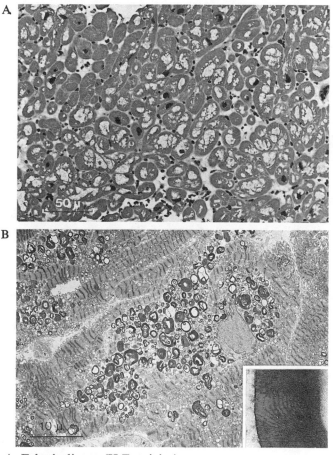

Fig. 4. A. Fabry's disease (H-E staining).
B. Fabry's disease (electron microscopy). The insert shows the perfectly laminar structure of a myelin figure (sphingolipid).

artery embolization (serum creatinine concentration of 190 μmol/l). In July 1988 the patient was admitted to hospital due to increasing dyspnea. On chest X-ray the cardiac silhouette was enlarged compared to previous investigations. At echocardiographic examination there was myocardial hypertrophy, and hypertrophic cardiomyopathy was suspected. Furthermore, a pericardial effusion was demonstrated and pericardiocentesis was undertaken with evacuation of 1,000 ml of sanguinolent fluid. Cardiac catheterization and endomyocardial biopsy were performed 10 days later and the following pressures were obtained: mean right atrial pressure 17 mmHg, right ventricular pressure 36/5 mmHg, pulmonary arterial pressure 39/18 mmHg, and pulmonary capillary wedge pressure 14 mmHg. Cardiac output was 2.7 l/min.

Paraffin sections on morphogic examination showed large irregular clear spaces in the perinuclear regions of the myocytes (Fig. 4a). Frozen sections stained with PAS stain showed darkly stained globoid structures shown electron microscopically to consist of large, round, or somewhat irregular inclusions with regular lamellar organization typical of sphingolipid (Fig. 4b).

The patient has regained her habitual condition, *i.e.*, functional class IIIa. A son died at the age of 44 years from a disease described as hypertrophic cardiomyopathy. However, review of paraffin sections showed exactly the same pattern of myocardial inclusions as those found in his mother.

Carnitine Deficiency

The patient was an 18-month-old girl who developed signs of congestive heart failure and general muscular atrophia. After an episode of long-lasting upper airway tract infection, chest X-ray showed severe enlargement of the heart. She was initially treated with digitalis and diuretics and underwent metabolic deficiency screening including endomyocardial and skeletal muscle biopsy. The diagnosis of carnitine deficiency was established by radiochemical analysis of plasma L-carnitine concentration, which was less than 1 % of the reference value.

The girl was treated with carnitine 0.6 g/day p.o. After only 3 weeks she became more active, with rapid clinical improvement and with complete normalization of heart function as evaluated roentgenologically, noninvasively, and hemodynamically. Endomyocardial biopsy specimens showed mild endocardial fibrosis with accumulation of smooth muscle cells, but no elastofibrosis. The myocytes were moderately hypertrophied with a diameter of 18.8 μm $\pm$ 4.3 μm (Fig. 5a). A few vacuoles were seen in the paraffin sections, but lipid accumulation was not found in cryostat sections or by electron microscopy.

In subsequent endomyocardial biopsies after 6 months of treatment with carnitine the endocardial thickness was within normal limits. There was no longer accumulation of smooth muscle cells, and myocyte diameter had returned to normal (10.6 μm $\pm$ 2.8 μm) (Fig. 5b).

An elder brother had died suddenly from pneumonia. At autopsy severe cardiac hypertrophy was found with endocardial fibroelastosis of the left ventricle and perinuclear vacuolization of several myocytes (Fig. 5c). The liver showed extreme steatosis. Blood collected for phenylketonuria screening after his birth has subsequently been investigated and a very low concentration of L-carnitine was found.

Calcification

Roberts and Ferrans[12] have stated that the fibers infiltrated by calcium are always necrotic and that calcification of myocardial cells is therefore always of a dystrophic

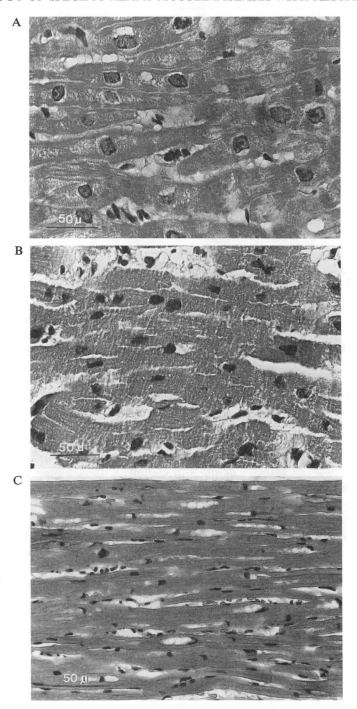

Fig. 5. A. Carnitine deficiency, patient before treatment. Myocytic hypertrophy (H-E staining).
B. Carnitine deficiency, patient after treatment. The myocytic hypertrophy has decreased, especially of nuclei (H-E staining).
C. Carnitine deficiency. Perinuclear vacuolization of several nuclei (H-E staining).

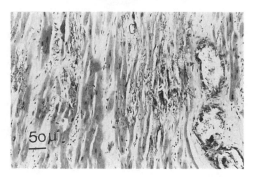

Fig. 6.   Calcified myocytes in myocardial section from patient with hyper-
parathyroidism (H-E staining).

nature. This is definitely the most frequent event. Terman *et al.*,[13] however, found
metastatic calcification in 10 of 26 patients on chronic dialysis. They had proven hyper-
calcemia, and early calcification was seen as a fine granular basophilia in small areas of
otherwise intact fibers. Parathyroid hyperplasia was noted in all of these patients. Figure
6 represents another example: the patient was a 53-year-old woman developing hyper-
parathyroid crisis over a 2-day period due to parathyroid adenomas. Severe calcification
in this otherwise healthy patient was found in many organs at postmortem examination.

RESTRICTION CAUSED BY THERAPEUTIC MEASURES

Chronic Anthracycline Cardiotoxicity[14]

Of 38 patients referred with suspected cardiotoxicity after administration of antineoplastic drugs, 11 patients with signs of manifest or latent anthracycline cardiotoxicity
were selected for heart catheterization with endomyocardial biopsy (Table 4). Ultrastructural abnormalities of the myocytes with myofibrillar loss and cytoplasmic vacuolation were present in most patients, and these findings were more pronounced in biopsy
specimens from the left ventricle.

Surprisingly, results from all but one patient showed pronounced fibrous thickening
of the endocardium, a disorder that was more pronounced in the left ventricle (mean
48 μm and 138 μm in the right and left ventricles, respectively) (Fig. 7, Table 5). This
observation had already been made indirectly at biopsy when it was rather difficult to
excise tissue specimens with the bioptome. Until now endocardial fibrosis has been
described in only a few case reports, and such damage may have been attributed to
radiation damage. Only one of our patients (patient 3) had received radiation therapy;
however, this patient had the most pronounced endocardial fibrosis. Methysergide has
been reported to cause endomyocardial fibrosis,[15] as has long-term treatment with
certain antineoplastic drugs such as busulfan.[16]

Cyclosporine

Restriction changes may be expected in some heart transplant patients with side
effects in the endomyocardium after treatment with cyclosporine (Quilty phenomenon;
interstitial fibrosis).[17,18] Cyclosporine-associated microfibrils have recently been
described[19] in 8 of 21 heart transplant patients. The fibrils had an ultrastructural composition similar to that of amyloid fibrils but light microscopic stains were uniformly

TABLE 4. Clinical Details of 11 Patients with Anthracycline Cardiotoxicity (Reproduced, by permission, from *Br. Heart J.*)

Patient no.	Age	Sex	Diagnosis	Risk factor	Total dose of anthracycline	NYHA class	ECG	Chest X-ray	Outcome
1	33	F	Pancreatic carcinoma	—	Doxorubicin 550 mg/m²	I	ST	No cardiomegaly	Died of cancer
2	49	M	Lung carcinoma	—	4-epidoxorubicin 360 mg/m²	II	Negative T waves	No cardiomegaly	Died of cancer
3	55	F	Breast carcinoma	Irradiation, cyclophosphamide	Doxorubicin 575 mg/m²	IV	ST and low R waves	Cardiomegaly	Sudden death
4	59	F	Parotid carcinoma	—	Doxorubicin 550 mg/m²	I	ST and low R waves	No cardiomegaly	Died of cancer/ CHF
5	29	F	Soft tissue sarcoma	Cyclophosphamide	Doxorubicin 550 mg/m²	IV	ST and low R waves	Cardiomegaly	Alive NYHA I
6	58	F	Ovarian carcinoma	Cyclophosphamide	Doxorubicin 530 mg/m²	IV	ST and low R waves	(Cardiomegaly)	Alive NYHA II
7	55	M	Lung carcinoma	—	4-epidoxorubicin 1533 mg/m²	III	ST and low R waves	No cardiomegaly	Died of cancer/ CHF
8	57	F	Ovarian carcinoma	Cyclophosphamide	Doxorubicin 564 mg/m²	II	SR and low R waves	No cardiomegaly	Alive NYHA I
9	53	F	Ovarian carcinoma	Cyclophosphamide	Doxorubicin 550 mg/m²	II	ST and negative T waves	(Cardiomegaly)	Sudden death
10	60	M	Lung mesothelioma	Arterial hypertension	Doxorubicin 550 mg/m²	II	ST and low R waves	(Cardiomegaly)	Alive NYHA I
11	53	F	Lung carcinoma	—	4-epidoxorubicin 645 mg/m²	II	SR and negative T waves	(Cardiomegaly)	Died of cancer?

ST: sinus tachycardia, SR: sinus rhythm, CHF: congestive heart failure, NYHA: New York Heart Association. Parentheses indicate presence of slight cardiomegaly.

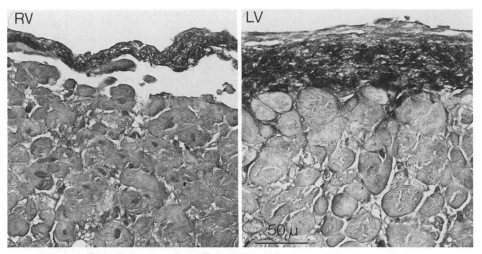

Fig. 7.   Adriamycin cardiotoxicity. Normal endocardium in the right ventricle (RV) and fibrous thickening of the endocardium in the left ventricle (LV) (elastic van Gieson staining). Reproduced, with permission, from Br. Heart J.

negative. However, it should be stressed that the restrictive pattern is most certainly due to other causes of altered hemodynamics.

Irradiation

Restrictive heart muscle disease has been reported after therapeutic mediastinal irradiation, notably in young patients with Hodgkin's disease.[20,21] More frequent, however, are constrictive symptoms due to chronic pericarditis and/or (organized) pericardial effusions or heart failure due to vessel damage ("enhanced atherosclerosis").

NEOPLASIA

Obliteration/restriction is a common finding in both primary and secondary heart tumors. Primary myocardial tumors are rare, with a reported incidence between 0.002% and 0.3%. In a study over a period of 20 years we found an autopsy incidence of 0.06%. A total of 34 patients (Table 6) during that period were diagnosed either at autopsy or in surgical specimens. Most common were myxomas; angiomatous sarcomas were most common among the malignant tumors.[22]

Metastases/infiltrations of the heart by malignant tumors occur in about 12%.[23] Nearly one-third are confined to the pericardium; the rest include the endomyocardium as well. Metastases from lung and mammary carcinomas are observed most frequently in Europe; however, in relative terms leukemias and malignant melanomas are seen most frequently, in 47.5% and 56.6%, respectively.

Although outside the scope of this paper, we want to point out that the eosinophilia and release of cationic proteins that occur in several forms of cancer, notably carcinomas arising from mucin-secreting epithelium,[24,25] could be associated with the development of endomyocardial disease.

ELECTRIC DISORDERS

All of the aforementioned disorders and many others may result in arrhythmias, the

TABLE 5. Endomyocardial Biopsy Data in 11 Patients with Anthracycline Cardiotoxicity

Patient no.	Sampling site RV	Sampling site LV	Morphological grade	Endocardial thickening RV (m)	Endocardial thickening LV (m)	Mitochondriosis	Myofibrillar drop out	Sarcotubular swelling	Deformation of nuclei
1	+	+	1 (focal LV)	—	—	Slight	Slight	—	Moderate
2	+	+	1 (focal LV	—	60–100	Slight	Slight	—	Slight
3	+	+	3 (widespread LV)	60–100	>100	Moderate	Slight	Slight	Severe
4	+	+	1 (focal LV)	20–60	60–100	Severe	Moderate	Slight	Moderate
5	+	+	1.5 (focal RV and LV)	—	60–100	Moderate	Moderate	—	Slight
6	—	+	2.5		60–100	Severe	Moderate	Slight	Moderate
7	+	+	2.5 (widespread LV)	20–60	>100	Moderate	Severe	Moderate	Moderate
8	+	+	3 (focal LV)	—	60–100	Moderate	Moderate	—	Moderate
9	+	+	1* (focal LV)	20–60	60–100				
10	—	+	2.5*		>100	Moderate	Slight	—	
11	—	+	1		20–60	Moderate	Slight	—	Slight

* Light microscopy.
RV: right ventricle, LV: left ventricle.
(Reproduced, by permission, from *Br. Heart J.*)

TABLE 6.   Primary Cardiac Tumors

	Total	Number Operated	Autopsy
Myxoma	14	9	5
Pericardial cyst	6	6	0
Teratoma	2	2	0
Papillary tumor of the leaflet	4	3	1
Rhabdomyoma	1	1	0
Lipomatous hypertrophy	2	0	2
Hemangiosarcoma	2	1	1
Others (including ectopic thyroid tissue of right ventricular outflow tract)	3	0	3

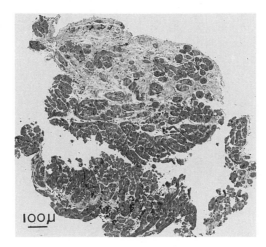

Fig. 8.   Electrical injury. Left ventricular endomyocardial biopsy showing endo- and subendocardial fibrosis. Single myocytes are encased by dense collagen tissue (elastic van Gieson staining). Reproduced, with permission, from *Br. Heart J.*

character of which depends on the area involved and the extent of changes. As has been reported by other investigators of endomyocardial biopsies, we have often observed abnormal structures in patients with arrhythmias of various types: frequently a picture consistent with dilated cardiomyopathy, sometimes with myocarditis both specific, like sarcoidosis and giant cell myocarditis, and nonspecific, like lymphocytic myocarditis (probably of viral origin), or metabolic disorders. Not infrequently, however, the only structural change is increased interstitial fibrosis and slight to moderate hypertrophy of myocytes with the clinically important information that active myocarditis is not present.

Anecdotally, we can report on "dangerous" or long-lasting ventricular arrhythmias that developed in 3 patients who had sustained electric injury in which current passed through the thorax.[26] In all there was a delay of 8–12 hr between the injury and the onset of symptoms. In 2 of the 3 patients, ventricular tachycardia, or ventricular fibrillation, or both occurred, and in one patient ventricular parasystoles developed. No en-

TABLE 7. Characteristics of Patients with Suspected Heart Muscle Disease and Restrictive Contraction Pattern (Echo and/or Angio)

Patient no.	Age/ sex	Clinical diagnosis	Echo EDD	LA	MUGA EF%	CATH Dip	Plateau	Biopsy findings
16	41M	Amyloidosis	42	40	36	+	+	Amyloid
42	36F	RCM	52	34	27	+	+	Myocarditis active
53	53F	Polymyositis	52	41		−	−	Myocarditis active
56	32M	RCM	45	50	56	+	+	Myocarditis healed
77	7M	RCM or HCM	36	32	63	−	−	Endocardial fibrosis
79	22F	RCM/ataxia	55	35	35	−	−	HCM-like
85	32M	RCM/diabetes	49	38	20	+	−	Myocarditis active
98	42F	RCM/angina	53	49	56	+	+	Small vessel disease
121	56M	Amyloidosis	41	40	47	+	−	Amyloid
124	59M	HCM	52	45	42	+	−	Amyloid
143	61M	HCM or RCM	37	36	48	+	−	Amyloid
148	26F	Constrictio cordis	47	48	50	+	+	Sequelae peri-myocarditis
162	50F	HCM	40	39	67	+	−	Amyloid
165	20M	Right ventr. dysplasia	37	44	69	+	+	Myocarditis healed

Echo: echocardiography, Angio: left ventricular angiocardiography, MUGA: radionuclide angiocardiography, CATH: diastolic pressure curves, EDD: left ventricular end-diastolic diameter (mm), LA: left atrium (mm), EF%: left ventricular ejection fraction, RCM: restrictive cardiomyopathy, HCM: hypertrophic cardiomyopathy.

zymatic evidence of myocardial necrosis was found, but the results of an endomyocardial biopsy carried out in 2 of the 3 patients showed focal myocardial fibrosis (Fig. 8) and increased numbers of Na, K-pumps. The 2 patients with ventricular tachycardia became symptom-free after appropriate antiarrhythmic treatment, and in the third patient ventricular parasystoles disappeared spontaneously within 2 years.

A CONSECUTIVELY COLLECTED GROUP OF PATIENTS

In 14 of 151 patients (9%) with suspected myocardial disease (anthracycline patients not included) a restrictive pattern was found. In Table 7 various data, including diagnoses before biopsy are listed. It is noteworthy that amyloidosis was suspected in only 2 of 5 patients before biopsy. In this series of patients the occurrence of active or healed myocarditis was substantial. Neither before nor later have we diagnosed small vessel disease. This patient—a 42-year-old woman (patient no. 98 in Table 7)—did not have diabetes. Two general points can be deducted from Table 7: a) most of the metabolic disorders, except for amyloidosis, are rarely seen; and b) restrictive heart disease is certainly not a well-defined group of disorders in terms of pathology.

This brief review of the main groups of specific heart muscle disorders where restriction may be found has emphasized the useful information that can be obtained by endomyocardial biopsy. Further insights into pathophysiologic mechanisms can be achieved by appropriate investigation of biopsy material.

REFERENCES

1. Report of the WHO/ISCF task force on the definition and classification of cardiomyopathies. *Br. Heart J.* **44**: 672–673, 1980.
2. Schoenfeld, M.H., Supple, E.W., Dee G.W., Jr., Fallon, J.T., and Palacios, I.F. Restrictive cardiomyopathy versus constrictive pericarditis: Role of endomyocardial biopsy in avoiding unnecessary thoracotomy. *Circulation* **75**: 1012–1017, 1987.
3. Eishi, Y., Takemura, T., Sone, R., Yamamura, H., Narisawa, K., Ichinohasama, R., Tanaka, M., and Hatakeyama, S. Glycogen storage disease confined to the heart with deficient activity of cardiac phosphorylase kinase: A new type of glycogen storage disease. *Hum. Pathol.* **16**: 193–197, 1985.
4. Bergsma, D. (ed.), Birth Defects Compendium. The Macmillan Press Ltd., London and Basingstoke, 1979.
5. Olson, L.J., Reeder, G.S., Noller, K.L., Howell, R.R., and Michels, V.V., Cardiac involvement in glycogen storage disease III: Morphologic and biochemical characterization with endomyocardial biopsy. *Am. J. Cardiol.* **53**: 980–981, 1984.
6. Glenner, G.G. Amyloid deposits and amyloidosis. The β-fibrilloses. *N. Engl. J. Med.* **302**: 1283–1292, 1333–1343, 1980.
7. Frederiksen, T., Gøtzsche, H., Harboe, N., Kiær, W., and Mellemgaard, K. Familial primary amyloidosis with severe amyloid heart disease. *Am. J. Med.* **33**: 328–348, 1962.
8. Husby G., Ranløv, P.J., Sletten, K., and Marhaug, G. The amyloid in familial amyloid cardiomyopathy of Danish origin is selected to prealbumin. *Clin. Exp. Immunol.* **60**: 207–216, 1985.
9. Nordlie, M., Sletten, K., Husby, G., and Ranløv, P.J. A new prealbumin variant in familial amyloid cardiomyopathy of Danish origin. *Scand. J. Immunol.* **27**: 119-122, 1988.
10. Reske-Nielsen, E., Baandrup, U., Bjerregaard, P., and Bruun, I. Cardiac involvement in juvenile amaurotic idiocy— A specific heart muscle disorder. *Acta Pathol. Microbiol. Scand. Sect. A.*, **89**: 357–365, 1981.
11. Baandrup, U., Rosenskjold, B., and Bjerregaard, P. Hypertrophic cardiomyopathy in combination with juvenile amaurotic idiocy. Chance or fundamentally related findings? *Br. Heart. J.* **51**: 674–675, 1984.
12. Roberts, W.C. and Ferans, V.J. Pathologic anatomy of the cardiomyopathies. *Hum. Pathol.* **6**: 287–347, 1975.
13. Terman, D.S., Alfrey, A.C., Hammond, W.C., Donndelinger, T., Ogden, D.A., and Holmes, J.H. Cardiac calcification in uremia. A clinical, biochemical and pathological study. *Am. J. Med.* **50**: 744–755, 1971.
14. Mortensen, S.A., Olsen, H.S., and Baandrup, U. Chronic anthracycline cardiotoxicity haemodynamic and histopathologic manifestations suggesting a restrictive endomyocardial disease. *Br. Heart J.* **55**: 274–282, 1986.
15. Mason, J.V., Billingham, M.E., and Friedman, J.P. Methysergide-induced heart disease. A case of multivalvular and myocardial fibrosis. *Circulation* **56**: 889–890, 1977.
16. Weinberger, A., Pinklias, J., Sanabank, U., Shaklai, M., and DeVries, A. Endomyocardial fibrosis following busulfan treatment. *JAMA* **231**: 495, 1975.
17. Billingham, M.E. Diagnosis of cardiac rejection by endomyocardial biopsy. *J. Heart Transplant.* **1**: 25–30, 1980.
18. Stovin, P.G.I. and English, T.A.H. Effects of cyclosporine on the transplanted human heart. *J. Heart Transplant.* **6**: 180–185, 1987.
19. Myles, J.L., Ratliff, N.B., McMahon, J.T., Tubbs, R.R. Golding, L.R., Hobbs, R.E.,

Rincon, G., Sterba, R.W., and Stewart, R. Cyclosporine-associated microfibrils in cardiac transplant patients. *Am. J. Cardiovasc. Pathol.* **2**: 127–132, 1988.

20. White, D.C. An Atlas of Irradiation Histopathology. Technical Information Center, Office of Public Affairs, U.S. Energy Research and Developmental Administration, Washington, D.C., 1975, pp. 93–105.

21. Gottdiener, J.S., Katin, M.J., Borcr, J.S., Bacharach, S.L., Green, M.V., and Lipsow, L.C. Identification of subclinical cardiac abnormality 5–15 years after therapeutic mediastinal irradiation. *Am. J. Cardiol.* **45**: 475, 1980. (abstract).

22. Ardest, S., Baandrup, U., and Lund, O. Primary tumours of the heart. A material from a period of 20 years. *Ugeskr. Laeger* **148**: 2280–2282, 1986.

23. Fiala, W. Herz Metastasen maligner Tumoren. *Schweiz. Med. Wschr.* **112**: 1497–1501, 1982.

24. Beeson, P.B. Cancer and eosinophilia. *N. Engl. J. Med.* **309**: 792, 1983.

25. Fredens, K., Dybdahl, H., Dahl, R., and Baandrup, U. Tissue damaging effect of the eosinophil cationic proteins ECP and EPX. *APMIS.* **96**: 711–719, 1988.

26. Jensen, J.J., Thomsen, P.E.B., Bagger, J.O., Noergaard, Aa., and Baandrup, U. Electrical injury causing ventricular arrythmias. *Br. Heart J.* **57**: 279–283, 1987.

Chagas' Disease: Overview and Perspectives

J.J. Puigbo, H. Acquatella, H. Giordano, C. Suarez, I. Combellas, and I. Mendoza

Caracas University School of Medicine, University Hospital, Caracas, Venezuela

ABSTRACT

Epidemiological studies carried out during a period of 20 years (1961–1984) have allowed a better understanding of the natural history of Chagas' disease, particularly of the early presymptomatic stages, and to assess the results of the Chagas' control program. A changing pattern of the disease has been established. Electrophysiological abnormalities are very frequent, and the association of RBBB with LAHB and premature ectopic beats is usually found. Progressive ECG patterns have been described. Functionally, the disease leads to systolic and diastolic dysfunction.

INTRODUCTION

Chagas' disease evolves mainly in 2 stages: acute and chronic. The acute stage is characterized by local signs caused by the *Trypanosoma cruzi* penetration through the skin and mucous membranes, systemic manifestations, visceral involvement (myocarditis, meningoencephalitis), and parasitemia during the first months of evolution. It is generally found in children, and the course of the disease is favorable in nearly 90% of the cases. After spontaneous remission of the clinical manifestation and parasitemia, the disease enters a prolonged latent stage that has been called the latent or "indeterminate form," characterized by: a) the absence of clinical manifestations and b) immunologic changes expressed in positive serological reactions (98% of patients) and low parasitemia (30–50%). A variable percentage (15–20%) of patients with latent or indeterminate infection develop a chronic visceral, cardiac, or digestive (megaorgans) form. Chagas' heart disease (Ch'HD), a secondary disease of the myocardium, is the most frequently found pathologic consequence, which affects most individuals and causes the greatest economic and social burden. Once it has set in, it often causes congestive heart failure, arrhythmias and conduction disturbances, thromboembolic phenomena, and sudden death (Fig. 1).

The purpose of this paper is to discuss epidemiologic, electrocardiographic, and functional aspects of chronic Ch'HD.

EPIDEMIOLOGIC ASPECTS

The Changing Pattern of Chagas' Disease (a 20-year study, 1961–1984)

It has been estimated that some 20 million persons living on the South American continent have been infected by *T. cruzi* and are exposed to the risk of contracting Chagas' disease.[1,2] The first epidemiologic studies in different countries aimed at

CHAGAS HEART DISEASE' SPECTRUM

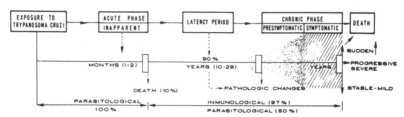

Fig. 1.   Ch'HD spectrum showing the classic evolutional pattern.

determining the rates of the disease (of infection by *T. cruzi* with or without involvement of the myocardium), its distribution among the population, studying the natural history of the disease, and confirming the clinical and experimental hypothesis of an etiological association with *T. cruzi* as a specific agent of the disease. Emphasis was placed on studying the preclinical stages, evaluation of the progress of the disease, and implementation of preventive measures that could have a favorable effect on the course of the disease.[1,2] Infection by *T. cruzi* causes a humoral and a cellular immunologic response in the host. The humoral response made it possible to develop serologic tests that could be used for both clinical research and surveys of the affected population.[3]

Results

The results of the epidemiological studies[4,5] in 2 endemic areas (population studied 1,210; 395 subjects) during the 1960s showed:

a) A high rate of infection (47.3%, 39.7%). Using the serologic survey as an indicator, the population was divided into 2 subgroups (seropositive and seronegative) and followed for 10 years. Most of the seropositive population showed no signs of heart disease (76.1%, 83.6%) when the study began.

b) A high rate of myocardial disease associated with seropositive individuals; it was thus possible to determine the etiology of the heart disease since other types of cardiac disease had been excluded. Some of the patients with Ch'HD were asymptomatic (33.7%). Others were symptomatic (66.3%). Most of the patients with symptoms had good functional capacity (class I or II, 94.5%).

c) Electrocardiographic abnormalities, including a high rate of conduction disorders: advanced right bundle branch block, whether or not associated with left anterior fascicular block (LAFB) (52.3%), and multifocal ventricular ectopic activity (43.2%). Serial electrocardiograms (ECGs) showed progression from apparent normality to incomplete or advanced forms of conduction abnormalities. Wall motion abnormalities were found during physical examination and kymographic X-rays.

Follow-up

a) Serologic evolution and mortality: The rate of both infection (18.4%) and heart disease (10.2%) during the 10 years of the study was high. The mortality rate of the survey during this period was 9.5% (81 deaths among 853 patients). Fifty-five percent of the deaths were due to chronic Ch'HD (45/81), heart failure (35), and sudden death 10). In 4 (5.1%) death was due to a cerebrovascular accident. In 25 cases (30.8%) it was unassociated with heart diseases. The cause of death was unknown in 7 (8.6%).

b) The clinical progression of Ch'HD could be assessed on the basis of the initial examination of patients and new cases in the initial or presymptomatic stage, without cardiomegaly but with bundle branch block and ectopic ventricular beats. These cases could also be assessed in the intermediate stage with arrhythmias, with discrete to moderate cardiomegaly, right bundle branch block, and LAFB up to the advanced stage with heart failure, extreme cardiomegaly, life-threatening arrhythmias, and an ECG pseudoinfarct pattern (electrically inactive zones).

c) The electrocardiographic progression showed a pattern frequently consisting of the following elements:

1) progressive conduction delay in the right bundle branch;
2) progressive left axis deviation (LAFB);
3) progressive abnormalities of ventricular repolarization (V_2-V_6);
4) increasingly severe arrhythmias; and
5) progressive appearance of abnormal "Q" waves (pseudopattern of myocardial infarction).

The rate of Chagas' infection after 4 years was 16.3%, with the highest rate in the older age-group (45–64 years old, 30.0%). The rate of heart disease was higher in the seropositive than in the seronegative group (4.2% vs. 0.7%). Recently Maguire et al.[6] have corroborated that the rate of conduction disorders is significantly higher in sero-positive subjects than in seronegative subjects. These investigators found, however, that the rate of new cases with intraventricular conduction disorders was highest in the 10- to 14-year-old age-group. Seropositive persons with LAFB showed an incidence rate of RBBB of 43.5 per 1,000 person-years. Seropositive individuals with conduction disorders had a higher risk of developing ventricular extrasystoles. There were multifocal and paired extrasystoles between the ages of 20 and 60. Mortality among seropositives was higher in the 20- to 59-year-old age-group. Seropositive persons with the combination of RBBB with fascicular block and ventricular extrasystoles had a higher mortality rate than those with normal ECGs.

The Results of the Control Program (20 years later)

The control program consisted of improving housing, educating community, and antivectoril measures such as spraying with insecticides. The purpose of these measures was to reduce transmission by *T. cruzi* and control superinfections. The area chosen was representative of the implemented national control program.

1) Serologic evolution: The serologic surveys undertaken before and after the control measures showed a marked reduction in the rate of seropositive cases, from 47.8% to 17.1% (p < 0.01). This was even more pronounced among children and adolescents, among whom the rate dropped from 29.9% to 1.9%. This indicated a fall in transmission of the disease. A similar drop has also been found in other national regions and in other South American countries.[7-11]

2) Clinical and age differences: a) The acute form has not been found in the population survey in the area following implementation of the control program. Results in other countries, such as Brazil (Bambui), have been similar; acute cases have disappeared following antivectorial measures.[8,9]

b) The average age of the seropositive population in the 3 groups, defined as asymptomatic with normal or abnormal ECGs and no cardiomegaly (A), arrhythmic (B), and with heart failure (C), rose (average age: A 45.1 ± 14.2, B 53.9 ± 12.0, C 58.7 ± 12.3). Patients under the age of 50 years showed fewer symptoms, only 12% vs. 32% in patients over that age. These figures differed markedly from the previously recorded figures of 66% of symptomatic patients under the age of 50. The average age of the seropositive population studied was higher (46.7 ± 15.1 years old) (p. <001 vs. others) than the age found in precontrol studies (34.9 ± 17.3; 32 ± 17.5; 31.1 ± 15.9).

3) Electrocardiographic findings: In group A, ECGs were normal in the majority of the cases, 61% of the subjects, and abnormal in only 27%. In groups B and C they were abnormal in the majority of the patients (89%). This confirms many earlier studies, that the most frequent and significant association is associated RBBB, LAFB, and ectopic ventricular activity. However, there was no significant difference between the proportion of electrocardiographic abnormalities in the studies before and after implementation of the control programs.

4) Mortality study: This showed statistically significant differences in survival between the 3 clinical groups in a 3- and 5-year follow-up, except for A vs. B after 5 years ($p < 0.5$). The cause of death was heart failure (19 patients), sudden death (19), cerebrovascular accident (4), cancer (4), cirrhosis of the liver (1), and unknown (6).

Comments

Epidemiological studies on Chagas' disease done over a period of 2 decades were fundamental for providing information of the natural history of the disease and proved to be especially useful for recognizing early stages; they made it possible to describe the gradual progression of electrocardiographic abnormalities. Progress was made in defining a type of myocardial disorder in human beings in which the affected population can be followed by means of an immunologic marker. Epidemiologic studies have shown geographic differences,[4,5,13–17] variations in visceral involvement (megaorgans), and variations in the average age of the age-groups most affected. Little is known regarding the causes of these differences, except in one important area of research, and that is the difference in the strains of *T. cruzi*, the host-parasite factor, including variations in immunologic response.

The lower infection rate, changes in the clinical picture of the disease, and higher life expectancy are proof of the favorable results achieved by the control program.

ELECTROCARDIOGRAPHIC ASPECTS

The ECG, together with the serologic test, is one of the main tools used in epidemiologic surveys.[4,5,7,16,17] Dynamic electrocardiography has expanded the field of application for studying and treating arrhythmias. The frequency of the disorders found depends on the type of population being studied (field or hospital studies) and the method used (conventional or dynamic ECG). The use of a standard interpretation, such as the Minnesota code, have been useful for facilitating the comparison of population studies.[4,16]

Morphological Bases

The correlation between conduction system lesions and electrophysiological abnormalities has been important and useful in studying Ch'HD, but unfortunately the knowledge gained is still very incomplete.[18,19] Andrade has described the main, frequent findings in the conduction system consisting of focal fibrosis, fatty infiltration, and vascular lesions affecting the sinus node, the AV node (lower right half), main bundle of His (right half), bundle of His branches (RBB), and left anterior fasicule (LAFB) and Purkinje system. Benchimol reported[20] that the rate of sinus node involvement rises from 29.1% using conventional methods to 68.7% with special techniques. The fibers of the Purkinje cell system may be affected by the chronic inflammatory process, fibrosis, degenerative and ischemic lesions related to abnormalities of the microcirculation, and mural thrombosis, which are frequent and important factors leading eventually to arrhythmias.

Frequency

The frequency of clearly abnormal ECGs in patients infected with Ch'HD (seropositives) in endemic areas is variable and fluctuates between 6% and 20%.[4,5] The incidence during the 10 years before spraying was (10.2%), and in some series it was 2.4% per annum, vs. 1.2%.[16] The frequency of the electrocardiographic alterations differed in the population-based surveys from those in the hospital studies.

Most Frequent Electrocardiographic Abnormalities

Conduction disorders and arrhythmias. The progressive electrocardiographic changes from normal conduction to definite conduction disorders have been described.[4,5] The ARBBB alone or associated with LAFB,[12,21-23] *i.e.*, bifascicular block with VPBs, constitutes a very characteristic triad. This finding is a very useful guideline and suggests a diagnosis of Ch'HD in a young patient with serologic evidence of Chagas' infection without symptoms of coronary artery diseases. The rate for ECGs classified as abnormal in population-based surveys is close to 50%, whereas in hospital surveys it is near 70%. The rate of conduction disorders rises with age. The LPFB and the ALBBB are 2 uncommon electrocardiographic abnormalities.[23,24] Ventricular and supraventricular arrhythmias account for 45%; VPBs can be unifocal, although they are usually multifocal and can be paired (bigeminy). There can be sustained and unsustained ventricular tachycardia (VT), which is frequently the electrophysiologic basis of sudden death.[25] Electrophysiologic studies have shown that initiation of VT could be reproduced and terminated by programmed stimulation. This finding suggests that reentry is a possible mechanism for VT in this disease. In view of the high frequency of focal lesions with either incomplete or advanced block in Ch'HD, it is likely to be the most frequent mechanism. Atrial fibrillation is relatively rare, being around 10%; it increases with age and is associated with CHF. An electrocardiographic analysis of 775 ECGs from Chagas' disease patients (seropositive group) was recently carried out.[32] Abnormalities were found in 39%, whereas in 923 ECGs from seronegative subjects (control group), the abnormality rate was 14% (p<.001).

Bradyarrhythmias

Sick node syndrome or sinus node dysfunction: Chronic Ch'HD is one of the causes of sinus node dysfunction. Sinus node abnormalities caused by this disease include the same abnormalities prompted by other causes: a) spontaneous sinus bradycardia not related to drugs; b) sinus arrest or exit block; c) node dysfunction associated with conduction disorders; and d) bradycardia-tachycardia syndrome. Brasil[26] was the first author to describe its presence in this disorder (19% of 200 cases). The rate of sinus bradycardia (SB) fluctuates from 1% to 6%.[27,28] The involvement of the node is variable and depends upon the degree of myocardial involvement. In 143 Chagas' disease patients Carrasco *et al.*[29] found absence of sinus node abnormalities in patients classified as showing no heart disease; the presence of sinus automatism disorders (10%, 45%, and 22%), of innervation (3%, 12%, and 33%), and of infra-His AV conduction (14%, 37%, and 47%) in the groups with heart disease; and differing degrees of myocardial involvement. A high rate of sinus node disease had been described in electrophys-

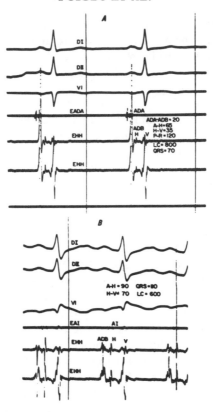

Fig. 2. Patient with Chagas' infection. Peripheral electrocardiogram and intracardiac electrogram.
A. Control time intervals before the Ajmaline test.
B. Time intervals after the Ajmaline test (0.75 mg/kg). RBBB and LAFB appear; H-V 70 msec.

iologic studies (52%).[20] The morphologic basis of the syndrome is the frequent involvement of the sinus node together with the AV node and the rest of the conduction system by the inflammatory and sclero-degenerative process. The symptoms are related to low cardiac output, periods of asystole which can cause sudden death, the onset of heart failure, or thromboembolic phenomena. A pacemaker must be implanted in symptomatic patients.

Complete AV Block

The frequency of any degree of AV block is low in population-based surveys (6%), first-degree AV block being the most common, and higher in hospital surveys (25%), where third-degree AV block is more common. In endemic areas this is the main cause of complete AV block and requires implantation of a pacemaker in persons under 50. The dynamic electrocardiogram and electrophysiologic studies are useful in cases of bifascicular block, which are very frequent in Ch'HD, and in the presence of suggestive symptoms. Temporary and/or permanent pacemakers are usually implanted for Mobitz type II second-degree AV blocks or for complete AV blocks. The prognosis will depend on the stage of evolution of the patient's disease: for patients in stages I and II (with no cardiomegaly or discrete cardiomegaly and with no ventricular dysfunction) it may be very good, whereas for those in stage III (extreme cardiomegaly plus ventricular dysfunction) the prognosis is poor.

Ventricular repolarization disorders. This is one of the most frequent and early disorders, found in 80% of the population-based surveys. Specificity is, however, low. It is characterized by the onset or progression of a ventricular repolarization abnormality from V_2 to V_6.[5] It may occur in isolation or together with an intraventricular conduction disorder. Accompaniment by a counterclockwise rotation of the precordial leads is frequent. At times the T wave morphology is symmetric, suggesting an ischemic factor (small vessel alterations) or inflammatory changes (underlying myopericarditis).

The less frequent abnormalities. Pathological "Q" Waves, or electrically, inactive zones (population studies 10.2%).[4,5] This abnormality usually develops gradually, and the most frequent locations are the diaphragmatic, posterior wall (D_2, D_3, aVF) or the anterior wall (V_1-V_2; V_1-V_4). This sign appears in the intermediate stage, but above all in the advanced stage, and is frequently associated with CHF, severe ventricular arrhythmias, and atrial fibrillation. As mentioned above, the underlying morphology of these alterations is not clear, but it has been related to extensive fibrotic patches, myocytolysis, or atrophy of the fibers, especially in the apical region.

Ventricular hypertrophy, atrial abnormalities, and low voltage. The frequency of left ventricular hypertrophy is low (13.6%) and the frequency of right hypertrophy is even lower (2.3%). Left atrial abnormalities are also more frequent (12.5%) than those of the right atrial abnormalities; they are an electric signal associated with advanced stages and ventricular dysfunction. Low voltage is relatively rare (18%).

Invasive Electrophysiological Studies

Moleiro and Mendoza[30] recently studied 15 patients with Chagas' infection and 9 patients without infection (control group). They were evaluated by means of recognized techniques for intracardiac recordings and programmed stimulation, using the Ajmaline (0.75 mg/kg) test on all the patients in the control group and on 7 patients with Chagas' disease. The basal H-V interval values were significantly longer in the Chagas group than in the control group (p < 0.01) (Fig. 2). The His-Purkinje refractory period was prolonged in 6 of the Chagas patients and in none of the control group.

In another study[31] the Ajmaline test was useful in detecting latent electrophysiological disorders (arrhythmia, conduction and repolarization disorders), and the difference between the toxic effect of the Ajmaline and a positive test was determined.

Using serial electrophysiologic studies in order to select antiarrhythmic treatment, Mendoza et al.[25] evaluated 16 patients with recurrent sustained VT resistant to conventional treatment (group 1), and 35 patients (group 2, control) who were evaluated using invasive electrophysiologic studies for arrhythmias other than VT. VT was artificially initiated and terminated in all of the patients in group 1 and in none of those in group 2. The most effective drugs in this group were Mexiletine and Amiodarone. The study also determined the site where the VT originated by analyzing the first ventricular endocardial recording during tachycardia. This was the left ventricle in 14 patients, the right in one patient, and 2 different places (one in each ventricle) in one patient. Determination of the location where the tachycardia originated provided the rational basis for aneurysmectomy in 2 patients.

Invasive stimulation and pharmacology studies make it possible to detect intraventricular conduction system abnormalities which are not evident by conventional ECGs. A positive test is not a specific indication of Ch'HD.

Sensitivity and Specificity

Ch'HD is the main cause of RBBB and third-degree AV block in individuals under the age of 50 in endemic areas. RBBB is a good indicator because it occurs in 52.9% of seropositive patients and high specificity due to its low rate (5.5%) in seronegative individuals in the same endemic area.[6,16] Specificity of the association of RBBB and LAFB is greatest in the 45- to 64-year age-group, and it was not found in any seronegative cases. As for AV conduction, this series showed[6,16] that the PR interval in the ECG is in the upper range in seropositive subjects. The ventricular arrhythmias lack specificity for the diagnosis of Ch'HD when a conventional ECG is used, but sensitivity is greater with a dynamic ECG. The predictive value, however, is high in the case of repetitive ventricular arrhythmias.

Prognosis

The frequency of arrhythmias, associated with conduction disorders and conduction system lesions, found at necropsy has often been related to sudden death.[17,24,27] Mortality associated with advanced isolated RBBB (33.3% in 5 years) is lower than with RBBB associated with LAFB (67.4% in 5 years, 80.6% in 10 years).[24,27] Tables 1 and 2 show the mortality risk and yearly survival according to ECG findings.[32] Added association of several electrocardiographic disorders is found in advanced forms with CHF. Concomitant 3rd degree block is associated with a high mortality rate: 51% in 5 years and 100% in 10 years.[33] Figure 3 compares the survival of patients with pacemakers and those from earlier controls without pacemakers.[24] If there is atrial fibrillation the prognosis is poor. Sustained VT is frequently found in Ch'HD, and electrophysiologic studies are useful in making the diagnosis and guiding the therapy.[25]

TABLE 1. Estimate of Mortality Risk in Seropositive Groups According to ECG Findings*

ECG	N°	Mortality per persons/year	Relative risk abnormal ECG/normal ECG
Normal	376	2.15 (2/928.2)	1
RBBB (isolated)	58	46.6 (6/128.7)	21 7
RBBB (all)	130	85.6 (22/257.0)	39.8
LAFB (isolated)	56	41.2 (5/121.3)	19.2
LAFB (all)	128	75.5 (19/251.7)	35.8
Abnormal (asymptomatic subjects)	238	11.9 (6/502.7)	5.5

* Includes all subjects, not corrected by age and clinical group.
Estimate of mortality risk in chronic Chagas patients. According to ECG findings, RBBB and LAFB associated with others ECG disturbances show the highest mortality risk.

TABLE 2. Yearly Survival (%) According to ECG Findings

ECG	Years of follow-up				
	1	2	3	4	5
RBBB (isolated)	94	91	87	87	76
RBBB (all)	87	81	78	78	71
LAFB (isolated)	92	89	89	89	89
LAFB (all)	87	82	82	80	80
Normal	99.7	99.7	99.2	99.2	99.2

Yearly survival according to ECG findings, showing the differences between RBBB and LAFB.

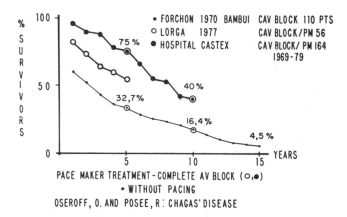

Fig. 3.   Survival rate of patients with Chagas' chronic heart disease with complete AV block. With and without pacing treatment.

Sudden Heart Death

In Ch'HD death is either heart failure or sudden death. The predisposing factors are age, male sex, the degree of cardiomegaly, exercise, life-threatening arrhythmias, conduction disorders, and, especially, complete AV block and apical aneurysm. Sudden death can be preceded by prodromes or these may be absent. Occasionally sudden death can be the first and last sign of the disease (forensic deaths). This generally happens in those under 50 years of age and within the first hour according to our definition. The rate of sudden death in Ch'HD is high, totaling close to 40%. Heart failure is the cause of death in 40%, with the remaining deaths being linked to other causes.[7] Hearts from patients who died suddenly usually weigh less than those of individuals who die of CHF (350 g vs. 500 g) and show less dilatation. The subepicardial lymph nodes located in the intrapericardial sac of the pulmonary artery are infarcted in nearly to 75% of those who die suddenly and in only 40% of those dying of heart failure.[33] The histological characteristics are usually similar in the cases of sudden death and in CHF, but Prata[33,34] noted a higher rate of granulomatous inflammatory process (50%) in cases of sudden death. Sustained and nonsustained VT[25] and ventricular fibrillation make up the electrophysiological substratum of sudden death. Little is known about the causes leading to sudden death, but it has been attributed to: a) arrhythmias and conduction disorders; b) vascular lesions affecting the irrigation of the sinus and the atrioventricular nodes; and c) autonomic lesions and cardiac denervation.

Antiarrhythmic drugs, especially the combination of amiodarone and mexiletine, have been used[25] to control arrhythmias; artificial pacemakers and aneurysmectomies are among the measures aimed at preventing sudden death.

FUNCTIONAL ASPECTS

Systolic and Diastolic Dysfunction

Left ventricular dysfunction has been related to several etiologic-pathogenic factors which lead to different structural lesions or to intrinsic myocardial damage. Left ventricular dysfunction in Ch'HD is related to intrinsic myocardial damage; wall motion

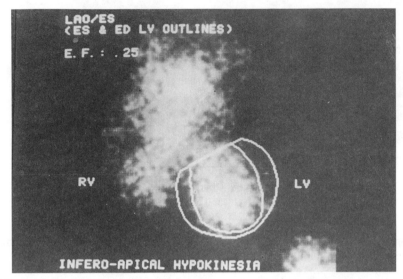

Fig. 4.   Radionuclide ventriculogram in early Chagas' disease: inferoapical hypokinesis.

abnormalities (segmental or global), cardiac arrhythmias and disorders of the conduction system, thromboembolic phenomena, and AV valvular incompetence can be contributing factors.

Systolic Function

In characterizing left ventricular function and its relation to other objective and clinical variables, LVEF was determined from the RV in 41 patients.[35] In the asymptomatic group, the ejection fraction (EF) was generally within normal limits; among patients with arrhythmias, EF was moderately depressed, and markedly subnormal values were seen in the congestive group (0.64 ± 0.6; 0.47 ± 0.15; 0.28 ± 0.08). In the same 41 patients right ventriculography was used for evaluation of left ventricular segmental wall motion. Normal LVWM was seen in the asymptomatic group (34% of the population); abnormal segmental wall motion was predominant in the arrhythmic group (37%), and abnormal global wall motion was predominant in the congestive group (29%). A good correlation was found between the severity of VWMA and depressed EF. The region most frequently affected was the inferoapical site (87%) (Fig. 4), and apical aneurysms were frequently detected (17%). Scintigraphic studies performed with 99m technetium pyrophosphate in Ch'HD, either in the latent phase or in the myocardial involvement stage, have shown diffuse uptake, at times intense (4+) and at other times discrete (1+) or negative.[36] Exercise thallium-201 perfusion scintigraphy (ergometry test) has shown the presence of fixed apical perfusion defects in a subgroup of Ch'HD patients.[37,38] Echocardiographic findings (64 patients)[39] show: a distinct pattern characterized by a hypokinetic or dyskinetic posterior wall motion with relatively well-preserved septal wall motion and apical aneurysm. The anatomical basis for this pattern is the presence of fibrotic changes of the apical posterior region. Wall motion studies by M-mode echo showed three patterns: 1) normal; 2) hypokinesis of the posterior wall, which is frequently accompanied by normal septal movement (septo parietal discrepancy); and 3) diffuse hypokinesis.

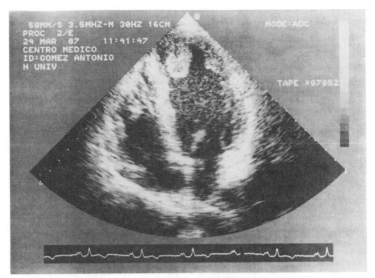

Fig. 5. Two-dimensional echocardiogram in a Chagas patient showing apical thrombus.

In symptomatic patients 2-dimensional echocardiography frequently showed the typical apical aneurysms of the left ventricle (19 of 33), and apical dyskinesis with or without thrombosis (Fig. 5). This is particularly important for early detection of apical dyskinesis in asymptomatic patients (3 of 7).

Diastolic Function

Digitized echocardiography (64 patients)[40] showed diastolic function abnormalities. Asymptomatic patients revealed prolongation of the isovolumic relaxation time (IVRT), delayed mitral valve opening and aortic valve closure, increased left ventricular dimension during IVRT, reduction of the peak rate of the increase in dimension, prolongation of the diastolic filling period, reduction of the peak rate of the posterior wall thinning, and prolonged thinning of the posterior wall (Fig. 6). Among patients with arrhythmias, more severe alterations were found. The presence of diastolic abnormalities is very helpful in the early detection of Ch'HD. Diastolic dysfunction precedes systolic dysfunction by a long period. We suggest that this evolving sequence should be taken into consideration for purposes of preventive, diagnostic, therapeutic, and rehabilitation programs, which should start before severe left ventricular systolic function deterioration develops.

The increased mitro-septal separation provided a simple method of using the M-mode echo to detect segmental contraction and diminished overall functions of the left ventricle.

To summarize, the echocardiogram is considered a useful, noninvasive technique for diagnosing evolutional Ch'HD and determining its severity. It discloses segmental dyskinesis which is common in Ch'HD in the ventricular apex and the posterior wall. It provides a very precise picture of morphologic and dynamic abnormalities, such as apical lesions or aneurysms. In some asymptomatic patients it may disclose the first indication of a contractile alteration in a heart which shows no other signs of heart disease. It provides a noninvasive method for monitoring chronic heart disease. What has yet to be determined is the value of this and the other diagnostic methods described

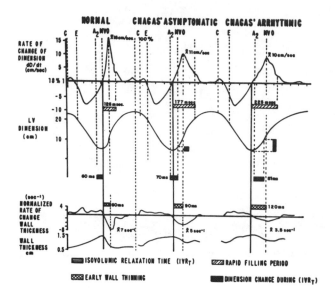

Fig. 6.   Diastolic abnormalities in Chagas' disease.

above in evaluating the efficiency of specific treatment of Ch'HD. Evaluating diastolic function is emphasized.

REFERENCES

1. World Health Organization: Sixth programme report. Chapter 6: Chagas' disease. UNDP, World Bank, WHO. Special programme for research and training in tropical disease. Document TDR, PR-6, 83.6-CHA, 1983.

2. World Health Organization: Workshop on epidemiological, social and economic aspects of present and future methods of Chagas' disease control. UNDP, World Bank, WHO. Special programme for research and training in tropical diseases. Document TDR, SER-CHA, 80-3, 1980.

3. Maekelt, G.A. Die komplementbidungsreaktion der Chagas krankheit. *Z. Tropemmed Parasit.* **2**: 152–156, 1960.

4. Puigbo, J.J., Nava Rhode, J.R., Garcia Barrios, H., Suarez, J.A. and Gil Yepez, C. Clinical and epidemiological study of chronic heart involvement in Chagas' disease. *Bull. WHO* **34**: 655–669, 1966.

5. Puigbo, J.J., Nava-Rhode, J.R., Garcia Barrios, H. and Gil Yepez, C. A 4-year follow-up of a rural community with endemic Chagas' disease. *Bull. WHO* **39**: 341–348, 1968.

6. Maguire, J.H., Hoff, R., Sherlock, I., Guimaraes, A.C., Sleigh, A.C., Borges Ramos, N., Mott, K.E. and Weller, T.H. Cardiac morbidity and mortality due to Chagas' disease: Prospective electrocardiographic study of a Brazilian community. *Circulation* **75**:(6): 1140–1145, 1987.

7. Acquatella, H., Catalioti, F., Gomez-Mancebo, J.R., Davalos, V. and Villalobos, I. Long term of Chagas' disease in Venezuela: Effects on serological findings, electrocardiographic abnormalities; and clinical outcome. *Circulation* **76**(3): 556–562, 1987.

8. Abreu-Salgado, A., Goncalves-Nogueira, P. and Mayrink, W. Comprovaçao em populaçao humana do controle da doenca de Chagas. *Rev. Bras. Mal. Doencas. Trop.* **20**: 109, 1968.

9. Vichi, F.L., Costa, Neto, M.M. and Romero, L.C. Declinio da prevalencia da molestia de Chagas en Ribeirao Preto (SP). Estudio epidemiologico. *Arq. Bras. Cardiol.* **34**: 347, 1980.

10. Perez, C., Stagno, S., Welch, E., Villaroel, F., Rojas, A. and Schenone, H. Infection chagasica humana y animal en viviendas rociadas previamente con insecticidas. *Bol. Chi. Parasitol.* **25**: 33, 1980.

11. Segura, E.L., Perez, A.C., Yanovsky, J.F., Andrade, J. and Wine de Martini, G.J. Decrease in the prevalence of infection by *Trypanosoma cruzi* (Chagas' disease) in young men of Argentina. *Bull. Pan. Am. Health Organ.* **19**: 252, 1985.

12. Moleiro, F., Mendoza, I. Miocardiopatia cronica chagasica. *Acta. Cient. Venez.* **31**: 66, 1980.

13. Rezende, J.M. Manifestacoes digestivas da molestia de Chagas. In Cancado J.R. Doença de Chagas. Im. of. Estado de Minas Gerais, Belo Horizonte, 1968.

14. Koberle, F. Patologia e anatomia patologica de la enfermedad de Chagas. *Bol. Ofic. Sanit. Panam.* **51**: 404–428, 1961.

15. Koberle, F. Cardiopatia chagasica. *Hospital* (Rio de Janeiro). **53**: 311–346, 1958.

16. Maguire, J.H., Mott, K.E., Lehman, J.S., Holff, R., Muniz, T.M., Guimaraes, A.C., Sherlock, I. and Morrow, R.H. Relationship of electrocardiographic abnormalities and seropositivity to *Trypanosoma cruzi* within a rural community in northeast Brazil. *Am. Heart J.* **105**: 287, 1983.

17. Laranja, F.S., Dias, E., Nobrega, G. and Miranda, A. Chagas' disease. A clinical, epidemiologic and pathologic study. *Circulation* **14**: 1035–1060, 1956.

18. Andrade, Z.A., Andrade, S.G., Oliveira, G.B. and Alonso, D.R. Histopathology of the conducting tissue of the heart in Chagas' myocarditis. *Am. Heart J.* **93**: 316–324, 1978.

19. Andrade, Z.A., Andrade, S.G., Sadgursky, M. and Maguire, J.II. Experimental Chagas' disease in dogs. A pathologic and ECG study of the chronic indeterminate phase of the infection. *Arch. Pathol. Lab. Med.* **105**: 460–464, 1981.

20. Benchimol, C.B., Kreuzig, R., Ginefra, P., Schlesinger, P. and Benchimol, A.B. A disfuncao do nodulo sinusal na cardiopatia chagasica cronica. *Arq. Bras. Cardiol.* **30**: 337–344, 1977.

21. Rosembaun, M.B. and Alvarez, A.J. The electrocardiogram in chronic chagasic myocarditis. *Am. Heart J.* **50**: 492–527, 1955.

22. Rosembaun, M.B., Lazzari, J.O., Kreis, A. and Ruos, H.O. The clinical causes and mechanisms of intraventricular conduction disturbances. In: Advances in Electrocardiography. Schlant, R.C. and Hurot, J.W. (eds.) Grune & Stratton, N.Y. 1972.

23. Rofeld, A., Fernandez, M.A.O.C., Camargo, N.B., *et al.* Electrocardiograma em individuos com reacao de Guerreiro Machado positiva. *Arq. Bras. Cardiol.* **31**: 191–194, 1978.

24. Dias, J.C.P. and Klowtzel, K. The prognostic value of the electrocardiographic features of chronic Chagas' disease. *Rev. Inst. Med. Trop. Sao Paulo* **10**: 158–162, 1968.

25. Mendoza, I., Camardo, J., Moleiro, F., Castellanos, A., Medina, V., Gomez, J., Acquatella, H., Casal. H., Tortoledo, F. and Puigbo, J.J. Sustained ventricular tachycardia in chronic chagasic myocarditis: Electropysiologic and pharmacologic characteristics. *Am. J. Cardiol.* **57**: 423–427, 1986.

26. Brasil, A. Autonomical sino-atrial block. A new disturbance of the heart mechanism. *Arq. Bras. Cardiol.* **8**: 159–212, 1955.

27. Porto, C.C. O electrocardiograma no prognostico e evolucao da doenca de Chagas. *Arq. Bras. Cardiol.* **17**: 313–346, 1964.

28. Fioroni, M.A.L., Vichi, F.L., Oliveira, J.S.M. and Poggi, J. Correlacao electrocardiografica-patologica em 90 pacientes falecidos pela cardiopatia chagasica. *Rev. Ass. Med. Bras.* **19**: 245–248, 1973.

29. Carrasco, H.A., Mora, G.R., Inglessis, G., Contreras, J.M., Marval, J. and Fuenmayor, A. Estudio de la funcion del nodo sinusal y de la conduccion atrioventricular en pacientes con enfermedad de Chagas. *Arch. Inst. Cardiol. Mex.* **52**: 245–251, 1982.

30. Moleiro, F. and Mendoza, I. Evaluacion electrofisiologica de los trastornos de conduccion en la miocarditis cronica Chagasica. In: Miocardiopatias, Salvat Editores, SA 1982. pp. 77–78,

31. Mendoza, I., Zaman, L., Moleiro, F., Medina, V., Myerbury, R., Castellanos, A. and Rozanski, J. Toxicity of the Ajmaline test used to expose latent atrioventricular block. *Clin. Res.* **30**: 255A, 1982.

32. Acquatella, H., Gomez, J.R., Catalioti, F., Davalos, V., Villalobos, L., Sequeda, M. de, Gonzalez, H., y Alvarado, M. de. Evaluacion de los efectos a largo plazo de la ,.campaña de control de la enfermedad de Chagas en Venezuela: Evidencia de cambios favorables en tasas serologicas, anormalidades electrocardiograficas y evolucion clinica obtenidos en el Distrito Roscio del Estado Guarico. (in press). Gac. Med. Caracas.

33. Prata, A., Lopes, E.R. and Chapadeiro, E. Morte subita na doenca de Chagas. In: Cardiopatia Chagasica. Romeu Cancado and Moises Chuster, Belo Horizonte, MG, Brasil, 1985.

34. Prata, A. Prognostico e complicacoes da doenca de Chagas. *Rev. Goiana Med.* **5**: 87–96, 1959.

35. Arreaza, N., Puigbo, J.J., Acquatella, H., Casal. H., Giordano, H., Valecillos, R., Mendoza, I., Perez, J.F., Hirschhaut, E. and Combellas, I. Radionuclide evaluation of left ventricular function in chronic Chagas' cardiomyopathy. *J. Nucl. Med.* **24**: 563–567, 1983.

36. Rocha, A.F.G., Meguerian, B.A. and Harbert, J.C. Tc-99m pyrophosphate myocardial scanning in Chagas' disease. *J. Nuc. Med.* **22**: 347–348, 1981.

37. Rotondaro, D., Castelletti, L.J., Rios, V., Di Nunzio, H.J., Mivayoulo, J.R., and Gallardo, E.A. Dianostico precoz de miocardiopatia Chagasica por perfusion miocardica con talio-210 (Abst.) *Arq. Bras. Cardiol.* **32**: 161, 1979.

38. Thom, A.F., Martins, L.R.F., Marioni Filho, H., Meneglelo, R.S., Silva, M.A.D. and Fragara Filho, A.A. Cicloergometria con talio-210 e cintilografia con pirofosfato-tecnecio-99m en pacientes com doenca de Chagas (Abstr.) *Arq. Bras. Cardiol.* **37**(1): 91, 1981.

39. Acquatella, H., Schiller, N.B., Puigbo, J.J., Giordano, H., Suarez, J.A., Casal, H., Arreaza, N., Valecillos, R. and Hirschhaut, E. M-Mode and two-dimensional echocardiography in chronic Chagas' heart disease. A clinical and pathologic study. *Circulation* **62**. No. 4: 787–799, 1980.

40. Combellas, I., Puigbo, J.J., Acquatella, H., Tortoledo, F. and Gomez, J.R. Echocardiograph c features of impaired left ventricular diastolic function in Chagas' heart disease. **53**: 298–309, 1985.

Summary

P.J. Richardson

King's College Hospital, London, U.K.

It gives me very great pleasure to be able to summarize this most successful meeting. We have had a very free and active discussion of many important aspects of heart muscle disease, cardiomyopathy, and myocarditis that have been engendered by the program which Professor Sekiguchi drew up.

The three important aspects we have covered relate to endomyocardial disease and the role of eosinophilia in its pathogenesis; arrythmias and conduction system disturbances in cardiomyopathy, myocarditis, and other specific heart muscle diseases; and restrictive cardiomyopathy and specific heart muscle diseases. I think it is particularly appropriate that we have had a feast of histopathological and clinical pathological correlations shown to us here in this building, since, as Professor Sekiguchi has shown us, this is where it all started with regard to myocardial biopsy. Drs. Konno and Sakakibara are responsible for a great deal that has taken place today, and will be responsible for a very great deal which is going to take place in the future.

In discussing all the various aspects that we have covered of myocardial disease, we must recognize their very important place, but at the same time Professor Sekiguchi has continued and carried on the impetus which was started by the development of the catheter biopsy method.

To summarize this meeting in great detail would be perhaps invidious; indeed it would be almost impossible. Omission of any particular individual from this summarization is simply a result of constraints of time, not any lack of importance of the particular paper presented.

On the first day we had the classification according to the WHO/ISFC laid down by Dr. Olsen. This was an important and very appropriate start to the meeting, since it became clear that we had to look at other aspects of the diseases we are discussing in relationship to this classification. We then followed the detailed classification by a session on endomyocardial fibrosis and hypereosinophilia, and we had papers by Dr. Vijayaraghavan from India and Dr. Andy from Nigeria relating to microfilaria and the role of the helminthic infestations in pathogenesis. Then Dr. Acquatella showed us how we can use echocardiography to look at the abnormal ventricle in myocardial disease, with Dr. Moraes summarizing his very great experience with regard to the surgical treatment of this condition. We subsequently focused on the role of the eosinophil in the pathogenesis of endomyocardial disease. Dr. Makino described the response of eosinophil in allergic asthma, and the clinical spectrum of hypereosinophilia in heart disease in Japan was described by Dr. Take who underlined the different incidence of this disease in this country as compared to that in the tropical equatorial countries. Dr. Spry described the beautiful clinical experimental data linking degranulation of the eosinophil to the pathogenesis of endomyocardial disease, and it was all tied up by Dr. Tai with further exposition relating to the experimental data. Radionuclide ventriculography in the hypereosinophilic syndrome was outlined by Dr. Hiroe. At the end

361

of the session we had a very important discussion in which it was——I think by con-sensus——decided that endomyocardial disease should now be classified as specific heart muscle disease whether or not it is associated with eosinophilia.

On the second day we began with papers related to arrhythmias and conduction disturbance in cardiomyopathy. Prof. Sekiguchi opened the session with his overview paper recounting his experience of biopsy in over 200 patients who had presented with arrhythmic or conduction system problems in his total population of 1500 patients. His data included patients without specific heart muscle disease but with definite biopsy changes which, although perhaps nonspecific, were consistent with a histopathological diagnosis of cardiomyopathy. He also described his experience with right atrial biopsy, and felt that a diagnosis of right atrial cardiomyopathy could be made with some certainty in some of his patients. He concluded that a separate group of electric disturb-ance type of cardiomyopathy appeared to exist, and in that context asked that we might consider that the WHO/ISFC classification might be modified to include this electric type of disturbance cardiomyopathy as a special entity.

Following this paper Dr. James presented his view of the pathology of the conducting system in cardiomyopathy and myocarditis, including an alternative definition of the term cardiomyopathy from that accepted by the WHO/ISFC. Professor Okada then presented a carefully documented pathological study of disease of the conducting sys-tem and Dr. Suwa delineated left ventricular false tendons by echocardiography and correlated their presence in normals with ventricular premature contractions.

The session continued with a description of the electrophysiological findings in the patients described by Dr. Mason, presenting the use of electrophysiology in the United States and trying to predict the use of electrophysiology in Japan on the basis of the different incidence of coronary disease: but in fact, as it turned out, it appeared that electrophysiology is performed almost as frequently in Japan as in the States.

We then followed with a paper by Dr. Hasumi, who described the findings on en-domyocardial biopsy in patients, with idiopathic ventricular tachycardia; significant pathology was found in a very high percentage of these patients, particularly when they had ventricular enlargement on angiography. The authors suggested that this might support the concept of an electric type disturbance cardiomyopathy. Fontaine then described transmitted and acquired right ventricular dysplasia as a cause for life-threat-ening ventricular tachycardia, and biopsy samples provided the tissue, reflecting what appeared to be typical findings of fatty infiltration fibrosis with some remaining myo-cardial cells being seen. These findings and the similarity that they have to dilated cardiomyopathy was discussed, and there was considerable discussion relating to whether in fact this entity represented a true separate pathological cause for ventricular tachy-cardia or whether it was really a normal finding.

Treatment of arrhythmogenic ventricular displasia and the potential value of elec-trophysiology were described by Dr. Kasanuki, and Professor Iwa described surgical experience and treatment of repetitive ventricular tachycardia in patients with ischemic heart disease in Japan. In his series he reported surgical biopsy findings in 34 of 38 patients; in eight of these the findings appeared to be consistant with arrythmogenic right ventricular dysplasia and in a further seventeen chronic myocardic changes were seen.

In the afternoon we continued with a further discussion of the role of myocarditis in the pathogenesis of conducting system problems and arrhythmias, and a large follow-up study was presented by Kawamura from Japan following up patients initially de-scribed in 1982 but followed up in 1985. What was of interest here was what appeared to be a very high incidence of complete heart block; of 67 patients described, 73 percent had important arrhythmic or other sequelae with regard to conducting system disease and 6 percent of these patients had died. Matsumori described his work on animal models; his demonstration of ventricular aneurysms induced by coxackievirus B in Syrian hamsters was of particular interest since it does mimic in some ways the clinical pattern of focal myocarditis, which may give rise in occasional patients to sudden death. We then followed with what might be regarded as very "high scientific" session, with Maisch describing immunologic changes in the conducting system and Schultheiss providing convincing evidence of the potential for the characterization of antibodies against the calcium channel in gap junctions as a potential pathogenetic mechanism for arrhythmias if not for impairment of cardiac function in cardiomyopathy. Camerini completed the session with a clinical paper on his experience with arrhythmiagenic left ventricular displasia.

The most important aspect perhaps of this whole section was the discussion which followed of the question of whether electric type disturbance cardiomyopathy should be classified as a separate entity or not. Following what I think could be described as a very lively and active debate, the consensus appeared to be that at the present time the WHO/ISFC classification should not be changed to include conduction disturbance or arrhythmogenic cardiomyopathy as a separate entity. However, the debate also reflected the fact that arrhythmogenic right ventricular dysplasia and possibly right atrial cardiomyopathy might be considered under the title of "unclassified cardiomyopathy." The meeting closed today with a very good session on restrictive cardiomyopathy and on the specific heart muscle diseases that may mimic restrictive hemodynamic patterns.

I think that we must recognize the very high standard of the posters that have been on display at this meeting; they do represent the high level of activity that is taking place with regard to detailed studies in cardiomyopathy both clinically and clinicopathologically. I think that we are left after meeting with plenty more to do. The last session for instance reflected the very great interest which is going to revolve around metabolic, immunological, and immunoreceptor aspects of heart muscle diseases as well as some aspects that have not been touched upon at all today——molecular biological aspects relating to the development of specific probes, for instance, for looking at viruses and so on in the pathogenesis of cardiomyopathy. There is therefore a very great amount of work to be done in the next few years, and hopefully some of what is at the discussion phase at the moment will become a practicality for the next meeting in four years.

In conclusion I would like to thank in particular, on behalf of us all, Prof. Sekiguchi and the organizing committee as well as the sponsors of this meeting for looking after us so well and for giving us such a full program. As always I think we must thank all of the people in the background——the secretaries, the general staff, projectionists, and others——who have made this meeting so successful. Before I close I would like to extend our best wishes to Prof. Yoshiike and also to Prof. Mukharlyamov who were unable to be present with us. Thank you, Prof. Sekiguchi.

Keyword Index